Contemporary Physician-Authors

This book examines the phenomenon of physician-authors. It focuses on the books that contemporary doctors write—the stories that they tell—with contributors critically engaging their works.

A selection of original chapters from leading scholars in medical and health humanities analyze the literary output of doctors, including Oliver Sacks, Danielle Ofri, Atul Gawande, Louise Aronson, Siddhartha Mukherjee, and Abraham Verghese. Discussing issues of moral meaning in the works of contemporary doctor-writers, from memoir to poetry, this collection reflects some of the diversity of medicine today.

A key reference for all students and scholars of medical and health humanities, the book will be especially useful for those interested in the relationship between literature and practicing medicine.

Nathan Carlin is Professor in the McGovern Center for Humanities and Ethics at the University of Texas Health Science Center at Houston (UTHealth), in Houston, Texas, where he holds the Samuel Karff Chair.

Routledge Advances in the Medical Humanities

Moments of Rupture: The Importance of Affect in Surgical Training and Medical Education
Perspectives from Professional Learning and Philosophy
Arunthathi Mahendran

Storytelling Encounters as Medical Education
Crafting Relational Identity
Sally Warmington

Educating Doctors' Senses Through the Medical Humanities
"How Do I Look?"
Alan Bleakley

Medical Humanities, Sociology and the Suffering Self
Surviving Health
Wendy Lowe

A Whole Person Approach to Wellbeing
Building Sense of Safety
Johanna Lynch

Rethinking Pain in Person-Centred Health Care
Around Recovery
Stephen Buetow

Medical Education, Politics and Social Justice
The Contradiction Cure
Alan Bleakley

For more information about this series visit: www.routledge.com/Routledge-Advances-in-the-Medical-Humanities/book-series/RAMH

Contemporary Physician-Authors

Exploring the Insights of Doctors Who Write

Edited by Nathan Carlin

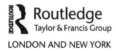

Routledge
Taylor & Francis Group

LONDON AND NEW YORK

First published 2022
by Routledge
2 Park Square, Milton Park, Abingdon, Oxon OX14 4RN

and by Routledge
605 Third Avenue, New York, NY 10158

Routledge is an imprint of the Taylor & Francis Group, an informa business

British Library Cataloguing-in-Publication Data
A catalogue record for this book is available from the British Library

Library of Congress Cataloging-in-Publication Data
Names: Carlin, Nathan, editor.
Title: Contemporary physician-authors: exploring the insights of doctors
who write / edited by Nathan Carlin.
Description: New York, NY: Routledge, 2022. | Series: Routledge
advances in the medical humanities | Includes bibliographical references
and index. |
Identifiers: LCCN 2021024112 (print) | LCCN 2021024113 (ebook) |
ISBN 9780367528805 (hardback) | ISBN 9781032131610 (paperback) |
ISBN 9781003079712 (ebook)
Subjects: LCSH: Physicians as authors. | Literature and medicine.
Classification: LCC PN492 .C66 2022 (print) | LCC PN492 (ebook) |
DDC 809/.933561–dc23
LC record available at https://lccn.loc.gov/2021024112
LC ebook record available at https://lccn.loc.gov/2021024113

ISBN: 978-0-367-52880-5 (hbk)
ISBN: 978-1-032-13161-0 (pbk)
ISBN: 978-1-003-07971-2 (ebk)

DOI: 10.4324/9781003079712

Typeset in Goudy
By Deanta Global Publishing Services, Chennai, India

For Barbara and William Carlin, with gratitude

Contents

Contributors

Nathan Carlin, PhD, is Professor in the McGovern Center for Humanities and Ethics at the University of Texas Health Science Center at Houston (UTHealth) in Houston, Texas, where he directs the Medical Humanities Scholarly Concentration for medical students. He has published seven previous books. He also holds the Samuel Karff Chair.

Andrew Childress, PhD, is Assistant Professor of medicine and medical ethics in the Center for Medical Ethics and Health Policy at Baylor College of Medicine and a Clinical Ethicist at Baylor St. Luke's Medical Center. He has written about physician–patient communication, integration of the humanities within medical education, and illness narratives within the context of clinical ethics consultations.

David Elkin, MD, MSL, codirects the Consultation Liaison Service at San Francisco General Hospital. He earned an MD degree from the University of Pennsylvania and an MSL (masters in the study of law) from UC Hastings, with specialization in bioethics. His academic interests include education, ethics, and the intersection of medicine, literature, and the arts.

Thomas D. Harter, PhD, is the Director of the Department of Bioethics and Humanities with Gundersen Health System in La Crosse, Wisconsin. His research focuses on ethical issues at the intersection of clinical practice, medical professionalism, and business.

Craig M. Klugman, PhD, is Professor of bioethics and health humanities in the Department of Health Sciences at DePaul University in Chicago, Illinois, where he teaches bioethics, health humanities, and death and dying, as well as codirects the Bioethics in Society minor. He serves on the ethics committee at Northwestern Memorial Hospital, is a member of the National Biosecurity Science Board, and was a founding cochair of the Health Humanities Consortium.

Tom Koch, PhD, teaches medical geography at the University of British Columbia, Vancouver, Canada, and is a consultant in chronic and long-term care at the Alton Medical Centre in Toronto, Ontario, Canada. He has authored more than 13 books, including the first works on elder care from the perspective of the caregiver, the first works on news and public information online, and, separately, 3 books on the role of cartography in mapping and understanding chronic and epidemic diseases.

Kaarkuzhali Babu Krishnamurthy, MD, was born in India and raised in the United States. She is System Director of Epilepsy for Steward Medical Group. She has developed a holistic practice dedicated to providing comprehensive care for people with epilepsy and seizure disorders; this includes a multidisciplinary program to minimize maternal and fetal risks for patients with epilepsy during pregnancy. She is a core faculty in the Center for Bioethics at Harvard Medical School in Boston, Massachusetts, and teaches medical students.

Carol Levine, MA, is a senior fellow of the United Hospital Fund (UHF) and former director of UHF's Families and Health Care Project. Before joining UHF in 1996, she directed the Citizens Commission on AIDS in New York City from 1987 to 1991 and The Orphan Project, which she founded, from 1991 to 1996. In 1993, Ms. Levine was awarded a MacArthur Foundation Fellowship for her work in AIDS policy and ethics.

Tony Miksanek, MD, is a family physician and the author of two collections of short stories: *Raining Stethoscopes* and *Murmurs*. He is Coeditor of the New York University Literature, Arts and Medicine Database. He teaches literature and writing to junior college students.

Abraham M. Nussbaum, MD, MTS, is Chief Education Officer at Denver Health and Associate Professor of Psychiatry at the University of Colorado School of Medicine in Aurora, Colorado. He maintains a website, www.abrahamnussbaum.com, where he writes brief book reports about, and curates playlists for, the strange worlds of medicine.

Keisha Ray, PhD, is Assistant Professor in the McGovern Center for Humanities and Ethics at the University of Texas Health Science Center at Houston (UTHealth) in Houston, Texas. Most of her works focus on bioethics, broadly construed, including the ethics of cognitive enhancement and the health of Black people, as well as incorporating race education into medical school curricula.

Lise Saffran, MFA, MPH, is Associate Teaching Professor at the University of Missouri in Columbia, Missouri, where she teaches Storytelling in Public Health and Policy. Saffran has served as cochair of the Health Humanities Consortium.

Sandhya Shetty, PhD, is Associate Professor of English at the University of New Hampshire in Durham, New Hampshire, where she teaches courses in post-colonial fiction, the nineteenth-century British novel, and medicine and literature. She has published articles on illness and nursing, colonial medical discourse, gender and nation, biopolitics, medicine and war, and postcolonial fiction from South Asia and the Caribbean.

Susan Stagno, MD, is Professor of Psychiatry and Bioethics and Medical Humanities at Case Western Reserve University School of Medicine (CWRU SOM). She holds the Sihler Family Professorship, focusing on physician–patient communication, and she is the founding faculty lead for the Humanities Pathway at CWRU SOM. She is also the Director of Education in the Department of Psychiatry at University Hospitals of Cleveland. Her clinical area of interest is in consultation-liaison psychiatry.

Jill Yamasaki, PhD, is Associate Professor in the Jack J. Valenti School of Communication at the University of Houston, where she teaches narratives of health and illness, communication in healthcare contexts, and doctor–patient interaction. Her research focuses on narrative inquiry and practice in health communication and aging, particularly in the contexts of humanizing care, creative engagement, the human–animal bond, and community connections.

Seema Yasmin, MB BChir, is an Emmy Award-winning medical journalist, physician, and assistant professor in the Department of Medicine at Stanford University in Stanford, California, director of the Stanford Health Communication Initiative, a health and science journalism lecturer at Stanford, and a medical analyst for CNN. Yasmin is the author of five books, including: *Viral BS: Medical Myths and Why We Fall For Them; Muslim Women Are Everything: Stereotype-Shattering Stories of Courage, Inspiration and Adventure; and If God Is A Virus: Poems.*

Foreword

Samuel Shem

Bravo to Nathan Carlin for putting together this massive undertaking with care and smarts. It is terrific. As a doctor, I would insert a warning: "If any readers have muscular-skeletal or cardiac issues, do not lift it alone, without permission from your doctor." (I first read this book when it was in a draft binder, and it was heavy!) But it's worth it—a marvelous volume, a labor of love of literature, with a broad purview and a deep digging. I am delighted to see this as a rainbow coalition of physicians dedicated to not only healing patients but also playing our part as leaders in healing a sick world.

Throughout this fine volume are analyses of *why* doctors write and *what* doctors write. Often we're not aware, at the time, of the unseen historical and cultural forces carrying us along. Huge forces start with the flicker of a butterfly's wing, barely noticed, often arising through a period of suffering. Looking back, things may come clearer.

This is certainly true in my own experience as a doctor-writer. I was a product of the 1960s. My generation in college did something rare: given the injustice of the Vietnam War, we protested. We learned that, if we stuck together, we could change things. We made strides in gender equality, helped put the voting rights act on the books, and ended the Vietnam War. That butterfly's wing lifted me to Oxford and, after three years as a Rhodes Scholar, changed my life. I wanted to be a writer, but I suddenly faced the choice between Vietnam or Harvard Medical School. I figured I would make my paying job a doctor, and somehow I would write.

Why and what I write? I got lucky. I did my internship in "The House of God," which in 1973 was the Number 1 medical match in America. But we interns were at the bottom of this huge hierarchy, and we were abused. After it was over, I recall hearing a little voice: "*Hey, wait a second, this is so bad, someone has to write it. I guess it's up to me.*" It started with our "resistance" actions during the internship. Afterward we six intern buddies gathered together and got drunk and talked and laughed until our sides hurt—what a catharsis! Sex, booze, and resistance. Much later I realized that the novel can be read as a primer for nonviolent resistance to an unjust system. As Chuck puts it at the end: "How can we care for patients, if nobody cares for us?"

For two years I never went out and publicized the novel—I was a purist. But one day I got a letter from the publisher: "I'm on call all night in a VA hospital in Tulsa Oklahoma and if I didn't have your book I'd kill myself." *Whoa. Maybe I have something to say, and make a difference?* From that day on, I accepted almost any invitation to speak, on every continent except Antarctica. I explain that what gets me writing is resistance to injustice. My topic is always the same: "Staying human in medicine: the danger of isolation and the healing power of good connection." What is a good connection? A mutual connection. If it isn't mutual, it isn't that good. As doctors, and as humans.

Often a first novel is easy, the second hard. Mine became a chore, then a depression. I thought of quitting writing. I already had one hard job—a psychiatrist for alcoholics and drug addicts. I myself started to drink more. My relationship with my wife got worse. For months I asked myself: *Why write?* Finally I heard another, kind voice: *Because I can't not.* I wrote out a sign for my desk: "Joy in the Process, Faith in the Work."

This time of suffering led me to join my wife Janet Surrey in shared work. We wrote two things together: one from her area of expertise, and one from mine. Janet was developing a new psychological theory at the women's Stone Center at Wellesley College. The dominant male-authored theories posited that psychological health and growth were in and of "the self." This did not ring true for women. Rather, women's psychological health and growth were in and of "the quality of their relationships, their connections." I was the only man at the women's institute. Janet and I did gender dialogues all over the world: bringing thousands of men and women (and boys and girls) together in dialogue and gender impasses: to shift from "I"/"You" to "We." Together we wrote *We Have to Talk: Healing Dialogues Between Women and Men*. My eyes opened to women's experiences. I wrote a companion paper on "Men's Relational Growth," and couples' therapy became my forte.

Our second writing endeavor, from my arena, was a play: "Bill W. and Dr. Bob", about the two founders of Alcoholics Anonymous in Akron in 1935. It too is a program for mutual: the only way an alcoholic can stay sober is to tell his or her story to another drunk. Eventually, we had productions all over the world. Writing is often solo. But writing *with* is a tremendous experience. Try it.

The latest flicker of that butterfly's wing was six years ago. Out of the blue, I got a call from NYU Medical School. "Do you want to be a Professor of Medicine at NYU?" I asked, why? "In medical humanities: We want you to teach a seminar on *The House of God*." I was stunned. I felt that Harvard hated me for the novel, but NYU wanted me to teach it? I jumped in.

Suddenly I was bringing fresh eyes to modern medicine and was stunned. On my first day on the wards I saw the miracles we can do. But I also saw, clear as day, the other side: money and screens. "*Hey wait a second—this is not just. Somebody's got to write about this, I guess it's up to me.*" I'd always wanted to write a sequel to *The House of God*, and now I had it. As narrator Roy Basch puts it: "Looking back, it was a time when medicine could go one way or the other: either toward more humane care or to money and screens—which means money and money (the machines are mostly billing)." *The House of God* was about the abuse of medical training; *Man's 4th Best Hospital* is about the abuse of the whole health-care industry.

We are no longer mainly a reading culture, but a watching culture. To those doctors who also want to be writers, you will have to be as dedicated and tough with your writing and publishing as you are with your medicine. The reasons that we doctors write—write seriously and comically and rivetingly and importantly—are because we can't not, and we want to bring our medicine to the reader. We want to change people's lives. So heal them with your stories, your words. Have fun—both as a doctor and as a writer—and do your part to heal not just our patients, our relationships, and ourselves but also our world.

January 2021

Acknowledgments

I would like to thank Grace McInnes, senior editor at Routledge, for believing in this project, as well as Evie Lonsdale, who helped move this book through the production process from start to finish. I would also like to thank my colleagues at the University of Texas Health Science Center at Houston (UTHealth), especially the core faculty and staff in the McGovern Center for Humanities and Ethics: Thomas Cole, Rebecca Lunstroth, Keisha Ray, Anson Koshy, Renee Flores, Alma Rosas, and Angela Polczynski. I am especially grateful to Anson Koshy for creating the frontispiece of this volume, a drawing of Fady Joudah, who did a reading of some of his poetry at McGovern Medical School on September 13, 2017.

I am grateful, too, to all of the contributors of this volume. They put in a lot of work to produce really wonderful essays. While I have always admired physicians for their intelligence, drive, and commitment, reading these essays produced in me some degree of regret for not having become a physician myself, for I have come to love them. It never occurred to me that I could have become a physician. Still, the lines have fallen for me in pleasant places (Psalm 16:6–8), something my mentor, Donald Capps, often said of his own life. Finally, I would like to thank Samuel Shem, who, because of this project, has become a friend.

This book is dedicated to my parents, Barbara and William Carlin. They provided me with unconditional love over the years, putting up with me when I was difficult. While maybe many sons are difficult, I probably was especially so, and so from them I have learned something about what it means to live by grace alone.

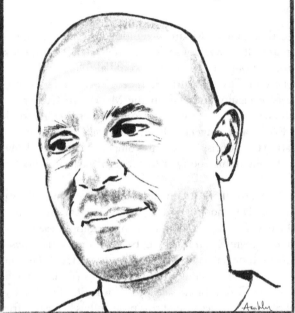

"One of the beautiful things about clinical experience that has enriched my life as a writer is the language of medicine."

Fady Joudah

Introduction

Nathan Carlin

When I mention to people that I teach medical humanities at a medical school, often they do not know what I mean. I go on by saying, "I teach medical students how to talk to patients, things like how to break bad news." Then their eyes light up and they say that this kind of work is *so* needed, sharing with me some story about how a family member received such news from a doctor poorly. Other times I explain to people what I do by saying that I teach medical ethics. This will open up a lively conversation as well, as people will ask my opinion on bioethics controversies in the news such as gene editing or rationing. Still other times I tell people that I read literature with medical students, things like short stories or physician memoirs. This, too, leads to an animated conversation, with people telling me about their favorite doctor-writer. This third type of conversation—conversations about physician-authors—is how I got the idea for this book.

For some, the writings of doctor-writers *are* what constitutes medical humanities. And this is for good reason, because this is what people see in bookstores when they spend time in the section on medicine. Yet, when I looked around for academic books about doctor-writers, I was surprised to discover that there are not any significant ones. There are, instead, anthologies, which are useful, but I saw a gap in the field and so decided to fill it by editing a scholarly (yet accessible) book about contemporary physician-authors.

When I sent out the call for proposals for this collection of essays, I asked academics in medical humanities, health humanities, and bioethics to submit to me three physician-authors about whom they would like to write. In compiling these submissions, I got a sense of whom the field is interested in. In making my selections for inclusion, my guiding criteria included diversity and balance. I wanted to have roughly an equal number of men and women represented in the book in terms of the contributors (this balance is harder to achieve with regard to physician-authors, for the tradition has skewed toward men). I also wanted to have close to an equal number of MDs and PhDs as contributors. Basically, I wanted to create the most diverse book I could in terms of training, race, gender, ethnicity, and sexual orientation, and this applied to both the contributors and the physician-authors. That said, while this book takes important steps on the path to diversity, these are only beginning steps. This book could be more global. In any case, based on the preferences of those who made submissions to me, and

DOI: 10.4324/9781003079712-101

given that each contributor only submitted three names, there is an element of randomness that emerged in the book, having taken this inductive approach guided by considerations of diversity.

Be that as it may, many of the physician-authors who would have been included if I were to have taken a more directive approach (i.e., by coming up with a list of doctor-writers myself) are, in fact, included. Oliver Sacks, Perri Klass, and Abraham Verghese, for example, are in this book. But, of course, no volume can cover everyone. Some prominent contemporary writers, therefore, are left out, such as Vincent Lam, Rafael Campo, and Sayantani Dasgupta.

One physician-author not included in the book due to this inductive approach is Stephen Bergman, whose pen name is Samuel Shem. He deserves special mention. Shem is undoubtedly one of the most successful of all of the contemporary doctor-writers, for he wrote *The House of God*,[1] which has sold millions of copies. *The House of God*, which is a satire,[2] focuses on the experiences of Roy Basch, exposing the dehumanizing forces of medical training as well as its hypocrisy. Because it focuses on intern year, the book continues to be bought by both those entering medical school and those graduating from it. In *The House of God*, Shem raised some of the core issues over which contemporary physician-authors are still struggling, especially with regard to the witnessing of suffering, the emotional toll of residency, the harms inflicted by medical bureaucracy, sexuality in clinical spaces, racism, sexism, and ageism on the wards, controversies about billing, and burnout. The book was scandalous when it was published; it remains controversial to this day.

In 2010, Shem wrote a new afterword for the book in which he notes that, when he began writing the book in 1974, he did so for reasons of "catharsis" so that he could "share with [his] buddies what had been the worst year of [his] life."[3] He adds: "I was just trying to express something about injustice and inhumanity that I knew to be true."[4] Shem sees himself as a product of the 1960s: "I and a core group of fellow interns … believed that if we saw an injustice, we could organize, take action, and change things for the better."[5] He continues:

> Our generation put the civil rights laws on the books and helped end the Vietnam War. We were pragmatic idealists. When we entered our internship, we were taught to treat our patients in ways that we didn't think were humane,[6]

so Shem and his colleagues used humor to resist and they "secretly treated people humanely."[7]

While Shem is somewhat of a celebrity for *The House of God*, he has written a number of other works as well. His other novels include *Fine, Mount Misery, The Spirit of the Place, The Buddha's Wife* (with Janet Surrey), *At the Heart of the Universe,* and *Man's 4th Best Hospital.* His plays include "Bill W. and Dr. Bob" (with Janet Surrey), which appeared on Broadway, "Napoleon's Dinner," and "Room for One Woman." He also wrote a nonfiction book on relationships, titled *We Have to Talk: Healing Dialogues Between Women and Men* (with Janet Surrey), as well as a curriculum for middle school and high school students on gender.[8] Because Martin Kohn and Carol Donley edited a scholarly book of essays reflecting on *The House of God*,[9] I felt okay about not including Shem in this book as the focus of one of the chapters.

A long tradition of physician-authors

I want to turn now to put the chapters of this book in a broader context. To do so, a few words need to be said about the historical tradition of physician-authors. In a sense, this tradition is almost as old as civilization itself. The Greek physician-author Hippocrates of Kos (460-370 BCE)—or, rather, his students—created the Hippocratic Corpus, which had a substantial impact on society in the West. Galen of Pergamon (129-210 CE), too, is a major physician-author of the Roman Empire, and Moses Maimonides (1135-1204 CE) was an influential physician and philosopher during the medieval period who had an enormous impact on Western thought. More recently, Sigmund Freud (1856-1939), who was trained as a neurologist, created psychoanalysis not only to address clinical problems but also to analyze culture. These are just four of the most well-known names; there are many others. During virtually all periods of recorded history, doctors have been writers, some impacting society in profound ways.

During the past 100 years or so, though, a new kind of physician-authors flourished. Anton Chekov (1860-1904), William Carlos Williams (1883-1963), and a number of others became known more as authors than as physicians, writing poetry, memoir, short stories, and novels. During the past 50 years especially, this writing became increasingly personal even as it focused on the clinical. This experiential emphasis coincided with the rise of pathographies where patients write about their journeys with illness. Incidentally, some have viewed the emergence of pathography as a response to industrialization, technologization, and the erosion of doctor-patient relationships.[10] It is a striking fact that the number of physician-authors has skyrocketed as well. It stands to reason that the rise in the number of physician-writers, along with the increasingly personal nature of this writing, could be seen as a reflection of physician dissatisfaction with their experience of modern medicine for many of the reasons that patients identify. It is worth pointing out that, as women joined the ranks of medicine, they, too, became physician-authors, but this happened relatively recently, and issues of gender are only now beginning to be explored.

Another aspect contributing to the personal quality of the writings of both patients and physicians includes the fact that people in the West now live in what Philip Rieff called a therapeutic culture, which emerged after—and because of—Freud.[11] Doctors and patients alike look inside themselves and write their lives. Moreover, we live in a time in history where it is easier to tell our story than ever, for we can post it on social media or the internet. "Ours," Ian Thomson writes, "is the era of Everybody's Autobiography."[12] The writings of contemporary physician-authors are a part of this cultural milieu.

While historians of medicine have focused on physician-authors such as Hippocrates and Galen, the subfield that has paid the most attention to the writing of doctors during the last century is literature and medicine. In an early essay outlining the contours of this tradition, M. Faith McLellan[13] notes that, on the one end of the spectrum, there are physician-writers, such as Freud, who have expanded the case history, which has been called "romantic science,"[14] and, on the other end, there are those who write about existential interests. In this regard, McLellan cites S. Weir Mitchell, a neurologist who wrote many novels and other stories, including "The Strange Case of George Dedlow."[15] This story is about a patient who was wounded during the American Civil War. He had all of his limbs amputated, and he subsequently experienced phantom pain in these limbs. McLellan suggests that the story is an "imaginative meditation on [an] altered sense of self."[16] A third form, which is a blend of the first two, is fiction that is informed by clinical practice. She cites Tobias George Smollett and Chekhov as representative figures.[17]

What is so special about doctor-writers? McLellan suggests that doctors have access to a variety of human experiences that most do not.[18] She adds that if doctors are serious writers, then they are deeply curious about what it means to be human: "For both [doctoring and writing] are ways of looking at [human beings] and both are, at heart, moral enterprises. Both must start by seeing life bare, without averting their gaze."[19] McLellan adds that another connection between being a writer and being a doctor is the attention to the technical craft. She cites Richard Selzer on this point, who describes writing as a suturing of words into sentences. Both doctors and writers also, she observes, have a need to communicate well, and both sustain a tension between identification and detachment. Finally, she points out that both attempt to formulate meaning in crafting (clinical) (hi)stories.

Why (else) do doctors write?

If one reason that doctors write is, as Shem suggested, catharsis, and another is, as McLellan suggested, that they are curious about what it means to be human, what are other reasons?[20] Tony Miksanek, a contributor to this volume, offers a list of seven reasons that doctors write.[21] Ranked in order of importance, he suggests:

1. Therapy
2. Exploration
3. Sharing
4. Joy
5. Honor
6. Atonement
7. Notoriety

In what follows, I will elaborate on this list, and I will offer four additional reasons that doctors write, labeled 8–11.

Commenting on "therapy" as a reason doctors write (which may be another way of saying catharsis),[22] Miksanek points out that being a physician can be stressful for lots of reasons. All too often doctors let this stress out on fellow coworkers, but writing can be an alternative path—or a way to advocate for change. Today, for example, I hear a lot of complaints about the electronic medical record. Doctors complain that writing notes in the electronic medical record takes up much of their time (often nights and weekends) and that this is uncompensated. Maybe writing about this in an accessible and compelling manner will lead to some kind of suitable solution for doctors.

By "exploration," Miksanek means that there are a lot of confusing (and curious) aspects of medicine, such as issues relating to medical ethics. For instance, in *Complications*, Atul Gawande writes about the necessary but ambiguous fact that surgeons learn by practicing on people. He adds, critically, that the uninsured often bear a disproportionate amount of this practice.[23] While it is true that someone has to be the first patient for each surgeon learning the trade, it does not have to be a poor person. This risk could be spread out more justly.

Also, outside of questions of ethics, writing for its own sake would fit under the category of exploration, as a way of getting to know (i.e., exploring) oneself. Some years ago, a medical student shared with me in a journal that he no longer felt disgusted by mangled bodies and that death really did not affect him anymore. This shift in him prompted his fiancé to ask him: "Who are you becoming?" By writing about this, if only for me and for himself, he was exploring his own answer to this question.

By "sharing," Miksanek suggests that doctors sometimes write for other doctors to share inside jokes as a form of bonding. This is close to exploration, but different in terms of audience and intent, for there are certain experiences that only doctors can appreciate. This is true, to some extent, of all professions, but most professions do not write about the nature of their work. I'm unaware of any memoir written by an accountant or a plumber, but I'm sure they have their own inside jokes that they share with each other.

By "joy" Miksanek rightly points out that medicine is full of happy moments, not just stress. The recently edited volume *Recognitions*[24] collects some of these narratives. I would add that I have read many student journals over the years that are joyful, especially when medical students help to deliver a baby for the first time, when a life is saved, or when patients respond quickly, positively, and dramatically to psychotropic medication.

"Honor" and "Notoriety" go together, as they are opposite sides of the same coin, for honor refers to honoring other people (such as patients or colleagues), while notoriety refers to seeking fame for oneself. These categories speak for themselves. "Atonement"[25] for Miksanek refers to writing in remorse after committing medical errors. A number of doctor-writers have written about this topic in recent years.[26] Usually these mistakes involve personal failures or systemic problems regarding patient care, but sometimes doctors will reflect on their families, when, for instance, they should have taken a child to the emergency room but didn't or when they overlooked a symptom.

If I could modify Miksanek's list, I would add several more reasons, without suggesting their order of importance. These include:

8. A desire to say more
9. Advocacy
10. A desire to create

I think implicit in a lot of the writings of contemporary physician-authors is that they have a desire to say more, especially in the context of medicine in the United States and elsewhere where visits are often limited to 10-15 minutes. The so-called golden age[27] of the doctor-patient relationship is something of the past, if it ever really was. Because things move so quickly in the hospital and care is so disjointed, doctors often do not get a chance to follow up with patients. In writing, they get this chance to say what they wanted to say previously but did not or could not.[28] (To me, the desire to say more recalls Sherman Alexie's *You Don't Have to Say You Love Me*, a memoir in which he writes everything he wished he would have said at his mother's funeral but didn't.[29]) The spirit of this impulse is a yearning after the fact.

Advocacy is another key reason doctors write, which I noted above, but it deserves its own category, for while both therapy and advocacy work for change, they are different. Gawande's *The Checklist Manifesto*[30] is a key example in this regard, though there is often a tone of advocacy in much of what doctors write, as they are addressing harms and wrongs that have happened to both patients and themselves.

I think creating simply for the sake of creating is a motivation as well, perhaps especially when doctors write poetry. Thinking of oneself as an author is very satisfying, not necessarily for reasons of fame (very few writers are famous) but because one can experience oneself as a creative person. My own hunch about physician burnout is that it is centrally about having a lack of creativity in one's life. Writing is a way of grabbing more out of what a life in medicine can afford.

One could also ask: why do people *read* doctor-writers? This is a little harder to answer without interviewing readers. Nevertheless, I think some reasonable guesses can be offered. The most obvious reason is that medicine is inherently interesting, like sex and crime. Just as there are many television shows that deal with medicine, there will be readers of these books. Another reason is that people may want to turn to doctors about their insights regarding disease and death as they struggle with illnesses of their own. In this sense, maybe people read doctor-writers for similar reasons that they read pathographies. Additionally, students may read doctor-writers because they want to know something about what their training will be like, both technically and emotionally. Just as there are many reasons that doctors write, there are likely a variety of reasons that people read.

Two insider critiques of physician-authors

While there are many doctor-writers, the critical discussion of physician-authors is limited, mainly confined to academic articles and chapters.[31] I would like to highlight two critiques of this genre, both raised by physicians who are committed to this work.

In "An Expostulation," published in 1991, Selzer reflects on a special issue of *Literature and Medicine*, published in 1984,[32] that was dedicated to doctor-writers.[33] He noted that, at the time, the theme of doctor-writers was very compelling because medical students could relate to such writings. After seven years, though, this volume seemed to Selzer to be "well-intentioned,"[34] which is another way of saying naïve. Why? Selzer suggests that, on the one hand, the writings produced by doctor-writers are often not very good. On the other hand, the weaknesses of their writings go unnoticed because literary critics are just too easy on doctor-writers.[35]

Selzer suggests that "a doctor is no better equipped to render art from suffering than an insurance salesman, a prisoner, or a patient."[36] Seeming to challenge the view that doctors have a special insight into the human condition by virtue of their work, Selzer points out that doctor-writer Walker Percy did his best writing on account of his suffering as a *patient*: "Nothing in his experience as a physician could have produced the profound insights that fill the pages of his novels."[37] While praising Percy as a patient-author, Selzer has harsh words for his fellow doctor-writers, in particular William Carlos Williams. Selzer attacks Williams's celebrated "The Red Wheelbarrow," which, Selzer writes, "is poem only because of the eccentric line endings and the cutting of words into separate parts."[38] Regarding Williams's stories, Selzer says that they "seem curiously devoid of craft."[39]

Selzer observes that key reasons that doctors write are because they are sentimental and because such writing can be therapeutic, as noted above. While there is nothing wrong with writing for sentimental or therapeutic reasons, Selzer's point is that such motivations in-and-of-themselves simply do not produce good *writing*. Selzer concludes his reflections by suggesting that we are *not* living in a renaissance of literature and medicine on account of the fact that there are so many doctor-writers now, for much of this work, in his assessment, is "mediocre."[40]

A more generous take on issues related to this kind of writing can be found in a brief commentary by Allan Peterkin. In "Why We Write (and How We Can Do It Better)," Peterkin conveys some of the lessons that he has learned about writing about patients, both as a doctor-writer himself and as an editor of a medical humanities magazine.[41] In educational settings, he notes that such writing is often encouraged with the hope that it will strengthen one's skills in empathy, thereby improving patient care. He also suggests that this kind of writing is a way to honor patients,[42] and he feels that it is "a welcome counterbalance to evidence-based practice, which emphasizes what is generalizable rather than what is unique, particular, and unpredictable."[43] All of these reasons that doctors write could be included in the above list of ten reasons, with the exception of the cultivation of empathy, which, of course, is a key objective of narrative medicine.[44] Thus, this should be added to the list of reasons doctors write:

11. The cultivation of empathy, both in oneself as a writer, and in readers

Peterkin goes on to identify five common errors that physician-authors make as writers. Three of them deal with the craft of writing itself. The other two are moral. The first is that physicians often fail to live up to the adage, "Show, don't tell," because they are accustomed to a terse style of writing and communicating in patient charts. The second is that doctors tend to favor tidy endings, but in real-life endings are not always tidy. Third, doctor-writers sometimes forget their intended audience, resulting in unfocused writing.

The fourth lesson is that the writings of doctor-writers can be narcissistic. Peterkin notes in this regard an anecdote in which Margaret Laurence, a very successful Canadian novelist, was

> at a dinner party, sitting next to a neurosurgeon who, without guile, told her he planned to write novels once he quit surgery. Without missing a beat, Laurence replied, "What a coincidence—when I stop writing, I plan to take up brain surgery."[45]

The fifth lesson deals with the ethics of writing about patients.[46] The key point for Peterkin is that doctors cannot think that what happens in their clinics or hospitals is *their* story. Rather, these stories are *co-created*. This leads Peterkin to suggest that doctors should get written permission to write about their patients from the patients themselves, and he notes that patients usually feel honored by these requests.[47] However, I would add that, even when permission is granted, some ambiguity remains, as has been noted in psychiatric and counseling literature where it has been pointed out that power imbalances always exist. Patients who provide written consent may be doing so in order to please their therapist.[48] While this issue will be taken up in various chapters in this book—different physician-authors handle this question differently—some further discussion is needed here.

The ethics of writing about patients

In "Not Whether but How," Arthur Frank notes that the telling of other people's stories in general is questionable but is especially so when telling the stories of patients. This is because, as noted above, there is a power differential between doctors and patients and also because confidentiality is assumed.[49] While some[50] feel that such writing should not be done at all, Frank does not share this view. Instead, Frank suggests that we focus on *how* these stories are told. In short, Frank calls for "narrative nuance."[51] What does this mean? He explains: "we need to understand how to tell respectful stories in which the characters are fully acknowledged fellow participants, not one-dimensional objects of a knowing gaze."[52]

Before addressing how to tell the stories of patients in an ethical manner, Frank also notes four key *benefits* of writing stories about patients. These include:

- Stories can enhance medical knowledge.
- Writing these stories can help clinicians improve their communication skills.

- These stories can help other doctors (and members of society at large) develop empathy for patients.
- These narratives can convey complexity and intersectionality, especially as related to access to care.[53]

Frank then proceeds to a discussion of the ethics of the telling of patients' stories. He points out that people tell different kinds of stories to different audiences via different media and that these different audiences have their own forms of speech. What may be ethical to say in one context (e.g., an academic journal article) may not be ethical in another context (e.g., *The New York Times*). Frank adds, though, that these boundaries bleed into one another. He also notes that "how people feel injured, usurped, or diminished by stories told about themselves is a complex issue."[54] The loss of privacy is key, Frank emphasizes, but he suggests that people may feel more upset over *how* they are represented in a story, not necessarily *that* a story was told about them. Or, he adds, patients may want to tell their stories themselves. In any case, while Frank concedes that "people are put at risk by having stories told about them, they can also gain comfort from having their stories told."[55] Frank points out that there is a fine line between appropriating (exploiting) and witnessing (honoring) the stories of patients. To guard against appropriating and exploiting, drawing on Mikhail Bakhtin,[56] Frank makes a distinction between monological and dialogical stories. Monological stories are singular and authoritative, unaware of perspective. Dialogical stories, in contrast, are "unfinalized."[57] Frank writes: "What matters—what constitutes the dialogue—is whether the character on the page is presented as exceeding what can be on the page."[58] In other words, the story on the page is *never* the full story.

Practically speaking, how can one tell if a story written by a doctor about a patient is dialogical? Frank suggests that if the story is written in such a way that it invites the patient to add to the story to enhance it (not to counter it), it is dialogical.[59] To put this less academically, when writing about oneself, the idea would be to write with a spirit of, "This is how I see things," and, when writing about someone else (such as a patient), the idea would be, "This is how I understand this person's experience—how do you see it from your perspective?" Readers are invited to assess the doctor-writers in this book along these lines, beyond the criticism offered by the contributors of this volume.

Books related to this one

While there are not any books exactly like this edited volume, there are several anthologies that are related, such as Lee Gutkind's *Becoming a Doctor*[60] and Leah Kaminsky's *Writer, M.D.*[61] Both of these books include a distinguished grouping of contributors. Likewise, *Doctors and Patients*,[62] edited by Cecil Helman, includes material from previously published works, from both doctors and patients, including from those who would be considered to be in the canon of physician-authors, if there is such a canon. *Recognitions*, edited by Carol Donley and Martin Kohn, is a little different, for the editors wanted to focus on "rewarding experiences" in the clinical lives of doctors, for too often "the struggle ... that is part of the calling to heal" has been depicted cynically.[63] The book itself contains new work by doctor-writers. Of note, the editors endorse the view that "physicians stand at a unique vantage point as observers of the human condition."[64] An especially good volume is *A Life in Medicine*,[65] edited by Robert Coles and Randy Testa, which provides experiential excerpts from doctors, nurses, patients, and others, and it is organized by four themes identified by the American Association of Medical Colleges as essential for the education of physicians: altruism, knowledge, skill, and duty. The most comprehensive of all of these anthologies is Iain Bamforth's *The Body in the Library*.[66] It includes physician-authors, but it is much wider in scope. This collection is also notable in that it begins to take steps toward a more global perspective.

How is this book different?

As noted, the main way that this book is different from the others is that it is not an anthology. It is a book *about* physician-authors. As such, this book is a work of original scholarship.

Another distinctive feature of this book is its use of introspection. In most of the chapters, the contributors write personally about why the particular doctor-writer is important to them. Some, such as Tom Koch, had a personal correspondence with the physician-writer. Others, such as Seema Yasmin, Susan Stagno, Craig Klugman, and Thomas Harter, conducted personal interviews with their subjects. Still others were drawn to their physician-authors because of personal congruencies in their lives. Carol Levine, for example, writes about her own role as a caregiver for her husband as she explores Arthur Kleinman's role as a caregiver for his wife.

I encouraged the contributors in this volume to write about themselves in their chapters because I have a particular interest in the relationship between one's personal experiences and public scholarship. Such connections have been a long-standing focus of pastoral theology,[67] one of my academic interests.[68] While open and honest reflection on one's feelings and identity is common practice in pastoral care courses in seminaries, such talk is less common in medical humanities circles, especially at colleges and universities unaffiliated with a health institution. I suspect that this is because humanities professors do not want to appear to be "soft" or, to use Selzer's word, "sentimental." Rather, humanities professors want to be perceived as serious and rigorous, especially next to their colleagues in science departments. I find such defensiveness unfortunate, unsatisfying, and uninteresting. Writing and teaching should be oriented toward experience and desire, and I'm unconcerned if this is perceived as lacking rigor. All of this is to say, this book has a personal dimension that is somewhat uncommon in academic publications.

Looking ahead

Part I focuses on two traditional representatives of the recent tradition of doctor-writers. In Chapter 1, Tony Miksanek focuses on Richard Selzer, a surgeon.

Miksanek has written extensively on Selzer's work, so he is in a unique position to offer this chapter. Miksanek analyzes three of Selzer's stories to demonstrate how Selzer writes about medicine and life in unexpected ways. In Chapter 2, Tom Koch writes about Oliver Sacks, a neurologist. Koch, who made a career as a professional writer, sees Sacks as standing in the Oslerian tradition of treating patients as persons.

Part II focuses on three contemporary favorites, all of whom are bestselling or award-winning authors. In Chapter 3, Seema Yasmin, an award-winning journalist herself as well as a physician, writes about Perri Klass, a pediatrician. Klass is distinctive not only for her talent but also for the themes that she addressed in her writing: life as a doctor, daughter, and mother. She explores female desire in her writing, making central women's perspectives and experiences in a profession that has been represented largely by men. In Chapter 4, Kaarkuzhali Babu Krishnamurthy writes about Abraham Verghese, an internist. Verghese was presented with the National Humanities Medal by President Barack Obama in 2015. In particular, Krishnamurthy focuses on two of Verghese's memoirs. In Chapter 5, Thomas Harter writes about Atul Gawande, a surgeon. He traces Gawande's interesting and meandering career, such as the time that he took out of his medical training to do work for Vice President Al Gore as well as time spent as a Rhodes scholar at Oxford University, studying philosophy. Harter stresses the role that philosophy plays in shaping the writings of Gawande.

Part III focuses on meaning and identity as related to medicine, broadly speaking. This section explores issues such as burnout, aging, death and dying, race, gender, ethnicity, liminality, and emotions and confusions in the lives of physicians, often raised by their clinical practice. In Chapter 6, Susan Stagno writes about Danielle Ofri, an internal medicine physician. Ofri cofounded the *Bellevue Literary Review* and writes regularly for major periodicals such as *The New York Times*. Stagno reports that Ofri's main motivation for writing is to make sense of her life in medicine. Following Klass, Ofri provides a much-needed female voice in this genre. In Chapter 7, Lise Saffran, who teaches storytelling in public health, writes about Paul Kalanithi's *When Breath Becomes Air*, a wildly popular book that focuses on the author's own experience of dying. Saffran reads the book critically as she questions Kalanithi's selectivity with regard to what he included. In Chapter 8, Abraham Nussbaum writes about Joanna Cannon, a psychiatrist. Nussbaum, himself a prominent physician-author, explores the theme of burnout in her work. Noting that burnout affects nearly two-thirds of practicing physicians, Nussbaum finds in Cannon's work that what are normally thought to be the causes of burnout are really the symptoms. Cannon left the practice of medicine, having become disenchanted with it, but Nussbaum wonders if medicine can be re-enchanted if the structural issues that Cannon identifies are addressed in meaningful ways.

In Chapter 9, Keisha Ray focuses on Damon Tweedy, a psychiatrist and the author of *Black Man in a White Coat*. As one of only a few professional African American female philosophers in bioethics, Ray provides an astute assessment of Tweedy's work in light of her own work on racial disparities in health, praising

Tweedy's use of stories in advocating for the health of African Americans. In Chapter 10, Andrew Childress writes about Fady Joudah, an emergency room physician who also is an accomplished poet. Joudah, born in Austin, Texas, is the son of Palestinian refugees. Issues of identity, politics, and marginalization emerge often in his poetry.

In Chapter 11, Craig M. Klugman writes about Louise Aronson, a geriatrician. She writes about a wide range of topics, all of which intersect with medical humanities in some way. Klugman focuses on two of her books, A *History of the Present Illness* and *Elderhood*, while also writing autobiographically about aging. In Chapter 12, Jill Yamasaki writes about Marc Agronin, a geriatrician and psychiatrist, by engaging two of his well-known books: *How We Age* and *The End of Old Age*. Yamasaki draws out key insights and arguments from Agronin to combat ageism. Without denying the real physical and social challenges of aging, Agronin is a champion of older adulthood, arguing that late life can be a time for growth and rejuvenation. I am pleased to include two chapters on aging in this book, for aging is so often neglected as a category of identity, as humanities scholars typically focus on race, gender, class, and sexuality.

Part IV of the book is a little different from the rest of the book. It shifts the emphasis away from the experiential to the academic, though experience is still engaged. In Chapter 13, David Elkin offers a close reading of two texts—one by David Watts, a gastroenterologist, and one by Frank Huyler, an emergency medicine physician. By comparing and contrasting these pieces, which themselves reflect different settings (the outpatient clinic and the emergency room), Elkin draws on medical humanities to explore unspoken norms and expectations to help understand both patients and physicians in richer ways.

In Chapter 14, Sandhya Shetty writes about Siddhartha Mukherjee, an oncologist who is well known for his Pulitzer Prize-winning *The Emperor of All Maladies*, which is a history of cancer and its treatment. Shetty engages Mukherjee's work as a literary scholar, making the case that there are different kinds of physician-authors. That is, one can be a physician-author without making one's own patients the focus of one's writing, or without writing poetry, novels, or short stories. She also lifts up the fact that Mukherjee is a physician who writes history, and that this is different from the work of academic historians. She provocatively suggests that a return to beauty (or aesthetics) can be a proper response to what is wrong with the world, in place of outrage or piety.

Finally, in Chapter 15 Carol Levine offers a thoughtful engagement of several key works by Arthur Kleinman, a psychiatrist and anthropologist, focusing in particular on his memoir *The Soul of Care*, in which he discusses becoming a caregiver for his wife after she developed Alzheimer's disease. Levine points out that Kleinman has been enormously influential in bioethics, medical anthropology, medical humanities, and related fields for his work in demonstrating the importance of social and cultural context in medicine. But she also takes him to task for neglecting the importance of individuals, for when the importance of the community is emphasized, it is often women who are forced to sacrifice the most for the common good.

Taken together, I hope these chapters demonstrate the richness of the writings of contemporary physician-authors and that this book will both inspire more such writing as well as more critical readings of these texts. Also, especially as Shetty emphasizes, there are a variety of ways one can be a doctor-writer, and so the possibilities for creativity are likely greater than has been fully recognized.

Teaching tips

While this book has been written with multiple audiences in mind, it is assumed that professors and students will be key constituents. Therefore, I offer here some suggestions for how to use this book in academic courses.

If this book is being used as the basis for an undergraduate course, I would recommend assigning selections from each of the physician-authors paired with the appropriate chapters of this book. For graduate seminars, whole books could be assigned alongside theoretical texts dealing with clinical ethics or life writing. For courses in medical schools, I would suggest focusing on the writings of the physician-authors themselves and gearing discussions toward clinical experience. This book, then, can be used to inform comments by professors in contextualizing this material for students. Alternatively, it could be used as the basis for a fourth-year elective for medical students, taught in the same way as a graduate seminar.

This book also could be used in parts. For example, in an introduction to medical humanities course, if there is a section on physician-authors, relevant chapters could be assigned along with selections from the physician-author. For all audiences, a quick search for recent TED Talks or podcasts, which are usually free, are very effective materials to use in class.

Discussion questions for each chapter

1. What are the reasons that this physician-author is writing?
2. What are the key themes that the physician-author is raising?
3. What is compelling about their writing?
4. What blind spots or limitations does this physician-author seem to have?
5. What connections do you see between life and work?
6. How does this author deal with the ethics of writing about patients?
7. If you are a clinician, in what ways does your experience align with the author? In what ways is it different?

Textbooks and pedagogy

Olivia Banner, Nathan Carlin, and Thomas Cole, eds., *Teaching Health Humanities*
Thomas Cole, Nathan Carlin, and Ronald Carson, *Medical Humanities: An Introduction*
Therese Jones, Delese Wear, and Lester Friedman, eds., *Health Humanities Reader*
Craig Klugman and Erin Gentry Lamb, *Research Methods in Health Humanities*

Useful websites

Literature, Arts, and Medicine Database:
http://medhum.med.nyu.edu/
Division of Narrative Medicine, Columbia University:
https://www.mhe.cuimc.columbia.edu/our-divisions/division-narrative-medicine
Life and Work, with Nathan Carlin:
https://med.uth.edu/mcgovern/life-and-work/
The Health Humanities Consortium:
https://healthhumanitiesconsortium.com/

Videos

Why Doctors Write, the Gold Foundation
TedMed: Danielle Ofri, "Deconstructing Our Perception of Perfection": https://www.youtube.com/watch?v=CaSv741Gjlg
TdExAtlanta, Rita Charon, "Honoring the Stories of Illness": https://www.youtube.com/watch?v=24kHX2HtU3o

Notes

1 Samuel Shem, *The House of God* (New York: Berkley Books, 2010).
2 The question of satire and *The House of God* requires some nuance. See Delese Wear, "*The House of God*: Another Look," *Academic Medicine* 77, no. 6 (2002): 496–501.
3 Shem, *The House of God*, 371.
4 Ibid., 380.
5 Ibid., 372.
6 Ibid.
7 Ibid.
8 See these books by Samuel Shem: *Fine* (New York: St. Martin's/Marek, 1985); *Mount Misery* (New York: Ballantine Books, 1997); *The Spirit of the Place* (New York: Berkley Books, 2012); *The Buddha's Wife* (with Janet Surrey) (New York: Beyond Words/Atria Books, 2015); *At the Heart of the Universe* (New York: Seven Stories Press, 2016); *Man's 4th Best Hospital* (New York: Berkley Books, 2019); and *We Have to Talk: Healing Dialogues between Women and Men* (with Janet Surrey) (New York: Basic Books, 1998).
9 Martin Kohn and Carol Donley, *Return to the House of God: Medical Resident Education, 1978–2008* (Kent, OH: Kent State University Press, 2008).
10 See, e.g., P. J. Kearney, "Autopathography and Humane Medicine: *The Diving Bell and the Butterfly*—An Interpretation," *Medical Humanities* 32, no. 2 (2006): 111–113.
11 Philip Rieff, *The Triumph of the Therapeutic: Uses of Faith after Freud* (Chicago, IL: University of Chicago Press, 1987).
12 Ian Thomson, "The Rise of the Literary Memoir: How Do You Balance Truthfulness with Drama?" *Independent*, February 12, 2015: https://www.independent.co.uk/arts-entertainment/books/features/rise-literary-memoir-how-do-you-balance-truthfulness-drama-10041988.html, accessed on August 20, 2021. Also see Alex Zwerdling, *The Rise of the Memoir* (New York: Oxford University Press, 2017).
13 M. Faith McLellan, "Literature and Medicine: Physician-Writers," *The Lancet* 349, no. 9051 (1997): 564–567.

14 On this point, McLellan cites: Debra Journet, "Forms of Discourse and the Sciences of the Mind: Luria, Sacks, and the Role of Narrative in Neurological Case Histories," *Written Communication* 7, no. 2 (1990): 171–199.

15 McLellan, "Literature and Medicine," 564.

16 Ibid.

17 Ibid.

18 Ibid., 565.

19 Ibid.

20 The Arnold P. Gold Foundation has supported a recent documentary, titled *Why Doctors Write*, on physician-authors: https://www.kbprods.com/portfolio/why-doctors-write/.

21 Tony Miksanek, "Seven Reasons Why Doctors Write," *LitMed Magazine*, accessed on August 20, 2021: https://medhum.med.nyu.edu/magazine/?p=151.

22 The notion that writing can be used as a form of therapy is widely recognized and advocated. For a recent example, see James Pennebaker and Joshua M. Smyth, *Opening Up by Writing It Down: How Expressive Writing Improves Health and Eases Emotional Pain* (New York: Guilford Publications, 2016).

23 Atul Gawande, *Complications: A Surgeon's Notes on an Imperfect Science* (New York: Picador, 2002), 18, 24.

24 Carol Donley and Martin Kohn, *Recognitions: Doctors and Their Stories* (Kent, OH: The Kent State University Press, 2002), xi.

25 Delese Wear and Therese Jones, "Bless Me Reader for I Have Sinned: Physicians and Confessional Writing," *Perspectives in Biology and Medicine* 53, no. 2 (2010): 215–230.

26 See, e.g., Danielle Ofri, *When We Do Harm: A Doctor Confronts Medical Error* (Boston, MA: Beacon Press, 2020).

27 Allan Brandt and Martha Gardner, "The Golden Age of Medicine?" in *Companion to Medicine in the Twentieth Century*, edited by Roger Cooter and John Pickstone (New York: Routledge, 2003), 21–38. Also see Jay Katz, *The Silent World of Doctor and Patient* (Baltimore, MD: Johns Hopkins University Press, 2002).

28 See, e.g., Pauline Chen, *Final Exam: A Surgeon's Reflections on Mortality* (New York: Alfred A. Knopf, 2007), 54.

29 Sherman Alexie, *You Don't Have to Say You Love Me: A Memoir* (New York: Little, Brown and Company, 2017).

30 Atul Gawande, *The Checklist Manifesto: How to Get Things Right* (New York: Metropolitan Books, 2010).

31 For example, a particular and exceptional such chapter on Oliver Sacks's work is in: G. T. Couser, *Vulnerable Subjects: Ethics and Life Writing* (New York: Cornell University Press, 2003), chapter 5.

32 William Claire, ed., *The Physician as Writer*, vol. 3 of *Literature and Medicine* (Albany, NY: SUNY, 1984).

33 Richard Selzer, "An Expostulation," *Literature and Medicine* 10, no. 1 (1991): 34–41.

34 Ibid., 34.

35 For a critical take on doctors writing poetry, see Alastair Gee, "Ode on a Stethoscope," *New Yorker*, January 14, 2015: https://www.newyorker.com/tech/annals-of-technology/ode-stethoscope.

36 Selzer, "An Expostulation," 35.

37 Ibid., 36.

38 Ibid., 39.

39 Ibid., 40.

40 Ibid., 41.

41 Allan Peterkin, "Why We Write (And How We Can Do It Better)," *CMAJ* 182, no. 15 (2010): 1650–1652.

42 Note the subtitle of Rita Charon's book, *Narrative Medicine: Honoring the Stories of Illness* (New York: Oxford University Press, 2008). Relatedly, in the Gold Foundation

documentary *Why Doctors Write*, physician-poet Rafael Campo notes that writing about patients gives doctors a chance to explore the social, personal, and cultural context of medicine, thereby expanding one's worldview. Also, specifically with regard to poetry, Campo points out that individuality and particularity can be honored.

43 Peterkin, "Why We Write," 1650.

44 Charon, *Narrative Medicine*.

45 Peterkin, "Why We Write," 1651.

46 There is a wide literature on the ethics of life writing, outside of medical humanities or discussions of physician-authors. Here are two significant recent texts: Paul John Eakin, ed., *The Ethics of Life Writing* (New York: Cornell University Press, 2004); and Mary Karr, *The Art of Memoir* (New York: HarperCollins, 2015).

47 This sentiment is supported by the move in clinical ethics toward joint decision-making, where doctors and patients make decisions together. For a scholarly discussion of this topic in bioethics, see Lars Sandman and Christian Munthe, "Shared Decision-Making and Patient Autonomy," *Theoretical Medicine and Bioethics* 30, no. 4 (2009): 289–310.

48 For a recent discussion on counseling literature, see Len Sperry and Ronald Pies, "Writing about Clients: Ethical Considerations and Options," *Counseling and Values* 54, no. 2 (2010): 88–102.

49 Arthur Frank, "Not Whether but How: Considerations on the Ethics of Telling Patients' Stories," *Hastings Center Report* 49, no. 6 (2019): 13–16.

50 For example, I have heard Rita Charon voice some degree of objection to this kind of writing on two occasions: once at the 2019 meeting of the American Society of Bioethics and Humanities, and another time during her visit with the McGovern Center for Humanities and Ethics, also in 2019. While she supports this kind of writing within closed professional circles, she has reservations about publishing this material out of a fear that this could exploit patients. To be sure, her reservations are not absolute. She just insists that great care be taken.

51 Frank, "Not Whether but How," 13.

52 Ibid.

53 Ibid.

54 Ibid., 14.

55 Ibid.

56 M. M. Bakhtin, *Speech Genres and Other Late Essays* (Austin, TX: University of Texas Press, 1986).

57 Frank, "Not Whether but How," 15. Frank cites Bakhtin, *Speech Genres*.

58 Frank, "Not Whether but How," 15.

59 Of interest, Frank, following Kathryn Montgomery and Steven Miles, sought to operationalize this way of thinking and writing in the journal *Second Opinion* (which is no longer published), and they framed such writing as "case stories" instead of "case studies."

60 Lee Gutkind, ed., *Becoming a Doctor: From Student to Specialist, Doctor-Writers Share Their Experiences* (New York: W. W. Norton & Company, 2010).

61 Leah Kaminsky, ed., *Writer, M.D.: The Best Contemporary Fiction and Nonfiction by Doctors* (New York: Vintage, 2012).

62 Cecil Helman, ed., *Doctors and Patients: An Anthology* (Boca Raton, FL: CRC Press, 2018).

63 Carol Donley and Martin Kohn, eds., *Recognitions: Doctors and Their Stories* (Kent, OH: Kent State University Press, 2002), xi.

64 Ibid., xii.

65 Robert Coles and Testa Randy-Michael, with Joseph O'Donnell and Penny Armstrong, eds., *A Life in Medicine: A Literary Anthology* (New York: The New Press, 2003).

66 Iain Bamforth, *The Body in the Library: A Literary Anthology of Modern Medicine* (New York: Verso, 2003).

67 For a description of this tradition of pastoral theology that focuses on individuals and introspection, see Robert Dykstra and Nathan Carlin, "At Home in the World: A Memorial Tribute to Donald Capps (1939–2015)," *Pastoral Psychology* 65, no. 5 (2016): 571–586; and Nathan Carlin, *Pastoral Aesthetics: A Theological Perspective on Principlist Bioethics* (New York: Oxford University Press, 2019), 13–33.

68 See Nathan Carlin, *Religious Mourning: Reversals and Restorations in Psychological Portraits of Religious Leaders* (Euguene, OR: Wipf and Stock, 2014).

Part I
Two traditional representatives

1   Richard Selzer

Three troubling tales of physicians' peculiar behavior

Tony Miksanek

What's so special about doctors who write?

The very best writers possess these six essential qualities: imagination, a keen power of observation, love of language, passion, vivid life experiences, and curiosity. Surgeon-writer Richard Selzer scores high marks in all these areas. Yet he is just one of many accomplished physicians turned writers. In addition to the authors discussed in this book, other celebrated doctor-writers include Anton Chekhov, William Carlos Williams, Mikhail Bulgakov, Arthur Conan Doyle, Lewis Thomas, and Khaled Hosseini.

So why do physicians as a group gravitate toward writing? And how come so many doctors are such effective writers? Physicians enjoy some built-in advantages as writers. Their work days are filled with drama, conflict (disease, difficult diagnoses, bureaucracy), colorful characters, and a fair share of irony. As for setting, physicians ply their craft in a high-stakes, sometimes life and death arena. Few venues can match the spectacle of the emergency room (ER), operating room, or ICU. Even the clinic exam room of a primary care physician can feel like a confessional booth. Regarding characterization, there's never a shortage of fascinating people in a physician's practice—silent and suffering, eccentric, stoic, crochety, resilient, jovial, stubborn. And for plot, how about a lengthy list of illnesses, trauma, and misfortune? A multitude of minute and momentous decisions and actions play out for dozens of patients every day. And those judgments often have ripple effects. Selzer is wise to acknowledge the inimitable realm available to physicians who write: "A doctor/writer is especially blessed in that he walks about all day in the middle of a short story."[1]

A doctor's encounter with a patient fits nicely into a short story's format. There are time constraints of a visit (limited word count), a protagonist (usually the patient, sometimes the physician), and antagonists (typically a disease but could be the health insurance carrier, a side effect of treatment, or even the doctor himself). Conflict (suffering, patient noncompliance, trouble inputting mounds of data into the electronic medical system) is rampant. And as for denouement, there is diagnosis and treatment (or sadly in some instances, failure to cure, disability, or death). Physicians get plenty of practice writing too—office notes, histories and physicals, consultations. And doctors may have special reasons to

DOI: 10.4324/9781003079712-1

write beyond a hope for fame and fortune: as a form of therapy and reflection, to honor and memorialize patients, as a sort of penance for bad behavior.[2] But physician-writers must be especially careful when translating real-life experiences into fiction. Safeguarding patient identity and protecting patient confidentiality are essential.

Selzer's start to a writing career and a brief biography

"Writing came to me late, like a wisdom tooth,"[3] Richard Selzer recalled. The general surgeon began writing seriously at age 40 and typically wrote between the hours of 1:00 and 3:00 AM. He dubbed his early efforts "nocturnal creatures" and those tales were mostly horror stories because he found that genre especially easy to compose. Even as years passed by and his literary output swelled, his affection for the macabre and the preternatural as subject matter did not diminish. Selzer frequently utilized morsels of the grotesque (and humor) in his stories.

Maybe his day job as a busy surgeon who regularly carved open fellow human beings, placed his gloved hands inside them, and removed diseased pieces of their bodies gave rise, in large part, to his affinity for horror. As a surgeon, to heal a patient meant he must wound them first—make an incision, cut out rotted flesh, slice away tumorous tissue. And then there's the living fluids and materials of nightmares—spilt blood, oozing pus, leaking contents of guts—that he is immersed in day-to-day. Selzer already knew much about fear before he even picked up a pen. How could terror not find a way to slink into many of his tales?

Rather than employing a typewriter or computer, Selzer relished writing out his stories in longhand using a fountain pen. He likened the writer's pen to the surgeon's scalpel—instruments of similar size. He remarked, "Wield a scalpel, and blood is shed. Wield a pen, and ink is shed upon a page."[4] It should come as no surprise then that Selzer had a fondness for the eerie compositions of Edgar Allan Poe, or that he was mindful of Emily Dickinson's line of verse: "Horror, Tis so Appalling, it Exhilarates."[5] He realized, "To make the flesh creep is an ancient and honorable literary endeavor."[6]

Selzer (1928-2016) was born and raised in Troy, New York. His father, Julius, was a general practitioner (GP). The family resided in the top floor of an old brownstone building, and his father's medical office occupied the first floor. Selzer recalled how he and his slightly older brother Billy were able to hear the moaning and wailing of his father's patients below their living unit. Selzer was only 13 years old when his father died. In his autobiography, *Down from Troy*, Selzer not so much recalls his youth as he reconstructs it. In a theme that he would revisit often, pain reverberates throughout his memoir—the pain of growing up in a town suffering through the Great Depression as well as the pain of loss.

Selzer obtained his MD degree in 1953, served in the US Army as part of a medical unit in Korea for a couple of years and later maintained his own surgical practice along with holding a volunteer teaching position at Yale School of Medicine in New Haven, Connecticut. He retired from the practice of surgery in 1985. Selzer invigorated the burgeoning field of medical humanities in the 1970s and 1980s with his unique style of writing, lectures, workshops, correspondence, and commencement addresses. He authored 13 books. Nine of them are collections of short stories and essays. In addition, he has written an autobiography (*Down from Troy*), an illness memoir chronicling his bout of Legionnaire's disease (*Raising the Dead*), a novella (*Knife Song Korea*), and his diary (aptly titled *Diary*).

Selzer's unique literary universe and his most important themes

Selzer's short story universe is expansive. While many of his tales occur in the places he knows best—the hospital, operating room, or interior of the human body—numerous other stories transpire in locales around the world. A sampling of distinct or distant settings includes the pampas of Argentina, a crematorium, a European monastery, a landfill, Korea, a library bathroom, Zaire, a convent of nuns, Moorish Spain, a cave, a military hospital in Germany, a slaughterhouse.

Understandably, doctors and sick folk abound in Selzer's stories and essays. His plots often incorporate an unexpected twist or injection of humor. For example, in one story, a woman about to have her gangrenous leg amputated draws a smiley face on the decaying limb prior to the operation. In another, a widow is fixated on listening to the transplanted heart of her deceased husband beating in someone else's chest. One tale poignantly details the innocent love between two teenagers who are doomed by tuberculosis.

Although Selzer incorporates a variety of themes in his stories, seven of them are recurrent throughout the majority of his work:

1. The experience of being a doctor;
2. The beauty of the human body and its marvelous anatomy;
3. The ritual of surgery;
4. The physician-patient relationship;
5. Pain;
6. Love;
7. How illness can sometimes elevate the sick and even make them holy.

Being a physician is simultaneously the most honorable and impossible occupation, the highest privilege and the heaviest burden. Medical training is lengthy and arduous. Perfection is the strived-for standard; a goal that is unattainable from the start. Selzer provides a peek at the mental, emotional, and physical toll physicians must withstand. His images of doctors highlight their strengths and fallibility. Peter Graham, in his essay about three particular doctor-writers, points out that the physicians portrayed in Selzer's stories "are neither angelic nor demonic," adding that these fictional doctors demonstrate ordinary human flaws and virtues but "are professionals first and last."[7]

As a surgeon, Selzer is privy to the exquisiteness of the body, especially its inner anatomy. Danger and dread lurk everywhere inside the opened chest or abdomen during an operation—a mistakenly nicked blood vessel or the detection of a previously hidden tumor metastasis, for example—but the splendor of how human bodies are designed and function is never lost on Selzer. On the other hand, flesh is transient and perhaps no one knows this more than a surgeon (or a mortician).

Selzer is smitten by the ceremony of surgery. One commentator, Enid Rhodes Peschel, notes Selzer's profound reverence for the ritual of surgery likening his depiction of operating on patients to "a metaphysical Mass." In her view, surgery is a kind of sacrament where Selzer can pursue grace.[8] The operating room is a temple where the devoted (patients) place all their faith in the surgeon and his acolytes (nurses, assistant, anesthetist). The patient is carefully cleansed and draped before being positioned upon the altar (operating table) with the anticipation that they will be cured, their body made whole again. Blood is often present in the proceedings—spilled from its vessels, sometimes replaced. Surgeons are priestly, outfitted in their vestments (sterile gown and gloves, cap and facial mask), who laboriously scrub their hands before beginning the solemn procedure. Prayers are usually offered up—by the patients themselves prior to the operation, their loved ones, and quite likely a considerable number of the surgeon-priests.

In any of his stories that feature a doctor and a patient, Selzer pays homage to the physician-patient relationship. It is a mystical bond—sacred and mighty, complicated and fragile. On the doctor's side, it draws its life force from his compassion, truthfulness, and advocacy for what is in the best interests of the patient. On the patient's side, the relationship survives and prospers mostly from faith in the physician, past experience with that doctor, and trust in him. Communication is the critical conduit.

Pain is obviously a universal experience. A sizeable portion of a doctor's workday involves confronting and managing the pain of his patients. The concept of pain (the physical and emotional pain of patients, the anguish of the physician) permeates the pages of Selzer's writing. He digs deep into its nature but decides that language and words are inadequate to convey its experience and depth. Love also has a heavy presence in many of his best stories, such as "Tom and Lily." Peschel believes that Selzer's stories express "a longing for love"—from God or from the physician's patients.[9] In Selzer's fictional universe, love is the greatest emotion of all. Love can serve as a remedy, but it might be a sort of contagion too.

Selzer believes that sickness and suffering can expose the soul. For him, disease sometimes has the potential to elevate, even beatify the ill and injured. In his essay, Charles Anderson explores Selzer's notion that illness has dual properties—the ability to harm, the potential to augment. He writes:

> If there is a single source of Selzer's power as a writer, it must be his ability to look unflinchingly at his patients and to see in their suffering that sickness both destroys and ennobles, wounds and heals, and creates the possibility of transcendence.[10]

Selzer has a wobbly affinity for the truth. In fact, he is forthright about how little he is concerned with facts. Rather, impressions are what matter most to him. On this matter, he spots no conflict between fact and fiction; each can be employed in the service of the truth:

> When the subject is that of the human body, how it's made, how it works, and what goes wrong with it, I have kept faith with the factual. In all other matters, I've committed the gentle treason of poetry and betrayed mere fact in search of truth, the real real that lies just beneath the real.[11]

For those individuals without the time or ambition to read the entire compendium of Selzer's stories and essays, which tales are must-reads?[12] A perfect place to start is his collection *The Doctor Stories*, which includes an informative "Introduction." Selzer's finest work includes the following five tales: "Tom and Lily," "Brute," "Imelda," "Luis," and "The Consultation." "Toenails" or "Fetishes" (kinder, softer stories) and "Sarcophagus" (a vivid, terrifying portrayal of an operation that goes very badly) could be added to the end of that list. "The Consultation," "Brute," and "Imelda" are a trio of cautionary tales that will be closely considered. Each one of them showcases a doctor who struggles to control the situation. The physician-patient relationship is atypical or flawed. Communication malfunctions.

A most unusual ménage à trois in "The Consultation"

"The Consultation," one of Selzer's earlier stories, effectively demonstrates how the author cleverly creates a lasting, singular effect by the tale's conclusion. The story displays his trademark knack for positioning an unexpected event (in this case, set to motion by a simple glimpse, then a touch) or moment in an otherwise ordinary or straightforward encounter. Here, he introduces a dash of humor to defuse the potential severity of the protagonist's unexpected finding and weighs in on what defines a physician-patient relationship. His nimbleness and economy with plot and dialogue are impressive as the story transpires in only five and one-half pages of text.

An unnamed surgeon attends a medical conference and abruptly becomes bored. He calls a prostitute to arrange a rendezvous. Gloria, a Polish prostitute, owned a virtuous voice on the telephone and a perfectly detached demeanor upon their meeting in a hotel. She had a small gesticulation—rubbing two fingers against the corner of her mouth—that reminded the surgeon of peasantry.

After an undescribed sexual encounter, the surgeon is the first to wake up the next morning. His eyes scan the pleasurable landscape of the prostitute's naked body. His gaze is interrupted, however, by a small elevation of her right breast along with some dimpling of the skin there. He proceeds to palpate and explore the breast with his fingers. The lump is irregularly shaped, hard, and immovable. He becomes alarmed, quickly removes his hand from Gloria's breast, and in the process, wakes her up.

He takes a long shower and gets dressed. The surgeon is troubled by his discovery and a bit frazzled. He places $100 on the hotel room table, payment for services rendered. Gloria senses something is awry. The conversation becomes terse and uncomfortable. He attempts to adopt his professional bearing and voice but becomes aware he is sweating. He blurts out the pronouncement: She has a breast lump. The surgeon guides her hand to the bulge in the right breast. He expresses the need for her to see a doctor.

They go back and forth in a cautious conversation that the surgeon does not want to have. Gloria asks the surgeon for his opinion. What might the lump be? He says he doesn't know for certain. Neither of them wants to be the first to say aloud what is on both their minds—that the lump could be cancerous. Finally, she says the word first. Cancer. For Gloria, breast cancer and a possible mastectomy could ruin her career. But the surgeon is secretly worried more about her life than her livelihood. As she dresses, he muses about the clout of the word, "cancer."

He is upset, not so much because Gloria has become a victim perhaps fated for future suffering, but because he pictures the breast lump as his challenger:

> But rather what sickened him was the thought that he and the lump had been rivals, each feeding on her flesh, reaching within her, that they had been competing for her in a kind of race to have her before the other could use her all up, leaving none.[13]

Before the surgeon could leave the room, Gloria plucks a $10 bill from the pile of cash the surgeon left as payment on the table. She thanks him for "the consultation" and offers him the money. With a dry mouth and slight smile, he declines the compensation, telling her he doesn't make house calls.

"The Consultation" is an unsettling story. One reason is the attitude and behavior of the surgeon. The other reason is sympathy for the prostitute. Her career and maybe her life are in great jeopardy. How she learns about her breast tumor is deplorable. And while the surgeon may have ultimately saved her life by finding the tumor, his total lack of empathy is appalling. Readers might wonder about Gloria's future. If the tumor is malignant (as the clinical description of the breast mass suggests), can she be completely cured? Will Gloria even pursue the recommendation to get the lump checked by a doctor? Would she ever consent to a biopsy or breast surgery?

Since the story unfolds from the perspective of the physician, consider his attributes and actions first. For starters, the protagonist is not your typical doctor. His name is not provided even though the prostitute's first and last name are supplied. His identity is guarded as might be expected for a john (the client of a prostitute). The fact that he is unnamed immediately sets up a kind of boundary, distancing him from Gloria and from readers of the story. Readers know next to nothing about him other than he is a bored surgeon—no specified age, physical appearance, or marital status are given.

His fix for boredom is soliciting a prostitute. That action says a lot about the man. Granted, doctors have needs and desires like other people do, but the idea of a doctor as a john is a bit off-putting. The thought of your doctor soliciting sex from a prostitute is likely to trigger a reaction ranging somewhere between disappointment and disgust. And that reaction is without even considering that he could be married. The surgeon also seems judgmental. He presumptuously attributes Gloria's fingers-to-mouth gesture as an indication that she comes from peasant stock.

When the surgeon detects her breast lump, he is initially distressed. That discovery makes the one-night stand awkward and complicated. He seems more interested in a hasty exit. He does instruct Gloria of the necessity of visiting a doctor, but cannot summon the decency to speak the truth that the lump very well might be cancer, necessitating an urgency to have it checked and biopsied. Medical humanities scholar Suzanne Poirier explores this type of blunt objectivity and desire to distance oneself that seems inherent to the medical profession as represented in the depiction of fictional physicians. She concludes: "But even when the [white lab] coat is not there, the [medical] profession itself provides an invisible coat of armor."[14]

The surgeon engages in some evasive conversation that ultimately forces Gloria to announce the word that the surgeon lacks the courage to speak: cancer. That slippery exchange and his deliberate avoidance of the truth further diminishes his image as a physician and his humanity. But his utter lack of empathy can only fully be comprehended when he imagines the tumor to be *his* competitor, not the enemy of the woman. He pictures a sort of race between himself and the almost certainly malignant tumor to see which of the two can use up Gloria's body. That moment makes the MD more than just merely sleazy, but truly malignant. Now the two of them—surgeon and tumor—are not merely rivals but peers.

The surgeon is done with Gloria. He is no match for the presumably cancerous lump. Of Gloria's "devourers," the surgeon is the more evil of the two. He is driven by lust, enabled by a lack of conscience. The tumor is only following its mutated genetic reprogramming. The surgeon's flippant joke before he leaves accompanied by a little smile further cements our opinion of him.

The story invites consideration of the ethical obligation and potential pitfalls that a doctor might encounter in providing an unsolicited diagnosis to a stranger or someone who is not an established patient. By refusing payment for the uninvited diagnosis that he makes in "The Consultation," the surgeon absolves himself of any responsibility. Is he correct? Can there be a genuine physician-patient relationship where there is no emergency obligation to treat or if there is no compensation accepted for the diagnosis rendered? Can physicians truly ever be "off-duty?"

"The Consultation" features some of Selzer's favorite themes: the life of an MD, the beauty of the body and the allure of the flesh, and the definition and complexity of the physician-patient relationship (or the minimum amount of responsibility required of any doctor in a nonemergency situation). The story additionally displays the intricacies of communication, the weight of the truth, and just how ugly an absence of compassion can get.

Bad behavior abounds in "Brute"

"Brute" is a cautionary tale centering on a physician's anger and the mistreatment of a patient. Over time, it has ignited considerable controversy as many readers have raised concerns that the story has stereotyped racist tones. Selzer has pleaded innocent to that charge, responding, "'Brute,' written some twenty-five years after the event described, is an act of atonement. It has been woefully misread as racist by some and by others as a 'missed opportunity for Grace.'"[15] Regardless of your stance on this issue, the story is a furnace of feelings—rage and remorse, humiliation and honesty. In fewer than 1,700 words, "Brute" condenses a night in the ER noteworthy for sheer exhaustion, bad choices, noncompliance, and a regret that can never be pardoned.

A weary physician-narrator working in the ER has dealt with a shift of myocardial infarctions, motor vehicle accident victims, and traumas. It's 2:00 AM when four police officers bring a gigantic black man into the ER. He is handcuffed, very drunk, belligerent, and has a deep gash across his forehead almost 5 inches in length. The ER doctor speculates as to the origin of this large facial laceration: was it from police brutality, or maybe a fight with another man? The narrator views the patient as a wild animal: "a great mythic beast broken loose in the city" and a "netted panther."[16] Yet the doctor senses the patient possesses a substantial amount of dignity too.

The police proceed to restrain the man's arms with straps. The doctor confesses to a strange attraction to this patient: "I am ravished by the sight of him, the raw, untreated flesh, his very wildness which suggests less a human than a great and beautiful animal."[17] As the physician cleans the wound, the patient does not hold still, swearing and spitting, and moving his head from side to side. The doctor implores the man to cooperate, but the patient does not oblige. The worn-out doctor proceeds to tightly suture each ear lobe of the man to the stretcher mattress and warns the patient not to move less the ears will tear off. Even more maliciously, the MD leans directly over the patient's face and grins. The doctor decides, "It is the cruelest grin of my life. Torturers must grin like that, beheaders and operators of racks."[18]

The patient no longer resists and now remains still. It takes 90 minutes for the ER doctor to suture the laceration. The restraints are removed. A wound dressing of bandages wrapped around his head makes the patient look like he is wearing a white turban. A drop of blood remains in each earlobe, remnants of where they were stitched to the mattress. A metamorphosis has occurred—no longer an unruly creature, now a magnificent maharaja. The police forcefully escort the man out of the ER. Years later, the doctor-narrator still cannot erase memories of that patient encounter and his own bad behavior. He will always remain apologetic for his unprofessionalism and that malevolent grin.

"Brute" is a brief story propelled by fury and tension. Anyone who has ever worked in a hospital emergency department can attest to the tale's genuine flavor. The ER is commonly a chaotic, volatile, and exhausting place. Patience can run thin there. Agitated and difficult patients are not uncommon in the ER and present unique challenges to the doctors caring for them. Two significant problems permeate the story. First is the doctor-narrator's view and depiction of his noncompliant patient, which for many readers seems racist. Second is the doctor's use of cruel treatment as his "solution" to dealing with the combative patient. Most readers equate the MD's actions with torture. The title "Brute" implies only one bully in the story, but the tale could just as easily have been named "Brutes" (plural). The primary beast is indeed the ER doctor who is mean and angry, abuses his power, and then gloats about his action. But there are additional bullies present in the tale: the aggressive patient and the police officers.

The moral of the story is evident: doctors need to keep their emotions in check. Anger is a particularly dangerous reaction for physicians. Dreadful acts can give rise to regret that may be difficult or impossible to expunge. It appears that writing "Brute" functioned as a form of therapy for Selzer, an effort to make amends, a public penance of sorts. Yes, the MD likely does feel bad about his "care" in this case, professing his torment even many years later over how he misbehaved and his nastiness. But it can certainly be argued that composing a short story for the inhumane treatment of a patient is not the most appropriate form of apology rendered.

Selzer's reverence for the human body and his homage to wounds are front-and-center. The doctor-narrator notes that "by the addition of the wound, his body is more than it was, more of a body."[19] By the time the laceration is stitched up and the wound dressed, the doctor admires the man. The patient has been transformed from a beast to a dignified, regal maharaja in the eyes of the physician. Here, Selzer illustrates how illness and injury can alter those who are afflicted. In *The Exact Location of the Soul*, he proposes, "Again and again, in patients ravaged by disease, or deformed, we are stunned by a sudden radiance."[20] And in "Textbook" (*Letters to a Young Doctor*), Selzer instructs that "disease raises the sufferer, granting him from out of his fever and his fret an intimate vision of life, a more direct route to his soul."[21]

The physician-patient relationship that must be forged on the spot in the emergency room starts out poorly and proceeds badly. But by the conclusion of the tale, both men have reached a détente of sorts. Robert Leigh Davis in his essay "The Art of the Suture: Richard Selzer and Medical Narrative" offers an especially kind explanation of the MD's bad behavior: "The doctor's inability to compose or control the afflicted body may lead to the violent suturing in 'Brute,' but it may also lead to a powerful kind of love."[22] The doctor-narrator early on does admit to an attraction to the wildness and strength of the man. Later, the physician becomes protective of him, expressing a concern that perhaps the police might get too rough with the patient. Still, readers should rightly question the narrator's sincerity along with his actions. The doctor proclaims his greatest regret to be his grin. He professes more shame over his gloating than his torturous treatment of the patient. Has the brute really learned his lesson?

Perfection, obligation, and postmortem plastic surgery in "Imelda"

"Imelda" is a heartbreaking and haunting story about the pursuit of perfection and its toll, unexpected loss, coping, and burnout. What are the consequences for a truly gifted surgeon (who is numb to the emotional needs of his patients) when a young girl dies? "Imelda" serves as a jarring reminder that despite its science and technology, its precision and rigor, the practice of surgery and medicine can be unpredictable with random events influencing or dictating outcomes.

The doctor-narrator (no name provided) learns that a prominent plastic surgeon, Dr. Hugh Franciscus, has recently passed away. The narrator was a third year medical student when he first encountered Franciscus and remembers him as a model of professors of surgery—dynamic, a skilled operator, and dedicated. Even heroic. Yet he was standoffish with staff and viewed as arrogant by some. Franciscus volunteered every year to lead a medical mission. He was heading to Honduras and recruited the narrator to accompany him and serve as an interpreter of the Spanish-speaking population and to take photographs of patients before and after their surgical procedures.

With only a few days left in their three-week stay, the narrator greets the last patient to be seen that day, a thin 14-year-old girl named Imelda Valdez who is accompanied by her mother. Imelda clutches a dirty pink cloth against her mouth. Her chart documents a complete left-sided cleft lip and palate. Imelda will not voluntarily remove the rag from her face so that she can be examined. Franciscus abruptly jerks the cloth off. The narrator's initial impression of her congenital defect is "utterly hideous—a nude rubbery insect that had fastened there." Slightly later though, he revises his assessment of Imelda: "She was a beautiful bird with a crushed beak."[23]

In the operating room the following morning, Imelda is under general anesthesia and Franciscus is ready to begin the surgical repair of her cleft. Suddenly, the anesthetist stops him from starting. Imelda's blood pressure is elevated, her pulse rapid. Her temperature is 108 degrees. She is experiencing malignant hyperthermia, a very serious reaction to the anesthesia medication. Ice is ordered to cool her down, but none is available in the hospital. The EKG tracing flatlines. Imelda is dead on the operating table. Franciscus finds the girl's mother. She is holding the cloth Imelda used to conceal her facial defect. He struggles to announce Imelda's death and explain how it happened. The mother tells Franciscus that Imelda's death was God's decision. She expresses a mistaken belief that Imelda's cleft has been fixed, and now the girl can ascend to Heaven without the disfigurement.

The next day, Imelda's wrapped dead body is loaded into a wooden cart headed for her burial site. The mother tells the narrator that Franciscus "has finished the work of God" and that Imelda "is beautiful."[24] When the narrator removes part of the covering of the corpse, he is astonished that the cleft lip and palate have indeed been mended, a track of small sutures marking the repair. He speculates why Franciscus finished the operation and imagines how such a postmortem surgery might have transpired in the hospital morgue late at night.

Weeks later, Franciscus gives a presentation in the medical school auditorium about surgeries performed in Honduras. The narrator operates the slide projector. Unexpectedly, a photograph of Imelda and her cleft defect is projected on the screen. A long silence follows. It is finally broken with Franciscus saying only, "Imelda." The narrator removes the next slide featuring a picture of Imelda in the morgue following correction of the cleft. He determines that the teenage girl was

Franciscus's "measure of perfection and pain—the one lost, the other gained."[25] Franciscus taught surgery for another 15 years but operated less often and then stopped altogether. He quit embarking on medical missions. The narrator still thinks of Imelda from time to time and now realizes that Franciscus's impractical surgery on the dead girl "was one of goodness."[26] Unfortunately, he never told his teacher that, and now it's too late.

"Imelda" reads like a fractured fairy tale with a most unhappy ending. The teenage girl dies, a ceremonial surgery is performed in a morgue, the surgeon's life force seriously ebbs, and the now much older narrator continues to live with regret (the girl's tragic demise and the failure to express to his surgery professor that his act was virtuous). The story lends itself to a consideration of the nature of the physician-patient (and patient's family) relationship, the quest for perfection in a doctor's daily work, the reaction of a doctor to a patient's death, and the causes of physician burnout.

What it *means* to be a surgeon. That is certainly one of Selzer's prime aims in many of his stories. Not so much the mastery and execution of the technical skills, but rather the intellectual, philosophical, ethical, and emotional components of the occupation. The responsibility, demands, and expectations. The long hours and complex decision-making. The awareness that calamity is never far-removed. How does the stress of being a surgeon spill into his private life?

In Dr. Franciscus, Selzer molds a complicated character with plenty of praiseworthy traits and a few serious faults. Perhaps his supreme attribute is also his paramount weakness—an obsession with perfection. It's understandable why a plastic surgeon might be a perfectionist. Unlike a hernia repair or a coronary artery bypass operation, the majority of a plastic surgeon's work product will be viewed externally. Cosmetic results count greatly.

Readers become acquainted with Dr. Franciscus through the eyes of the biased narrator. The plastic surgeon's clinical knowledge, precise operative skills, and devotion to the profession and his patients are rated by the narrator as exemplary. And Franciscus is also altruistic, volunteering his surgical services annually to inhabitants of needy nations. But the narrator admits that Franciscus lacks affection for the people he treats. In a passage that foreshadows the major event of the story, he makes this assessment about Franciscus and his relationship with patients:

> He did not want to be touched by them. It was less kindness that he showed them than a reassurance that he would never give up, that he would bend every effort. If anyone could, he would solve the problems of their flesh.[27]

Upon meeting Imelda, Franciscus finds her reluctance to remove the cloth covering her face "silly" and threatens to dismiss the girl. And then he suddenly and unsympathetically yanks the rag from her face. That act encapsulates some of what is lacking in the doctor—no proper bedside manner, a dearth of compassion, impatience with people. How can any doctor (no matter the excellent results of his surgical work) be considered perfect or admirable where there is a deficiency of empathy? But Poirier suggests a reason for the heartless behavior of the surgeon: insulation. She writes, "Selzer's characters sometimes use authoritarianism to provide a defense against their vulnerability."[28] Peschel provides an alternative explanation postulating that the insensitivity and callous actions demonstrated by physician characters in literature by some doctor-writers (including Selzer) may "in effect be a supreme exercise in self-control."[29]

Such behavior and the surgeon's personality set up the central question of the story: exactly why did Franciscus repair the cleft lip and palate of the dead girl? Who did he do it for—Imelda, her mother, the student narrator, or himself? Perhaps he ultimately felt pity for the girl, empathy for Imelda's mother, a responsibility to teach the narrator, an obligation to complete the promised surgery. At first, the narrator wonders if the surgeon's action arises out of arrogance or madness. But later he comes to believe Franciscus had his own need to finish the work. Indeed, the strongest case can be made that he did the surgery on Imelda's corpse for his own accomplishment—a professional duty to finish the job, his pursuit of perfection, or avoidance of any shame resulting from not fulfilling the task. In her essay "Richard Selzer: The Rounds of Revelation," M. Teresa Tavormina contends that performing surgery "upon another human being is a simultaneous act of love and violation."[30] Perhaps suturing the dead girl's defect was indeed a feat of love.

When a doctor loses a patient, especially someone young or when the death is unexpected, coping can be very hard. Reactions can range from sadness to self-questioning to guilt. French surgeon René Leriche wisely addressed this subject of loss in his book *The Philosophy of Surgery* in 1951: "Every surgeon carries within himself a small cemetery, where from time to time he goes to pray—a place of bitterness and regret, where he must look for an explanation for his failures."[31] Other worthy issues contained in the story include problems with communication and the potential for burnout. Downsides of medical training are also noted. The narrator alludes to his "terrifying" experience while in his third year of medical school and also submits that "[t]he opportunity for humiliation was everywhere."[32] Shame and spirituality, failure and accomplishment have dueling presences in "Imelda." Does Franciscus save his soul or lose his mind in performing the macabre surgery on a deceased patient? Is his postmortem operation on Imelda an act of penance or the pursuit of grace? Maybe a bit of both.

Seeing the big picture

Selzer is arguably the most important doctor-writer in the last 40 years. It is impossible to imagine what the discipline of medical humanities would be like without his literary contributions and influence. Selzer's writing style is distinctive—confessional, instructive, blunt, affectionate, and imaginative. As an author, he is the ultimate excavator, a meticulous forager. In a literary landscape littered with disease, suffering, and lives on the precipice of disaster, he unearths the splendor in the simplest things, finds meaning in the mundane. But he does not ignore the malicious and the horrible.

How does it *feel* to be a doctor? What is it *like* to be sick? In what manner do doctors and patients interact with one another? Over and over again, Selzer addresses these fundamental questions in his stories. The majority of his doctor-characters are good physicians, caring human beings with frailties and quirks who try to do the best they can for patients. Yet he is mindful that doctors can act badly (cruel, angry, insensitive) and make poor choices. Even in those instances, a plausible path to repentance and reform often exists.

Advances in medicine and surgery have made many of Selzer's stories seem outdated. There is no electronic medical record (EMR) in any of his tales. Mid-level providers (physician assistants, nurse practitioners) have no presence in these stories. Access to healthcare and the enormous might of health insurance companies don't pop-up as frequent concerns. Sophisticated technology is mostly missing in Selzer's tales—no MRI or PET scans, no robotically assisted surgery, or even laparoscopic surgery. Rather, his doctor-characters are most comfortable holding a stethoscope or a scalpel or a patient's sweating hand. Commentator Charles Schuster calls Selzer a "committed idealist" who "addresses the issue of how medical practitioners can maintain their humanity amid the welter of tests, data, and quantitative measures."[33] Selzer's stories are timeless precisely because they don't rely on the ever-advancing technology and science of medicine. His focus on healing and the consequences of individual relationships keeps them relevant.

Like all fine writers, Selzer loves language and the sounds of words. And although he can stitch together beautiful sentences, at times it feels like he can't help himself from trying too hard to be elegant. Graham acknowledges the two-edged sword that is Selzer's obsession with turning a phrase or being extra clever: "This love affair with literary technique … is sometimes a distinctive strength and other times the greatest weakness of Selzer's art."[34] A review of Selzer's *Letters to a Young Doctor* that appeared in *The Washington Post* specifically targets his style of sometimes strained, overly fancy writing.[35] The reviewer finds fault with Selzer's "idiosyncratic word order," wordiness, and "stilted, artificial tone of some-one who is compulsively literary." The critic decides that "Selzer lets himself be too tempted by the sounds of phrases." That judgment might be a tad harsh, but there can be little dispute that no one is going to mistake Selzer's lyrical and lush brand of writing for the succinct, concrete prose of Hemingway. Selzer defends himself, countering: "It is my pleasure to use as much of the English language as I can rather than as little."[36]

Some readers and critics may deem Selzer's physician-characters too paternal-istic (and perhaps even authoritarian in the stories discussed). Shared decision-making (weighing patient's choice with doctor's advice) is generally absent from the stories. Scholar David B. Morris finds the narrators in Selzer's stories "share a curious detachment as spectators" and even the empathetic doctor-narrators struggle mightily "to penetrate *inside* the suffering of another human being."[37] Still, suffering seems to be very much on Selzer's mind as both doctor and writer. And if his benevolent doctor-characters appear to some as incapable of breaching a patient's pain (physical or emotional), it's certainly not for lack of effort.

The three disturbing stories highlighted here reveal a dark side of the medical profession; physician behavior that is outside the norm, out of control. Yet these cautionary tales potently remind all doctors of three lurking dangers in the practice of medicine: lack of empathy ("The Consultation"), abuse of power in the physician-patient relationship ("Brute"), and professional burnout ("Imelda"). Make no mistake though. For Richard Selzer, good doctors require equal parts of clinical competence and compassion, the talents of well-honed observation and astute listening, courage and integrity. And that formula applies just as much to real-life physicians as it does for most of his fictional ones.

Notes

1 Richard Selzer, "A Worm from My Notebook," *Taking the World in for Repairs* (New York: William Morrow and Company, 1986), 153.
2 Tony Miksanek, "Seven Reasons Why Doctors Write," *Lit Med Magazine*, January 4, 2009: https://medhum.med.nyu.edu/magazine/?p=151.
3 Richard Selzer, "Introduction," *The Doctor Stories* (New York: Picador, 1998), 11.
4 Ibid., 11.
5 Ibid., 8.
6 Ibid., 3.
7 Peter W. Graham, "A Mirror for Medicine: Richard Selzer, Michael Crichton, and Walker Percy," *Perspectives in Biology and Medicine* 24, no. 2 (1981): 231.
8 Enid Rhodes Peschel, "Richard Selzer and the Sacraments of Surgery," in *Medicine and Literature*, edited by Enid Rhodes Peschel (New York: Neale Watson Academic Publications, 1980), 73.
9 Ibid.
10 Charles M. Anderson, "It Is the Poet Who Heals": Richard Selzer's Literature of Wholeness," *Bioethics Forum* (Summer 1993), 40.
11 Selzer, "Introduction," *The Doctor Stories*, 15.
12 Tony Miksanek, "Richard Selzer and Ten Terrific Tales," *Lit Med Magazine*, July 20, 2016: https://medhum.med.nyu.edu/magazine/?p=13493.
13 Richard Selzer, "The Consultation," *Rituals of Surgery* (New York: Harper's Magazine Press, 1974), 22.
14 Suzanne Poirier, "The Physician and Authority: Portraits by Four Physician-Writers," *Literature and Medicine* 2 (1983): 33.
15 Selzer, "Introduction," *The Doctor Stories*, 17.
16 Richard Selzer, "Brute," *Letters to a Young Doctor* (New York: Simon and Schuster, 1982), 60.
17 Ibid., 61.
18 Ibid., 62.
19 Ibid., 61.
20 Richard Selzer, "Introduction," *The Exact Location of the Soul* (New York: Picador USA, 2001), 14–15.
21 Selzer, "Textbook," *Letters to a Young Doctor*, 14.
22 Robert Leigh Davis, "The Art of the Suture: Richard Selzer and Medical Narrative," *Literature and Medicine* 12, no. 2 (1993): 181.
23 Selzer, "Imelda," *Letters to a Young Doctor*, 27.
24 Ibid., 31.
25 Ibid., 35.
26 Ibid., 36.
27 Ibid., 23.
28 Poirier, "The Physician and Authority: Portraits by Four Physician-Writers," 33.

29 Enid Rhodes Peschel, "Callousness or Caring: Portraits of Doctors by Somerset Maugham and Richard Selzer," *Mosaic: An Interdisciplinary Critical Journal* 15, no. 1 (1982): 77.

30 M. Teresa Tavormina, "Richard Selzer: The Rounds of Revelation," *Literature and Medicine* 1 (1982): 71.

31 René Leriche, *La Philosophie de la Chirurgie* [*The Philosophy of Surgery*] (Paris: Flammarion, 1951).

32 Selzer, "Imelda," *Letters to a Young Doctor*, 22.

33 Charles I. Schuster, "Passion and Pathology: Richard Selzer's Philosophy of Doctoring," *Perspectives in Biology and Medicine* 28, no. 1 (1984): 65.

34 Graham, "A Mirror for Medicine: Richard Selzer, Michael Crichton, and Walker Percy," 230.

35 "A Little Surgery Needed," *The Washington Post*, August 14, 1982: www.washingtonpost.com/archive/lifestyle/1982/08/14/a-little-surgery-needed/6a4b03ce-9bff-466f-925a-f659be6e567f/.

36 Selzer, "Introduction," *The Doctor Stories*, 14.

37 David B. Morris, "Beauty and Pain: Notes on the Art of Richard Selzer," *The Iowa Review* 11, no. 2 (1980): 129.

2 Oliver Sacks

A kind of reminiscence

Tom Koch

In 1985, a local literary magazine asked me to write a short review of an unusual book, Oliver Sacks's *The Man Who Mistook His Wife for a Hat*. A year earlier I had lost my career as a medical reporter when visual limits resulted in my inability to use the newspaper's ill-maintained computers—with unstable characters bouncing, green on black—in a newsroom overwhelmed by glaring, florescent lighting. A successful Workers Compensation Board complaint of "unsafe work conditions" set a precedent for computer office ergonomics. It cost the newspaper $350,000 to upgrade their system. The result pretty much ended my news career.

To complicate matters further, in 1985 I had returned only recently to Vancouver, Canada, after an intense period of hands-on, often 18-hour-a-day parental care in Buffalo, NY. I needed work, and any assignment was welcome, even one whose pay was a $50 gift certificate from *The Reader's* publisher, Duthies Books.

The review began with what in retrospect was an inspired if flawed pairing:

> Oliver Sacks and Diane Arbus would seem to have much in common. Arbus photographed a seemingly endless parade of physically and emotionally deformed subjects who stare at the viewer with a sullen, knowing look. ... There is about Arbus' work something of the surreal but it does not heighten a sense of humanity, nor inform one. We are all twisted, her photographs proclaim, isolated in some fundamental sense. Oliver Sacks's *The Man Who Mistook His Wife for a Hat* deals with what most would see as the equally bizarre. His subjects are medical patients with organic, neurologic disorder who often manifest their symptoms in truly outrageous and outré ways. The title subject has lost the ability to perceive the whole of a figure and does, indeed, mistake his wife for a hat; another patient whose sense of balance is affected walks on a tilt as if the world were a ship permanently heeling to port; and there is an elderly lady who gets positively "kittenish," not from normal dementia but from the effects of venereal disease. ... Like Diane Arbus he sees each subject as a manifestation of human will, as a human being in the greater community. For Sacks, however, that is not an accusation but a benediction, and he begs us to accept these unusual people, and ourselves, warts and all.[1]

DOI: 10.4324/9781003079712-2

With my gift certificate I bought two detective novels and ordered an earlier book by Sacks. Eventually, I would read them all.

I later wished I could rewrite the piece. It didn't do justice to Arbus' work that, as a former photographer (another career lost to visual limits), I admired. Her subjects were a mélange of strippers, carnies, nudists, dwarfs, and giants, shot in their homes and workplaces, on the street, or in a park. She neither gawked nor censored but quietly celebrated her subjects, and in doing so, "lent a fresh dignity to the forgotten and neglected people in whom she invested so much of herself."[2] The comparison *was*, at least in some ways, apt. What was said about her could equally be said of Sacks and his subjects: "The world, in spite of its terrors, is approached as the ultimate source of wonder and fascination, no less precious for being [or appearing] irrational and incoherent."[3]

I sent Sacks a copy of *The Reader* review with an admiring note that mentioned, I think, my experiences caring for my father as a kind of membership badge that might permit me to comment on his cases. He responded with a polite but brief note thanking me for my review—he liked the comparison to Argus—while pleading obligations that prohibited a longer reply. Over the next ten years we exchanged occasional notes and letters as I found myself drawn into his world as patient, hands-on caregiver, and writer.

Outsiders: artists and subjects

If I had known the phrase, then I would have described the works of both Arbus and Sacks as "Outsider Art," a term coined in 1972 to describe images created beyond the boundaries of accepted, official culture. Its origins lay with Jean Dubuffet's *art brut* (raw art), which used as examples the work of psychiatric patients and children.[4] The word can refer equally to the artists themselves.

Arbus was no outsider except, perhaps, by choice. Her father, who owned a well-known New York department store, became a painter; her younger sister became a painter and sculptor; her older brother Howard Nemerov was an English professor and, later, a US poet laureate. She studied photography with Bernice Abbot and then with her first husband, Allen Arbus (who later portrayed Dr. Sidney Freedman on the TV show M*A*S*H), had a successful commercial career, working for was a slew of well-paying magazines, including, in a partial list: *Glamour*, *Seventeen*, and *Vogue*.

Arbus then gave up commercial photography, finding it stultifying, and spent the rest of her career photographing only those subjects she found interesting. In the 1960s, she developed an influential following, but that growing recognition did not result in financial security. Her photographs rarely sold, if at all, for more than $75 or $100. That said, she was less an outsider than its documentarian, a compassionate fellow traveler in the world, her photographs revealed.

Sacks *was* an outsider not merely uncomfortable in but often dismissed in the typically collegial world of standard medical practice and society. In the early years of World War II, at age six, he was sent from his family's London home to a residential school, where, it was hoped, he would be safe from the

German Blitzkrieg. The school was a brutal, dehumanizing, physically violent, and ultimately alienating experience. His autobiography begins with this memory: "When I was at boarding school, sent away during the war as a little boy, I had a sense of imprisonment and powerlessness, and I longed for movement and power."[5] That sense of estrangement did not leave him even after returning to his parents' home when he was ten years old.

Sacks realized in early adolescence that he was a homosexual in an era when same-sex relations were considered shameful as well as illegal. When his mother, an anatomist and surgeon, learned of her then young teenage son's predilections she responded violently: "'You are an abomination,' she said. 'I wish you had never been born.' After that she refused to speak to me for three days."[6]

Sacks read books on sexual pathologies shelved in his parents' medical library (his father was a family physician) but "found it difficult to feel that I had a 'condition,' that my identity could be reduced to a name or a diagnosis."[7] Throughout his career he would carry that skepticism forward, questioning accepted clinical assumptions that, he would argue, masked often complex responses to this or that underlying neural or physical state.

To add to this, in adolescence, Sacks was for a time covered in sores, making him feel as though, he later said, he were a leper. That period of "hideous self-consciousness,"[8] and debilitating migraines, added another layer to his alienation. And, too, his sense of skeptical difference was fueled by a love and sense of comradeship with his schizophrenic older brother, Michael. Treatments in the 1950s were at best only briefly successful. The deadening effects of Thorazine, a drug introduced in 1953, had little or no effect on Michael's schizophrenia while badly affecting his sense of place and being. With the failure of those treatments, Sacks later wrote, "Michael had begun to think of our parents, his older brothers [both physicians] and the entire medical profession as determined to devalue or 'medicalize' everything he thought and did."[9] As Sacks later wrote: "It is a question of not just medication but the whole business of living a meaningful and enjoyable life—with support systems, community, self-respect, and being respected by others, which has to be addressed. Michael's problems were not purely 'medical.'"[10] It was this sense of the clinical wrapped in the social that would be a keystone of his later writings.

What was said of Arbus after her death would be equally true of Sacks across his career: her aim has been not to reform life but to know it, not to persuade but to understand.[11] She was an insider looking out, or perhaps, an honorary outsider looking in. Sacks was an outsider from the start, inherently different and as a result suspicious of easy answers to complex clinical occurrences. At a deeper level, Arbus was a documentarian with no responsibility to her subjects and needed no long-term relationship with them. Sacks wrote about patients for whom he was clinically responsible. Their interactions were active, sometimes intense, and carried out over weeks or months of often intense diagnosis, treatment, and care. His description of their cases, and his involvement in them, were grounded in the medicine he sought to practice on their behalf.

Medicine

Sacks championed a kind of medicine that was fading even as his medical vocation began. Like most physicians of his era, Sacks was trained in an Oslerian approach defined by a closely personal, patient–physician relationship. William Osler taught a system of careful, hands-on diagnosis in which a physician's demeanor "should be one of 'good natured optimism' ... and should reflect 'infinite patience' and 'ever-tender' clarity.'"[12] It was *with* the patient and *in* the patient's life that Osler's medicine was carried out. As Sacks would put it in his autobiography:

> As medical students, we were not overloaded with lectures or formal instruction, the essential teaching was done at a patient's bedside, and the essential lesson was to listen, to get the 'history of the present condition' from the patient and ask the right questions to fill in the details. We were taught to use our eyes and ears, to touch, to feel, even to smell.

All this was in service of creating a "bond of a deep, physical sort; one's hands could themselves become therapeutic tools."[13]

Osler's magnum opus, *The Principles and Practice of Medicine*, was prefaced with quotations from Hippocrates—"Experience is fallacious and judgment difficult," and Plato's *Gorgias*: "I said of medicine that this is an art that considers the constitution of the patient and has principals of action in each case."[14] Later, Sacks similarly would use classical quotes in his consideration of not simply symptoms and their manifestation but the patient's whole constitution. In doing that he turned the clinical case report into a literary art form grounded in an extraordinary command of medical history and literature.

Sacks did not credit Osler as an inspiration, but A. R. Luria, a founder of modern neuropsychology, whose case histories combined "the classical and the romantic, science as storytelling" became Sack's model.[15] it was a type of narrative he first learned at his family's dinner table where a Hippocratic sense of the difficulties of medical judgment and a Platonic focus on the patient were frequent topics of discussion. Nightly his parents would tell

> stories sometimes grim and terrifying but always evocative of the personal qualities, the special value and valor, of the patient ... my parents' sense of wonder at the vagaries of life, their combination of a clinical and a narrative cast of mind, were transmitted with great force to all of us.[16]

Migraine

Sacks's sense of being an outsider and a resulting clinical skepticism freed him to see a complex of symptoms from a different and often therapeutically new perspective. Where others would simply diagnose and then prescribe, Sacks took a different route. He saw the limits to the state of medicine itself. This was true both of his technical writing—he published frequently in academic journals—and his longer narratives. I read his first book, *Migraine*, in the mid-1980s, during a period of my own frequent migraines which usually began with a light-headedness and proceeded to extreme photosensitivity, nausea, and incapacitating, violent headaches.

They were the consequence of surgery for strabismus, a genetically inherited neuromuscular condition in which, for extropics like me (wall-eyed persons), there is no binocularity, no depth perception. Before surgery I was having trouble reading, writing, and driving. After the correction—a complete success from the surgeon's point of view—the migraines began. They were eventually tamed after 18 months by an ophthalmologist who introduced Fresnel prisms into my prescription, forcing both eyes to more or less "play nice," vision alternating—near and far—from one to the other. There was something comforting, for me, about Sack's book, in which the complexity of the condition, and the varying effect on different patients, was considered.

At first, Sacks thought a 1966 posting to a migraine clinic in Bronx, New York, would be a simple matter of diagnosis and prescription for what, in those days, was assumed to be a perhaps temporarily debilitating, easily medicated, but otherwise clinically uninteresting condition. For Sacks, however, "no two patients with migraine were the same, and all of them were extraordinary. Working with them was my real apprenticeship in medicine."[17] In the diversity of their symptoms he found an encyclopedia of neurologies, in which the pain might be in the head but also could manifest elsewhere, for example, in the gut.

Not only were migraines a class of diverse symptoms but their onset was often embedded in psychosocial patterns. For many of Sacks's patients, treatment therefore was as much a matter of psychology—or psychiatry—as it was of a simple neuropharmacology. A young mathematician, for example, had weekly migraines every Sunday. He would begin to get nervous about their onset on Wednesday and by Friday would be unable to work. Saturday was a weekly torment and Sunday was given entirely to the migraine. Afterward he would feel calm and creative and then work Sunday night until Wednesday, when the pattern began again.

Sacks prescribed medication that tamed the migraines but, without that weekly cycle of experience, the patient was unable to continue with mathematics. The migraine cycle was so integrated into his daily life that losing the first, he then lost his ability to do the work he loved. Sacks came to understand the weekly migraine schedule as part of a complex that was at once neurological, personal, and social.

Migraine was a densely literate and massive text that redefined its subject and defined what would become his style of writing. In a review of the literature—from the Greeks to the modern—he focused less only on the science than the patients and their symptoms. "I delved into the literature of the subject, submerged, and then re-emerged, more knowledgeable in some ways but more confused in others," he wrote in the book's forward. "I [then] returned to my patients whom I found more instructive than any book. And after I had seen a thousand migraine patients, I saw that the subject made *sense*."[18] He detailed the range of neurologic, physiologic, and psychological conditions present in patients' repeated attacks. He paid full attention to then available clinical treatments ... and their limits. He was perhaps the first to pay close attention to the unusual "auras" that preceded some but not all onsets. And for those he could not help with drugs or therapies, he wrote in the book's forward, he could at least offer the balm of his personal attention and interest. Sacks showed the manuscript to his boss at the Bronx clinic, Dr. Arnold Friedman, then the head of the headache section of the American Neurological Association. Friedman hated the manuscript, called it trash, and warned Sacks that if he published it, he would be fired and blackballed, never to get another job in the field. Friedman was especially incensed by the idea that migraines might manifest as belly rather than headaches. Sacks persisted and the book was published in England by Faber and Faber to generally good reviews. He was then fired by Friedman, who, Sacks later learned, had taken some of the Sack's manuscript chapters and published them under his own name.[19]

For neither the first time nor the last, Sacks's sense of skepticism led him to listen to his patients rather than his superiors and then, as a result, rewrite medical knowledge. As a result, he was again unemployed in a field to which he had made a significant contribution.

A Leg to Stand On

The first draft of Migraine was written in a short burst of creative energy that followed an intense period of case work, research, and review. His next book took Sacks nine years to complete. It was the story of his own proprioceptive disorder, "a kind of paralysis and alienation of the leg," following a hiking accident in Norway begun "foaming with guilt, remorse and rage" after he had lost another posting after insisting upon innovative treatment for a patient and unrelated, and wholly unfounded, allegations of abuse.[20] When he wrote Luria (to whom he dedicated the book) about his proprioceptive disorder—one in which the injured limb seemed, after surgical repair, an object disassociated from his body—Luria replied that "Such syndromes are perhaps common, but very uncommonly described."[21]

That was the job he undertook in A Leg to Stand On, the most intimate of his clinical case studies. In it, he is at once a physician who understands his injury—a neurologist with a neurological disorder—and a patient who just wants a return to a normalcy he fears may be forever lost. He understands the therapies and like every patient is frustrated by them. He is outside and inside the story at once, handily describing as one his experience as physician, patient, and therapist. It became, for me, the model of how to write about personal experiences without letting a sense of the personal overwhelm.

Over the years, I have consulted for other physicians with serious chronic conditions, including cancer, dementia, Parkinson's disease, and stroke. They have almost uniformly masked their personal fears and sense of bodily dysfunction in a barrage of clinical verbiage. They know, at one level, what is going on. But most are unable to think about, let alone discuss what that clinical reality means to them as persons. My job has been to take them across that barrier to a personal and emotional rather than intellectual consideration of the effect of their disorders on their lives and, by extension, those of their loved ones. From time to time I have recommended A Leg to Stand On—and twice gifted it to patients—none of whom read it. For them, Sacks's book was simply too painful to endure, to close to a reality they experienced, at least until they came to see themselves not just as physicians but as medically educated patients.

Awakenings

In the fall of 1966, Sacks took up a post at Beth Abraham Chronic Disease Hospital, whose 500 residents included survivors of *encephalitis lethurgica* that, between 1919 and 1926, affected nearly five million people worldwide. These were the "long haulers," as we would call them today, whose symptoms followed survival during the influenza pandemic of 1918–1920. Its symptoms included high fever, headache, double vision, lethargy, and delayed physical and mental responses.[22] Its mortality rate was around 30% and to this day its origins remain unclear. In many survivors, a kind of postencephalitic stupor set in. These included Beth Abraham's long-term patients who were mired in "deeply parkinsonian states—some stuck in catatonic postures—not unconscious but with their consciousness suspended."[23]

Their supervision was presumably a dead-end, caretaker's job. "Chronic hospitals," Sacks was told by one senior physician, "you'll never see anything interesting in them."[24] The patients were assumed to be nonpersons, shells of humanness for whom no effective medical treatment could be offered. The post-pandemic patients were simply warehoused and forgotten as was, by all but the occasional medical historian, the pandemic itself.

The Beth Abraham nurses who cared for the patients believed that personalities remained in these bodies even if few others believed it, or cared if it was true. Sacks listened, observed, and agreed. Famously, Sacks began with a reorganization that brought these patients from different wards to one where they could be observed and then, perhaps, be treated as a group. Believing from the start that the patients were more than bodies, he found that they could be "activated." Thrown a ball, a "frozen" patient would catch and return it. That type of non-pharmacologic intervention was radical in itself.

Suspecting that L-DOPA (levodopa), then an experimental drug, might act upon their symptoms, he applied for its experimental use. That was an extraordinary clinical and intellectual leap that sought to define the patients' condition as the result of a deficit of neurotransmitters that might be replaced by the new drug. The effects were startling. Over time he observed a series of increasing side effects, until in time the efficacy of the treatment first diminished and then disappeared.

In short, Sacks took a group of forgotten patients for whom no treatment had been conceived and whose humanity had been discounted and discovered behavioral and pharmacological treatment approaches that resulted in dramatic if ultimately short-term improvements. As he had done with migraines, Sacks redefined the medical field's perception of a condition whose understanding was informed, in part, by the patients themselves.

For a book that was dryly clinical in its case reports, *Awakenings* was a surprising and unexpected success. It inspired a documentary film by Duncan Dallas of Yorkshire Television, a one-act play by Harold Pinter,[25] and then a ballet by Tobias Picker. But it was the 1990 movie that made the story, and Sacks, famous.[26] When first approached, he was ambivalent about the film whose script hewed close his book in the main but included as well fictional subplots introduced for dramatic effect.

> I had to renounce the notion that it was, in any way, 'my' file; it was not my script, it was not my film, it would largely be out of my hands. ... I would be able to advise and consult, to ensure medical and historical accuracy, I would do my best to give the film an authentic point of departure, but I would not have to feel responsible for it.[27]

He worked hard at that task, one that included both the patients themselves and their families. At actor Robert De Niro's request they visited the remaining patients at Beth Abraham. Sacks showed the actors portraying patients how to sit immobile—not an easy thing to get right—and the tremors and tics some would manifest on L-DOPA. Because Sacks saw a commonality between those and the convulsive acts of patients with Tourette's syndrome, he brought several persons with Tourette's to the set. The result was a film Sacks liked and so, too, did the patients' families. Sacks worried that for all this work, these were actors playing a role and not patients. He later noted with relief in his journal, one patient who observed them said approvingly of De Niro, whose character is the movie's focus, "He's okay—he's got it! He really knows what it's like."[28]

I doubt very many general readers read the book in its entirety. It's more than 300 pages are divided into three mostly scholarly sections. The first reviews the history of the pandemic, of Parkinson's disease, and the general state of those who survived the pandemic in a limited state of being. It then presents Levodopa as a critical biochemical precursor for the formation of a class of catecholamines (Dopamine, Norepinephrine, and Epinephrine), which had been used to treat some with Parkinson's. In the second section, Sacks presented rather dry, technical, individual case histories of 20 patients and their condition before, during, and after treatment. The final section includes a chapter titled "Perspectives" and an "Afterword" that together present his only sustained foray into the theory of medicine as a humanist vocation.

The case histories are a tough read. Miss A, for example, is described as a rather thin woman, appearing rather younger than her sixty-one years, with a greasy and rather hirsute skin, but without signs of acromegaly [a disorder in which the pituitary grand overproduces growth hormones in adulthood], thyroid or other endocrine disturbances.[29] For Sacks that level of clinical detail was necessary. In his "Perspectives" chapter, he quotes Goethe in what might later be seen as his own credo: "Everything factual is, in a sense, theory. ... There is no sense to looking for something behind phenomena: They are theory."[30] That said, the facts of these cases led Sacks, for the first and last time, to attempt to articulate a theory of medicine, its complexity, and its purpose. "The terrors of suffering, sickness, and death, of losing ourselves and losing the word are the most elemental and intense we know," he begins, "and so too are our dreams of recovery and rebirth, of being wonderfully restored to ourselves and the world."[31]

While his stated intention was to evoke Goethe's factual, the lesson of these patients and their care was as much moral and philosophical as it was clinical. To do his or her best, Sacks argued that the physician needs both science and an Oslerian dose of empathy and humanism. "We need in addition to conventional medicine, a medicine of a far profounder sort, based on the profoundest understanding of the organism and of life."[32] The lesson of *Awakenings* exemplified for him, "first and last, the utter inadequacy of mechanical medicine, the utter inadequacy of a mechanical world view."[33]

Had he known it, Sacks would surely have quoted playwright Eugene O'Neil: "I love life but not because it's beautiful. I'm a better lover than that."[34] Medicine, for Sacks, should have the same credo. He never saw himself as the hero of *Awakenings* but rather, perhaps, its muse. The real heroes, he wrote, where the patients themselves and the institutional attendants who cared for them and believed in their humanity.

Hat

Many assume that with *Awakenings*, Sacks became a doyen who could pick and choose his cases. Certainly, the book was generally well received on publication in the general press. Few neurologists commented, however, and those who did were skeptical of his case descriptions. At least one doubted there had ever been a pandemic. After its publication Sacks needed work beyond the few hours spent weekly with the patients at Beth Abraham. He did not abandon them and, indeed, remained close to their families and to them for years. But as they receded into a more frozen state, or died of old age, there was no need for a full-time neurologist.

He was offered a part-time position at Bronx State overseeing a ward whose young adults manifested a range of problems: from autism and early-onset schizophrenia (like his brother) to fetal alcohol syndrome and tuberous sclerosis. He hated the behavioral modification programs that were then a form of regimented treatment. They reminded him, he said in his autobiography, of his treatment as a child when sent away during the Blitz. "I felt myself falling sometimes into an almost helpless identification with the patients."[35]

After losing that job, Sacks gave up on the idea of a normal staff position anywhere and instead became a self-proclaimed "consulting neurologist." He did not become a writer about neurological patients but rather a neurologist who sometimes shared his and his patients' histories. Eight of the stories in *Hat* had been previously published in *The New York Review of Books*, and three in the *London Review of Books*. Several had begun as "clinical curiosities" in *The British Medical Journal*.

Perhaps the story of Witty Ticcy Ray best describes the Sacks who emerged as a neurologist-writer. A *New York Times* story he read had described the "astonishing topography of tics" manifested by the postencephalitic patients on L-DOPA. After that article, Sacks received letters from others with multiple tics who wanted attention, and perhaps treatment. Among them was Witty Ticcy Ray, who wrote to Sacks and asked for a meeting, after which he wrote, "I realized that Tourette's syndrome was another rare but somehow kindred malady similar to that of the post-encephalitis patients."[36]

In truth, it was not so much rare as forgotten. The next day, walking in New York City, Sacks saw two or three persons with Tourette symptoms. The day after, he saw others. Sacks's description of Witty Ticcy Ray in *Hat*, and more generally of Tourette's syndrome as a forgotten diagnosis of a prevalent condition, returned it to the world not only of diagnosis and treatment but also of public attention. Within months of *Hat*'s publication, Tourette characters were being featured on nighttime dramatic TV medical shows. From a rarely diagnosed oddity it became generally recognizable by any primetime TV viewer.

Sacks had no part in the popular presentation of this or other clinical states he described in his casebooks. Hugh Laurie's *House, M.D.*, for example, diagnosed a case of Korsakov's syndrome, a disorder in which short-term memory is destroyed. In the 1980s and 1990s, dramatic TV storylines followed a range of clinical disagreements from the treatment of anencephalic infants to the possibility of adverse events resulting from ectopic pregnancies. Some may sneer at these dramas although, in the main, they attempt to carefully balance the clinical and social issues involved. Like Sacks's writings, they serve as a public primer of issues of care that, otherwise, were cloistered in medical and bioethical literatures.

Anthony Fauci, the longtime director of the National Institute of Allergy and Infectious Diseases, once commented that as a teenager he debated between careers in literature and social study or medicine. Later he decided the tension between these would be best resolved with a career in medicine.[37] A generation earlier, Sacks similarly weighed the merits of the purely clinical with the literary and social. He attempted to balance those tensions in *Hat* by concluding each case with a sometimes-extensive postscript that put the balanced the broad narrative and the critical neurology needed to understand it.

"The Lost Mariner," for example, described Jimmy G., a resident at a New York City Home for the Aged. A genial fellow, Jimmy lived in a perpetual present, the events of moments or days before slipping away as the clock ticked forward. His memories seemed to have stopped—his ability to form them—in 1945. His best diagnosis was Korsakov's syndrome. The diagnosis is almost always differential, and therefore not definitive. There is no treatment. After nine years of patient-physician interactions, Jimmy showed no change. Still, this was not, for Sacks, a failure, and Jimmy G. was no object of pity. "Humanly, spiritually," he was "attentive to the beauty and soul of the world, rich in all the Kierggardian categories—and aesthetic, the moral, the religious, the dramatic."[38]

By the late 1980s, Sacks was receiving dozens of letters weekly from physicians, and independently from patients seeking consults and advice. Sacks became the insider for communities of outsiders, the doctor who was at once documentarian and neurologist, a writer-advocate and physician. The cases he put into books did not ignore the neurologies he documented. Their principal focus, however, was the person in the disease as it affected their very being. His neurology became an exploration of the ways in which people of difference could blossom, practically and personally, despite what others would think were handicapped barriers.

The result was a series of case reports appearing first in prestigious magazines—*The New York Review of Books, The New Yorker*—and later, in book-length collections. Most cases began with a review of the science to which he then added a description of symptoms, an exploration of treatments, and where available, the ways in which people of difference blossomed, practically and personally.

All of Sacks's studies were grounded in the somewhat radical assertion that "a mind is not just a collection of talents. One cannot maintain a purely composite or modular view of the mind, as most neurologists and psychologists do."[39] Things are more complex than that and the opportunities for different kinds of being result. In the late 1970s, a former mentor in neurology, concerned that Sacks had no formal position, and thus no salary or standing, worried about his future. Sacks replied he might not have a paying post but did have a righteous place. ... At the heart of medicine ... [t]hat's where I am."[40] What once might have seemed a vain boast became a reality.

Mirrored Lives

My reading of Sacks's work began during an intense period of parental care in 1984 that continued through my father's death in 1989. His clinical history was medically mundane, a "geriatric cascade," as I later called it, one complication after another, each resulting from treatments that, while necessary, carried difficult side effects. The cumulative effect was increasing fragility and diminished mental acuity. For most of that period I spent half the year caring for my father—eventually with the help of nurses and home aides—and the rest of my time scrambling to find work as a writer and researcher.

In 1984, I began a radio treatment for the Canadian Broadcasting Corporation's show *Morningside*. After the show's host and producers were changed the story was canceled. The early scripts were the beginning *Mirrored Lives*,[41] the first book on eldercare from the perspective of the familial caregiver. In its fashioning I often thought of Sacks and the manner in which he combined the clinical and the personal in presenting the potential of a life lived differently but still fully.

After its publication in 1990, I sent Sacks a copy with a note saying how he had both informed and inspired me. He wrote back, and at relative length, a typed letter that was pure Sacks—personal and professional at once. Like most of his correspondence, it was filled with underlines, cross-outs, and additions. Some writers work slowly, word by word. Sacks wrote at speed and then edited continuously, and sometimes obsessively.

He thanked me for the book which he read "with more-than-usual resonances, and more-than-usual pain." His father had recently died and "although so many specifics are different, I know, all too well of what you are talking." He praised the book as "almost-unbearably concrete, and candid—this made it painful to read—but, of course, gives it, will give it, its great value as an authentic document, and call to attention."

Politely, Sacks doubted his contribution to my writing, insisting the book reflected "a depth of lived experience that stands in no need of any 'outside' stimulus." He did not see himself as inspiring as making space in the literature for this kind of reportage. As well as his personal experience—the death of his father—Sacks had worked with patients with dementia-like disorders. Indeed, he wrote that in 1980, he had completed a volume based on four patients with Alzheimer's disease. It was lost when he lent it to his chief, who never returned it. A book of his posthumous essays does include a chapter on "The Aging Brain" and on dementia, but these were relatively perfunctory compared to his other detailed case presentations.[42]

Mirrored Lives was an unexpected success. I received readers' letters for 20 years and, in the first year, many from those who wanted to tell me their stories. *Mirrored Lives* spawned two other books, *A Place in Time*[43] and *Age Speaks for Itself*,[44] the first detailing the stories of a number of spouses, children, and grandchildren caring for their seniors. The second included the narratives of a set of fragile seniors themselves.

The narrative stories in each case were followed, *a là* Sacks, with a postscript on the clinical medicine and eventual outcomes. In addition, I included in each volume a discussion chapter, a "Chorus of Experience," in which I asked, "What do we know together that none of us can express alone?" I sent these volumes to Sacks, mentioning *Awakenings*' "Afterward" as my inspiration for the discussion chapters. Sacks liked the stories—patient and family—but distrusted the rest. "I admire your advance from narratives to debate," he wrote, "but for myself, will probably stick to the descriptive and leave the judgmental and the prescriptive to others to chew on." His was a medicine of the particular and the patient. Anything more to him, despite his deep familiarity with philosophy and philosophers, did not interest him after *Awakenings*.

Like Sacks, in those years, I soon found myself the recipient of an expanding volume of letters and queries from patients and family members facing a range of medical challenges—dementias, cancers, multiple sclerosis, strokes. Some, but by no means all, involved seniors. Sometimes I was consulted on care options because, as one person said, "I don't want one more damn doctor. You know what I'm talking about." Physicians would on occasion invite me into the case of a recalcitrant or "non-cooperative" patient hoping I might connect where they could not. A final volume in the series *Watersheds*[45] moved the narratives from gerontology to cases based on the narratives of a range of life-altering events—clinical, social, and spiritual—in adulthood.

I include the personal, here, not out of pride but as evidence of the broader influence of Sacks's writings on other authors. I later carried a Sacksian perspective of the potential for different, seemingly restricted lives into the fields of bioethics and disability studies. These led in turn to my entry into the then fierce debates over medical termination and euthanasia. I sent the occasional paper to Sacks, who, while complimenting my passion, refused to be drawn into a discussion of those issues.

Assessment

Over the years Sacks picked up detractors. Psychiatrist Arthur Shapiro argued Sacks erred in blurring the line between art and clinical science. Sacks, he concluded, was "a much better writer than he is [was] a clinician."[46] I have met neurologists who, uncomfortable with Sacks's intense engagement with patients, similarly disapproved. What Shapiro and those others ignored were the substantial contributions Sacks made to neurology. *Migraine* was a radical and critical addition to the field. So, too, were his contributions to the literature on autism, brain injury, *Encephalitis lethurgica*, Parkinson's, Tourettes, strabismatics,[47] and so on.

As a neurologist who wrote about cases, Sacks created what Mikhail Bakhtin called a "speech genre," a new kind of dialogical storytelling more common to fiction writers than clinical essayists.[48] Sack's narratives were at once deeply clinical and personal. The result, Thomas Couser wrote, was "too distinctively voiced and simply too finished to invite innovative thinking about how to write about someone."[49] But it was never Sacks's goal to teach others how to write. Rather, he encouraged others, like me, to write in the way they found comfortable. His focus was his patients, their diagnoses, care and treatment, and the nature of their being in the world.

This is exactly what some critics attacked. His writings included no "clinical payoff," and, occurring outside the normal therapeutic relationship of doctor and patient, were therefore unacceptable and perhaps exploitative. Some ethical breach must have occurred here, somewhere.

These were largely sneers from the literary sidelines, complaints from the academic bleachers. Neither patients nor their families complained about this. To attack Sack's use of cases is to attack all other physicians and nurses who write about their work. If Sacks was "exploitative" and "too polished," then the same might be said of physicians like Atul Gawande, whose essays in *The New Yorker* are peppered with the stories of patients he has seen.[50] The difference is that Sacks's patients *are* the story, front and center, not an anecdotal addition to a more general essay.

The "clinical payoff" was, I would argue, broad and huge. It provided a voice to individuals whose stories were unheard and who could not tell their stories themselves. In this, they were, indeed, like many of the Arbus photographs. And there is no doubt Sacks's writings changed public understanding—and acceptance—of those with a range of neurologies previously ignored.

Perhaps the most violent criticism came from disability rights spokesperson Tom Shakespeare, who dismissed Sacks as a "voyeuristic cognoscenti" because it is his voice rather than that of the patient that dominates.[51] It is a strange critique. Across his oeuvre Sacks is intensely personal both in his own stories—*A Leg to Stand On*, for example—and in the reports of his interactions with patients. His goal is that of the reformer who seeks to bring outsiders into the commons.

At the heart of these criticisms is the complaint that the writings of Sacks and other doctor-writers somehow transform patients into "texts" that can only be read by a physician. This gives the physician author "undue authority in assigning meaning to the human experience of another."[52] But the whole point of these writings is to present the patient to the public that is invited to comment and understand. The voice is the clinician's but the story is the patient's and, as we come to see the person beyond the symptoms, ours as well. The challenge at every point is to society at large, an invitation to perceive the person who lives with conditions manifest in ways that might seem strange, or make us uncomfortable.

Sacks sat at the cusp of an older, more personal medicine as it was giving way to a technological, too often impersonal science grounded in advanced imaging and genetic testing. In this shift, the patient has been too often forgotten, objectified, and depersonalized. Ignored has been a concern of and appreciation for "the endless forms of individual adaption by which human organisms, people, adapt and reconstruct themselves, faced with the challenges and vicissitudes of life."[53] Deeply rooted in the clinical, Sacks championed the person in the disease, the individual who adapted, adjusted, learned, and sometimes prospered despite infirmities. If academics did not understand, the greater public did. That's why Sacks's stories resonated among so many readers, including me. I was not the only one educated, informed, motivated, and inspired. I'm just one who wrote about it.

Postscript

Somewhere around 1997 I attended a lecture by Sacks at the University of Toronto. The auditorium was full and at the back were cartons of books waiting for him to sell and then sign. There was a sense of reticent shyness in his presentation and little of the passion his writing revealed. Public speaking was never his métier and the podium never his preferred location. Afterward, we talked briefly. "Are you ever going to return to writing about the 'romantic medicine,' the theory of a clinical and social union that you proposed at the end of Awakenings?" I asked. He looked at me with a smile and shook his head. "I think I've learned to tell a pretty good story, Tom," he replied. "I'll leave the theory stuff to others like you."

Notes

1 Tom Koch, "The Man Who Mistake His Wife for a Hat," *The Reader* 5, no. 1 (1986): 25–26.

2 M. Kimmelman, "The Profound Vision of Diane Arbus: Flaws in Beauty, Beauty in Flaws," *New York Times*, March 11, 2005: https://www.nytimes.com/2005/03/11/arts/design/the-profound-vision-of-diane-arbus-flaws-in-beauty-beauty-in.html.

3 J. Szarkowski, "New Documents Exhibit," *The Museum of Modern Art*, 1967: https://www.moma.org/momaorg/shared/pdfs/docs/press_archives/3860/releases/MOMA_1967_Jan-June_0034_21.pdf?2010.

4 R. Cardinal, "Outsider Art and the Autistic Creator," *Philosophical Transactions: Biological Sciences* 364, no. 1522 (2009): 1459–1466. His original book, *Outsider Art*, was published in 1972.

5 Oliver Sacks, *On the Move: A Life* (New York: Alfred A Knopf, 2015).

6 Ibid., 9–10.

7 Ibid.

8 S. Callow, "Truth, Beauty, and Oliver Sacks," *New York Review of Books*, June 6, 2019: https://www.nybooks.com/articles/2019/05/05/truth-beaut-and-oliver-sacks/.

9 Sacks, *On the Move*, 60.

10 Ibid., 63.

11 Szarkowski, "New Documents Exhibit."

12 Michael Bliss, *William Osler: A Life in Medicine* (Toronto, ON: University of Toronto Press, 1999), 262–263.

13 Sacks, *On the Move*, 32.

14 William Osler, *The Principles and Practice of Medicine* (New York: D. Appleton & Co., 1893).

15 Oliver Sacks, "Perspectives," in *Awakenings*, rev. ed. (London: Picador, 1982), 253.

16 Sacks, *On the Move*, 185.

17 Ibid., 150.

18 Oliver Sacks, "Introduction," *Migraine* (New York: Macmillan, 1971). Revised and Expanded edition, New York: Picador, 1995.

19 Ibid., 157–158.

20 Ibid., 214.

21 Oliver Sacks, *A Leg to Stand On* (New York: Summit Books, 1984), 9–10.

22 NIH, "Encephalitis Lethargica Information Page," Bethesda, MD: National Institute of Neurological Disorders and Stroke: https://www.ninds.nih.gov/Disorders/All-Disorders/Encephalitis-Lethargica-Information-Page. Accessed August 20, 2021.

23 Sacks, *On the Move*, 169.

24 Ibid.

25 Harold Pinter, "Another Kind of Alaska," in *Other Places* (New York: Grove Press, 1982).

26 S. Zallian, *Awakenings* [screenplay], Penny Marshall (Director), Columbia Pictures, 1990.

27 Sacks, *On the Move*, 304–305.

28 Ibid., 310–311.

29 Oliver Sacks. "Margaret A," *Awakenings*, 139.

30 Oliver Sacks, "Perspectives," in *Awakenings*, rev. ed. (London: Picador, 1982), 208.

31 Ibid., 202–204.

32 Ibid., 246.

33 Ibid., 240–241.

34 I read this quote when I was 17 in a book of O'Neil's letters at a local store. I couldn't afford the book then but, flipping through it, the line struck me with such intensity I never forgot it. When I had enough money to purchase it, the book was gone from the shelf.

35 Sacks, *On the Move*, 210.

36 Sacks, "A Matter of Identity," in *On the Move*, 3.

37 M. Specter, "The Good Doctor," *New Yorker*, April 20, 2020, 34–45.

38 Oliver Sacks, "The Lost Mariner," in *The Man Who Mistook His Wife for a Hat* (New York: Summit Books, 1985), 39.

39 Oliver Sacks, *An Anthropologist on Mars* (New York: Vintage, 1995), 227.

40 Sacks, *On the Move*, 222.

41 Tom Koch, *Mirrored Lives: Aging Children and Elderly Parents* (Westport, CT, and London: Praeger Books, 1990).

42 Oliver Sacks, "The Aging Brain," in *Everything in Its Place* (New York: Picador, 2019), 144–154.

43 Tom Koch, *A Place in Time: Caregivers for Their Elderly* (Westport, CT, and London: Praeger Books), 1993.

44 Tom Koch, *Age Speaks for Itself: Silent Voices of the Elderly* (Westport, CT, and London: 2000).

45 Tom Koch, *Watersheds: Crises and Renewal in Our Daily Life* (Toronto, ON: Lester Publishing, 1994).

46 Andrew Anthony, "Oliver Sacks: The Visionary Who Can't Recognise Faces," *The Observer*, October 17, 2010: https://www.theguardian.com/theobserver/2010/oct/17/profile-oliver-sacks-author-neurologist.

47 Oliver Sacks, "Stereo Sue: Why Two Eyes Are Better than One," *The New Yorker*, June 19, 2006, 64–73.

48 M. Bakhtin, *Speech Genres and Other Late Essays* (Austin, TX: University of Texas Press, 1986).

49 Thomas Couser, "Beyond the Clinic Oliver Sacks and the Ethics of Neuroanthropology," in *Vulnerable Subjects* (Ithaca, NY: Cornell University Press, 2018), 74–122.

50 Atul Gawande, "Letting Go: What Should Medicine Do When It Can't Save Your Life," *The New Yorker*, August 2, 2010, 36–49.

51 Tom Shakespeare, "Review: Oliver Sacks: *An Anthropologist on Mars*," *Disability and Society* 11, no. 1 (1996): 137–142.

52 Abraham Nussbaum, "'I Am the Author and Must Take Full Responsibility': Abraham Verghese, Physicians as the Storytellers of the Body, and the Renewal of Medicine," *Journal of Medical Humanities* 37 (2016): 389–399.

53 Sacks, *An Anthropologist on Mars*, xvi.

Part II
Three contemporary favorites

3 Perri Klass

Books are like stethoscopes

Seema Yasmin

Early life

Perri Klass was born in a Trinidadian village in the spring of 1958 while her father conducted doctoral anthropological research. By the fall of that year, Perri's parents, Morton and Sheila Klass, moved their family to a suburban New Jersey town. Sheila worked as a professor of English at the City University of New York, and Morton completed his PhD and became a professor at Barnard College and an editor of science fiction novels.

The *click clack* of Sheila's typewriter would descend from the attic at 4:30 each morning and wake Perri. Sheila would rise hours before the rest of the family to write novels, and only after writing would she fulfill the duties expected of a woman in the 1960s: she would set the table and cook a hot breakfast for her husband and three children. Writing came before breakfast, hours before the drudgery of the day would begin. Perri describes her mother as "evangelical"[1] about writing. "We knew she loved us but we also knew there was a powerful force that took her up to the attic each morning,"[2] she said. Writing was a significant act, important enough to conduct in the precious hours of the morning, worthy of losing sleep, worthy of delaying the chores or the dog walk when a plot idea had to be urgently jotted down, or inspiration struck and the last sentences of a short story had to be typed immediately. There was little else in life more important than writing and reading.

Sheila had grown up in Brooklyn during the Depression with Orthodox Jewish parents who believed education was a luxury not befitting girls. An ardent feminist, Sheila fought for her education, and as a professor and mother, she encouraged all of her children and creative writing students to write, believing that everyone had a story to tell. "If she were to talk to you she would say 'Oh what a book you could write,'" said Perri, who describes the *click clack* of her mother's typewriter and the daily demonstration of the importance of writing, as being "imprinted on us children, as if we were ducks."[3] All three of Sheila's children would grow up to be writers.

While Sheila demonstrated the importance of telling stories and establishing a daily writing practice, she believed writers should have day jobs. So, when Perri, who wrote her first short story at age four and continued to write throughout her

DOI: 10.4324/9781003079712-3

teens, applied to university, it was to study biology, not creative writing. And yet, the interest in telling stories never left her. Instead, it crept into her mostly scientific academic life. During the eight semesters at Harvard, Perri took eight creative writing classes, penned dozens of short stories, and earned close to 300 rejections from literary magazines. She saw her writing life and biology life as two disconnected interests. There was Perri, the parasite enthusiast, and Perri, the purveyor of narrative arcs.

Perri graduated magna cum laude from Harvard and continued to mail short stories to editors as she took Sheila's advice of finding a day job. She applied to graduate school for zoology, where she fell deeper into a fascination with parasites and the organism's evolution to adapt to new neighbors and environments. But the veterinary and medical aspects of parasitology became more interesting than the lab work, and Perri realized she was better suited to a clinical career than to research.

Perri matriculated medical school at Harvard in 1982, around the same time that her first short story was accepted for publication in *Mademoiselle*, a weekly fashion magazine that published stories by noted authors such as Sylvia Plath, Truman Capote, and Tennessee Williams.[4] Two years later, the same editor at *Mademoiselle* who had published Perri's first story began curating a series of columns by young women detailing their experiences in male-dominated fields such as law and engineering. The editor asked Perri to write about life as a woman at Harvard Medical School.

First foray into journalism

It was Perri's first foray into journalism. Employing the same narrative tools of fiction to describe life as a trainee doctor, writing essays on medical life brought together Perri's two distinct worlds of medicine and creative writing. The story ran in the June 1984 edition of *Mademoiselle*, and Perri began a long career writing biographical essays.[5] Suddenly, classes at Harvard, life in Cambridge, the medical jargon that tumbled out of the mouths of professors, and posturing male students who bragged of their clinical acumen became fodder for a writer who excelled at storytelling across genres.

When Perri became pregnant in her second year of medical school, it was only fitting that she would write about the stark differences between the health advice given to expectant mothers in her prenatal class in Cambridge and the science she learned in her Harvard Medical School reproductive pathology class. Perri pitched the story to an editor at *The New York Times* and became the youngest woman to write for *The Times*' Her column, a weekly offering from a rotation of women writers.[6] Over a series of columns in the late 1980s, Perri shared stories at the intersections of medicine, gender, and motherhood.

Perri describes the phenomenon of doctors becoming patients and writing about the patient experience as "one of the basic tropes of doctor-writing."[7] In a 2017 essay in the *Bellevue Literary Review*, she writes:

I have rung this bell myself, over and over (yes, never send; it tolls for thee), starting with my wiseass second-year medical student self, writing to the editor of *The New York Times Magazine* to say, here I am, pregnant and in medical school, and what they teach us in my reproductive pathophysiology class does not overlap in any way with what I learn in my birthing class, and wouldn't that make an interesting article?[8]

Trope or not, Perri's experiences offered a valuable and necessary perspective. As one of few women writers offering analysis of gender roles in the workplace, Perri's columns were widely read and shared. When she graduated medical school in 1986, fewer than one in three new doctors was a woman.[9] (Perri was one of 5,109 women to graduate as a doctor in the United States in 1986, compared to 10,728 men the same year. In 2018, that proportion had almost equalized: 47.9% of US medical school graduates were women.[10]) *People* magazine described Perri's *The New York Times* columns as striking "a nerve with the nation's women," in a 1985 article. Perri herself said, "mothers everywhere sent it to their daughters."[11]

Perri began to navigate the wards with the eye of a student and the hunger of a journalist. She had a "figurative press card," she said; license to seek out stories and a duty to observe clinical experiences with an eye for what would make a good column.[12] One of those early stories, "Baby Poop," is now required reading for her journalism students at NYU.[13] Perri uses "Baby Poop" to illustrate the potential myopia that occurs when physicians seek to transform patient encounters into compelling essays.

In "Baby Poop," Perri writes of being the only woman medical student, in fact, the only woman at all, on the pediatric neurology ward of a teaching hospital. During a ward round, Perri offers to change the diaper of a newborn, prompting a debate among her seniors about gender norms and the expectations of medical students. Her male superiors insist that Perri should not undertake what they presume to be a menial task, beneath the expectations of a soon-to-be doctor, even a female soon-to-be doctor. But Perri insists on changing the diaper, shunning fears of stepping into gendered roles in the hopes of demonstrating her practical nature and ability to take on any task. It is this discussion then, the back and forth between the male attendings and the female medical student, and the debate about gender roles and expectations, that becomes the central theme of "Baby Poop." The baby matters less. "But that's not the point," says Perri, explaining why she teaches the story 30 years after it was published. "The point isn't how enlightened *I* am. The point is that the *baby* might be hypoxic. But in the story, I made the baby peripheral."[14]

"Baby Poop" appears in the essay collection *A Not Entirely Benign Procedure: Four years as a medical student*, published in 1987 and republished with a new foreword in 2010. The collection chronicles the ups and down of a medical education, detailing Perri's interactions with cadavers, peers, and her entry into motherhood. The 2010 foreword offers a humble retrospective on Perri's 29-year-old self, the "wiseass" version of her that authored the book. Listing some of her accomplishments since the 1987 version was published, Perri includes teaching medical students, practicing pediatrics in a community health center, and caring for many patients. "I don't say this to offer up any profound statements about the circle of life," she writes in the updated foreword,

> but I do want to point out that my perspective on medical education and on medical students has, of necessity, changed quite a bit. But that's not really the point, is it? This is not a moment to climb up on the somewhat creaky soapbox of mature reflection, or to pontificate about the good old days, or the bad old days, or about the changing nature of American medical education. What value this book has—if it has value—lies in its immediacy. It was truly written during medical school by someone who had no idea of the choices she would eventually make and the lessons she would learn.[15]

The book does have value, both for the immediacy of the writing, as Perri points out, but also for its continued relevance 33 years after it was published. This time Perri refers to her younger self as a "smart ass," in the new foreword, and admits to wincing and cringing as she rereads essays written while in her 20s. "There were moments when I thought, well, who the hell does she think she *is*? That smart ass medical student writing in the mid-1980s seemed at times a little smug, a little self-righteous, a little superior and a little ingenuous."[16] But the lessons learned and the experiences detailed in 1987 remain as relevant today as they were then. Electronic Medical Records may be a modern doctor's headache, and physician burnout may have reached epidemic proportions in the twenty-first century, but sexism, power dynamics, and stress are all concerns that ring as true for the modern medical student as they did for Perri's original audience.

As Perri's nonfiction writing proliferated in the mid-1980s, so did awards for her fiction. While still in medical school, Perri won two prestigious O. Henry Awards for short stories. The awards, named after the American short story writer, signal a writer of great talent. Those accolades, alongside her publishing record in *The New York Times*, helped pave the way for the publication of Perri's first novel, *Recombinations*, in 1985. Written in only two months and published the year before Perri would step onto the wards as a doctor, the novel tells the story of Anne Montgomery, a young geneticist who works in a private New York laboratory. By day, Anne shuffles DNA, and by night, she toys with a string of male lovers. The novel explores themes of female desire, friendship, and social status. As well as her string of lovers, Anne navigates a network of friendships with characters including young parents, single mothers with jobs, artists, and other scientists.

Asked how she was able to write the novel so quickly and how she juggled the multiple commitments of studying medicine, parenting a young child, and spending time with her partner, Perri said: "I don't agonize over the typewriter. I don't have time."[17] A year after *Recombinations* was launched, Perri published her first short story collection, *I Am Having an Adventure*, which included O. Henry Award-winning stories.[18] Through 20 tales, Perri offered a commentary on relationships, including a piece of experimental fiction, "Nineteen Lists," which describes the dissolution of an affair through list items such as: "Five good reasons for Nicole and Matthew to break up,"[19] "Four things which have gone well while they lived together." Other stories in the collection deal with heartache, infidelity, and Perri's common themes of female desire and friendship.[20]

From fiction to journalism and back

Medical school offers students a new identity as much as it offers a taxing course load and a preponderance of exams, but Perri sought refuge from her identity as a medical student in fiction, deploying narrative to experience different ways of being a woman in the world. "You come across so many good stories on rotations," she said. "Short stories were my escape fantasy, a way of escaping medical school. When you write fiction you get to live all these other lives."[21]

Residency at Children's Hospital, Boston, and a fellowship in pediatric infectious diseases at Boston City Hospital changed that. An intense workload and the duties of working as a qualified doctor limited Perri's ability to write fiction, to imagine fantasy lives. "In residency I couldn't imagine any life outside of a children's hospital," she said. "I lost my fantasy life. Residency is all-consuming. I'd been imagining all these other lives and then, I couldn't."[22]

In 1990, during her infectious disease fellowship, Perri followed in her mother Sheila's footsteps and published a young adult novel. (Sheila published nine young adult novels during her lifetime.) In *Other Women's Children*, pediatrician Amelia Stern struggles to balance work and home-life commitments, working all hours in a Boston children's hospital to keep her patients alive, while neglecting her own four-year-old child.[23] Of course, Amelia's struggles mirrored the same challenges faced by Perri at that time, as she embarked on the long hours of postgraduate medical training, but these were challenges shared by many women of the 90s, across professional fields.

While sexism played out in Perri's own life and the lives of women the world over, Perri, who identifies as a feminist, argues that the scarcity of women in medicine and publishing presented her with opportunities to be the voice of a generation. "When I started doing journalism there were fewer women and I probably profited from being more of a curiosity,"[24] she said. But Perri offered more than a female perspective. Besides being a woman writer, she was one of few physician-writers who could command the readership of *The New York Times* and a weekly fashion magazine, bringing a lay audience into the wards of a children's hospital. "I think we all still [profit from being more of a curiosity] in this field in this sense that people are glad to have a little bit of inside expertise,"[25] she said, of editors wanting to work with physician-writers.

Those insights into the life of a newly qualified pediatrician continued in Perri's next two books, *Baby Doctor: A Pediatrician's Training*,[26] published in 1992, and *Taking Care of Your Own: Parenthood and the Medical Mind*, published the same year.[27] *Baby Doctor* takes readers through the tribulations of residency at Boston Children's Hospital in a series of essays about end-of-life care, sleep deprivation, children with AIDS, child abuse, and her own family issues. The collection tracks Perri's evolution from frightened intern to calm and capable pediatrician, in command of her charge and confident in her abilities. *Taking Care of Your Own: Parenthood and the Medical Mind* connects clinical care with parenting, asking questions about personal and professional boundaries, detailing the angst and confusion of a pediatrician whose own child becomes some other pediatrician's patient. "Will I ever forget what it was like watching my own daughter get fluoroscoped—watching her heart beat inside her ribs, and thinking with confusion of what I knew about systole and diastole," she writes in *Taking Care of Your Own*.[28]

Perri's fourth book of fiction was published a little more than a decade after her third. *Love and Modern Medicine*, a short story collection, was published in 2001.[29] Again, medical themes, issues of parenting, balancing work pressures with home demands, and the complex emotional landscapes of female desire and friendships emerge. Pregnant obstetricians, high school biology teachers, geneticists, and anesthesiologists are some of the scientist characters in *Love and Modern Medicine*. The characters grapple with the same issues affecting Perri, as detailed in her biographical essays from *Her*.

Between the publication of her third and fourth books of fiction, Perri completed her postgraduate medical training and established herself as both a capable clinician and a literary success. With five critically acclaimed books under her belt and a string of columns in *The New York Times*, she had achieved Sheila's wildest dreams for her children, that they become published authors, committed writers, and hold down reliable day jobs. Literature was as much a part of Perri's daily routine as ward rounds. The two passions she once viewed as separate had fused to form a medico-literary loop encompassing her talents for truth-telling in fiction, journalism, novels, short story collections, and autobiographical essays.

Literacy for well-being

This medico-literary connection solidified further when literature surpassed its role as Perri's personal refuge, fantasy land, and family inheritance, to become a tool in her clinical toolbox. As Perri completed her subspecialty training in pediatric infectious disease, she embarked on a new parallel career as an advocate of childhood literacy. In 1993, Perri became a leader of *Reach Out and Read*, transforming the small literacy program from a single project to a national network of more than 3,000 program sites.[30] *Reach Out and Read* is a nonprofit organization that merges well-child doctor and nurse visits with literacy advocacy. Healthcare providers at more than 5,000 sites across 50 states promote reading skills and the love of books to young children and their families. In 1998, the American Academy of Pediatrics officially endorsed the literacy model used by *Reach Out and Read*.[31] Perri has continued her work at the organization ever since the early 1990s, combining her love of literature with her role as a healthcare provider. The American Academy of Pediatrics awarded Perri its Pediatrics Education Award in 2007 for her leadership and commitment to childhood literacy. In 2011, she received the Alvarez Award from the American Medical Writers Association.[32]

Perri frames literature as sustenance. Just as food and warmth nurture a child, so do books and pictures. Klass equates growing up in a home without books as growing up without the most basic of needs.

> When I think about children growing up in homes without books, I have the same visceral reaction as I have when I think of children in homes without milk or food or heat: It cannot be, it must not be. It stunts them and deprives them before they've had a fair chance.[33]

Journalism professor and journalistic peers

Perri is a professor of journalism and pediatrics at New York University and practices pediatric infectious disease medicine in NYU's Bellevue Hospital. She directs the Arthur L. Carter Journalism Institute and, as well as teaching journalism, writes a weekly column on child health for *The New York Times* called *The Checkup*. The column covers topics as far ranging as childhood masturbation, teenaged period pain, childhood trauma, and young athletes, among many other issues.

As a professor of journalism, Perri is able to draw on her earlier columns from the beginning of her writing career in the 1980s, including stories such as "Baby Poop," to extract lessons learned about voice and perspective over her almost 40 years as a journalist. In the classroom, she explores issues of patient confidentiality, boundaries, and ethics with her journalism students, reflecting on writing techniques she has employed to tell clinical stories while protecting patient identities. Her fiction and nonfiction works sometimes use composite characters that draw on multiple patient stories to make a point, but this is a technique she no longer wishes to use. "I wouldn't do that now and I wish I hadn't done that then," she said. "There's a distinction between journalism and fiction and once you start taking out too many parts of the truth, you can veer from non-fiction into fiction."[34]

Despite her wealth of experience, hundreds of published essays, and a faculty position at a journalism institution, Perri doubts her journalistic credentials. "I've never made a living off journalism," she said.[35] Few medical practitioners who practice journalism have formal training in journalism. Among Perri's physician-journalist peers are Sherri Fink, staff writer at *The New York Times*, and former reporter for investigative news outlet *ProPublica* and *Public Radio International*. Fink earned Pulitzer Prizes for innovative and deep medical reporting for newspapers and magazines and is author of *The New York Times* best-selling book, *Five Days at Memorial: Life and Death in a Storm-Ravaged Hospital*, which tells the story of the medical decisions made at a New Orleans hospital in the aftermath of Hurricane Katrina. Fink graduated from Stanford University School of Medicine in 1999 and did not complete postgraduate medical training or attend journalism school. *The New Yorker* writers Atul Gawande and Jerome Groopman are physician-journalists who report on health and science topics drawing on their respective expertise in surgery, for Gawande, and hematology and oncology for

Groopman. Neither attended journalism school but since joining *The New Yorker* in 1998, both doctors have contributed written journalism on health and science, building credibility across disciplines.

Perri's peers go beyond journalists to those physicians who write fiction, including novelists such as Abraham Verghese, Daniel Mason, Irene Mathieu, and Nawal El Saadawi. Of these, Mathieu is known for writing across genres, and Verghese has formally studied writing in an academic writers' program, as a 1991 graduate of the Iowa Writer's Workshop. Perri notes her lack of formal creative writing training as much as she questions her credentials as a journalist. "I was a biology major so I didn't know a thing that English majors knew about,"[36] she said, despite winning a James Beard Journalism Award[37] for writing on diet, nutrition, and health in 2000, and a Women's National Book Association Award in 2006.[38] Yet, among modern physician-writers, none is as prolific an author or as accomplished across genres as Perri.

Conclusion

It is likely Perri's humility and questioning of her credentials that continues to draw readers to her books, short stories, essays, and newspaper columns. Champion of childhood literacy, longtime executive board member, and former chair of literary organization PEN New England, merger of successful careers in pediatrics and literature, Perri is the role model for doctors, especially women doctors, barraged with mixed messages about "having it all." Referring to a full work life and a happy family life, "having it all" is often leveraged against women as a way of demanding they excel at one or fail at both. Perri has defied societal expectations of women and of doctors. Multi-hyphenate, writing across genres, publishing sometimes two books a year, Perri models the successful merging of a medical career with a literary one. Beyond the personal gratification of fulfilling a childhood dream as a writer, Perri considers literature a tool much like a stethoscope, using words to heal and books to change the world.

Notes

1 This chapter draws extensively on an interview with the author on February 11, 2020.
2 Personal interview with the author, February 11, 2020.
3 Ibid.
4 Perri Klass, "The Secret Lives of Dieters," *Mademoiselle*, July 1982.
5 Perri Klass, "Essay," *Mademoiselle*, June 1984.
6 Perri Klass, "Bearing a Child in Medical School," *New York Times*, November 11, 1984.
7 Perri Klass, "I'm Not Talking to Anybody," *Bellevue Literary Review* 33 (Fall 2017): 39–50.
8 Ibid.
9 Perri Klass, "Are Women Better Doctors?" *New York Times*, April 10, 1988.
10 "Diversity in Medicine: Facts and Figures 2019," AAMC, accessed August 20, 2021, https://www.aamc.org/data-reports/workforce/interactive-data/figure-12-percentage-us-medical-school-graduates-sex-academic-years-1980-1981-through-2018-2019.

11 Cable Neuhaus, "A Touch of Klass Is All It Takes to Be a Successful Author, Mom and Med Student at the Same Time," *People*, November 18, 1985.
12 Interview with the author, February 11, 2020.
13 Perri Klass, "Baby Poop," in *A Not Entirely Benign Procedure: Four Years as a Medical Student* (New York: Plume, 1987, revised 2010).
14 Ibid.
15 Ibid.
16 Ibid.
17 Neuhaus, "A Touch of Klass Is All It Takes to Be a Successful Author, Mom and Med Student at the Same Time."
18 Perri Klass, "The Secret Lives of Dieters," in *Prize Stories 1983: The O. Henry Awards* (New York: Doubleday, 1983).
19 Peri Klass, "Not a Good Girl," *Mademoiselle*, July 1983.
20 Perri Klass, *Recombinations* (New York: Putnam's, 1985).
21 Interview with the author, February 11, 2020.
22 Ibid.
23 Perri Klass, *I Am Having an Adventure* (New York: Putnam's, 1986).
24 Interview with the author, February 11, 2020.
25 Ibid.
26 Perri Klass, *Baby Doctor: A Pediatrician's Training* (New York: Kaplan, 1992).
27 Perri Klass, *Taking Care of Your Own: Parenthood and the Medical Mind* (Knoxville, TN: Whittle Communication, 1992).
28 Ibid.
29 Perri Klass, *Love and Modern Medicine: Stories* (Boston, MA: Mariner Books, 2001).
30 "About," Reach Out and Read, accessed August 20, 2021, https://www.reachoutandread.org/about/.
31 "American Academy of Pediatrics Education Award," American Academy of Pediatrics, accessed August 20, 2021, https://www.aappublications.org/content/28/10/31.1
32 "Fellowship and Award Recipients," American Medical Writer's Association, accessed August 20, 2021, https://www.amwa.org/page/Award_Recipients#Alvarez.
33 See her personal website: https://www.perriklass.com/bio#:~:text=In%20an%20essay%20on%20the,ve%20had%20a%20fair%20chance.%22.
34 Interview with author, February 11, 2020.
35 Ibid.
36 Ibid.
37 "Reach Out and Read: Award Winner," James Beard Foundation, accessed August 20, 2021, https://www.jamesbeard.org/chef/perri-klass
38 "WNBA Award," Women's National Book Association, accessed August 20, 2021, https://wnba-books.org/wnba-award/.

4   Abraham Verghese

The power of storytelling

Kaarkuzhali Babu Krishnamurthy

Abraham Verghese is a prolific writer, a talented infectious disease specialist, and a gifted educator. He is a product of multiple worlds, born in Ethiopia to Indian immigrant parents and trained in medicine in India, with many of his formative postgraduate years spent in rural Tennessee. His penchant for storytelling has propelled him into literary fame, guiding another generation of physician-authors along the way.

As an educator, Verghese promotes humanism in medicine, encouraging physicians to recognize the person beyond the disease. He has devoted his career to demonstrating how to see patients at the bedside, eliciting a primary history, and performing a comprehensive clinical examination that allows doctors to hone in on the process causing the patient's symptoms. He coined the term "chartoma" to refer to the practice of cutting and pasting data and previous diagnoses into current notes, thereby propagating error and propelling the diagnostician away from the true diagnosis.[1] He frequently writes about the benefit of having a clinical skills assessment as part of a certification process before residents can graduate, stating that this would improve diagnostic accuracy, and would move physicians closer to the goal of patient-centered care.[2] Verghese uses narrative to demonstrate the diagnostic value of listening to patients' stories. While he has authored one novel, the majority of his work is nonfiction. This chapter will explore in detail the two book-length memoirs that he has written while dipping into some of his shorter writings.

Stories written about the medical profession have always been popular. For the lay public, the mysteries of medical diagnosis and treatment can be both titillating and reassuring. Some narratives read as grippingly as mystery novels, providing us with unusual symptoms and challenging us to play detective; only rarely do they offer an experience that may be considered transformative. Verghese's first memoir, *My Own Country*,[3] fulfills both possibilities; his second, *The Tennis Partner*,[4] explores the boundaries of curiosity and professionalism in the practice of medicine. What makes these two volumes unique is that the reader is allowed to bear witness through the intertwined narratives from the professional side of Verghese's life (e.g., doctor–patient), and, to a variable extent, the personal side (e.g., husband–wife, father–son, mentor–mentee). We are privileged to see that doctors can be vulnerable and fallible. Verghese provides a tremendous service to patients

DOI: 10.4324/9781003079712-4

and doctors alike, showing us with lyrical prose that we are linked through our "humanness," and that both doctors and patients have important stories to tell.

After he and his family moved to the United States, Verghese spent some time working as a medical orderly before finishing his medical education in India. *My Own Country* represents the period from his medical residency in Tennessee, through his fellowship in Boston, and his subsequent return as an infectious disease specialist to small town Tennessee. The second memoir, *The Tennis Partner*, covers the years he spent as a physician-educator at the Texas Tech School of Medicine. These two memoirs have similar subtitles: *A Doctor's Story of a Town and Its People in the Age of AIDS* for the former and *A Doctor's Story of Friendship and Loss* for the latter. Like many books in this genre, each volume contains a wealth of detail about a specific medical condition, written in language understandable to nonphysicians. They provide insight into how doctors evaluate and interpret medical information and how this information leads to an understanding of prognosis and recommendations for treatment.

The mellifluous description Verghese presents in *My Own Country* when providing details of his family's geographic relocation gives the reader a preview of the eloquent language that will be found throughout the narrative:

> In their herald migration, my parents individually and then together reenacted the peregrination of an entire race. Like ontogeny repeating phylogeny – the gills and one-chamber heart of a human fetus in the first trimester reenacting man's evolution from amphibians – they presaged their own subsequent wanderings and those of their children.[5]

The facility with words and the ability to evoke powerful and lingering images are features that set Verghese's memoirs apart from the more typical expositions of the curiosities of medical practice.

As a neurology resident, I was a reluctant member of the medical profession, having applied to medical school as a cultural expectation; no one was more surprised than I when I was admitted. I disliked most of the medical school, finding the rote memorization impossible, and rigid hierarchy stifling. While internship and residency were marginally better, I continued to feel like an outsider, uncommitted to the idea of dedicating the entirety of my life to a profession that seemingly gave lip service to the concept of humanism. Had there been any period of time during those years when I wasn't physically, cognitively, and emotionally spent, perhaps I would have mustered up the activation energy required to leave medicine. As it was, I simply endured.

For me, spending time in proximity to physical books can be restorative, even if time does not permit lengthy reading. I came across *My Own Country* by chance, when an errand took me past the bookstore in the heart of our medical campus. With no time to browse, and little money to spare, I grabbed the first paperback I found on the discount rack and headed for the checkout.

Later that evening, with eyes bleary from lack of sleep and too many hours at the computer, I opened the book, and read:

Summer, 1985. A young man is driving down from New York to visit his parents in Johnson City, Tennessee. I can hear the radio playing, I can picture his parents waiting, his mother cooking his favorite food, his father pacing.[6]

Verghese's skill as a narrator was such that, instantly, I could "see" that young man, too. I was driving with him when, 300 miles from home, his chest became tight. When he developed chills, indicating the presence of a fever and likely a serious infectious condition, I wondered how he was going to make it through the Virginia mountains where the "road rises, sheer rock on one side."[7] When he finally got to the Johnson City Medical Center, the imagery of doctors and nurses trying to help him breathe was very familiar, but I could no longer conjure up a picture of the young man himself. In a moment of clarity, I realized that when I provided so-called bedside care, I was so busy thinking about the patient as a series of organ systems that I never had the presence of mind to look up and make eye contact. My fear of being inadequate to the task of healing, of being unprepared for the questions I would face during morning rounds, and of making a mistake that could have catastrophic consequences prevented me from properly considering patients as people.

I cried in my apartment that night, horrified that, from the hours I had been on call the night before, I couldn't remember one face or one fact about any patient that didn't have an immediate connection to the medical problem that brought them to the hospital. My rudimentary attempts at offering comfort had been perfunctory and algorithmic. They were never specific to what an individual patient needed or wanted. How could they be? I never saw them as individuals. The power of Verghese's prose is such that even now, rereading these first pages of *My Own Country*, I can still see this young man on the mountain highway, and my eyes again tear up with recalled pain and anguish.

Returning to the memoir, we find the emergency room staff racing to save this young man's life, but considerations change when the intensive care unit doctors and nurses realize that they are treating their first patient with AIDS. After the young man dies three weeks later, Verghese tells us, his readers, that he is "astonished [by the ICU nurses'] indignation. In their opinion, this 'homo-sex-shual' with AIDS clearly had no right to expect to be taken care of in our state-of-the-art, computerized ICU."[8] Further, "[all] those involved in [the patient's] care in the ER and ICU agonized over their exposure."[9] Just like that, we are catapulted into the heart of the AIDS pandemic.

In June 1981, the US Center for Disease Control (CDC) published an article documenting the diagnosis of *Pneumocystis carinii* in five previously healthy gay men in Los Angeles.[10] By the end of 1985, the CDC reported that there were almost 16,000 patients with Kaposi's sarcoma and/or *P. carinii* pneumonia, thereby meeting the criteria for AIDS; 26 of those patients were in Tennessee.[11]

On that memorable first evening of reading, my misery over my perceived deficiencies briefly receded as I was drawn further into the world of the Johnson City Medical Center, where intelligent, hardworking, and caring clinicians revealed their biases and worried about their personal safety. For those of us who were not clinicians at the onset of the AIDS era, it seems unbelievable that hospital staff contemplated disposing of the respirator used for the young man with AIDS, but Verghese shows his readers that, at that time, when very little was known about HIV, when its modes of transmission were unclear, and no specific treatment was available, thoughtful doctors and nurses struggled with their own beliefs and fears.

While our current residents and students are too young to remember any of that era, we are now living through the coronavirus pandemic, for which there are parallels. Worrying about whether one might have been exposed to a pathogen is a daily occurrence to any clinician providing direct medical care in 2020. The physician's duty to provide care must take priority over self-preservation, although the fear of acquiring a disease for which there is no cure and which confers a high morbidity and mortality risk is never far behind.

It may seem naïve to readers of this chapter that my training included two very palpable lessons: (1) having fear is not acceptable for physicians because it leads to expression of other emotions; and (2) being "emotional" or "emotionally invested" prevents doctors from having the objective perspective necessary to provide good clinical care. In moving on to Chapter 2 of *My Own Country*, I was, therefore, astonished to find Verghese giving the reader free access to his inner thoughts and feelings along with a description of how these influenced his decision-making. I had never previously been privy to either how or why my colleagues thought the way they did; I just felt as though my perspective was, somehow, quite different than theirs.

In medicine, as with many professions, there's always too much to do and not enough time to do it. In addition, the hidden culture of medicine leads many of us to believe that we're always one step behind our colleagues, that we were given our pass to medical training through some accident rather than because we deserved it, and that we're only one step away from public exposure. Some physician-authors inadvertently add layers to this emotional burden. They show us their successes, without allowing us to see the obstacles or barriers that impeded their progress.

Refreshingly, Verghese spoke honestly about his need to consider residencies that accept foreign doctors, and about the conditions he expected to encounter there: "At hospitals that took foreign physicians the work was grueling, the conditions appalling—but only by American standards—and the supervision and teaching often minimal because of the sheer volume of work."[12] He described learning about a new medical school in rural East Tennessee, with a new internal medicine residency and deciding to go because "it seemed a beautiful place to bring [his] bride."[13] He recognized that it was

difficult to entice young American medical school graduates into these isolated and often depressed rural areas where reimbursement depended heavily on the health of the coal mines and on being willing to have a large proportion of Medicaid patients in the practice.[14]

Verghese exuded a natural curiosity that seemed to endear him to his new community: "Essie and the rest of the gang took it on themselves to not only feed me but also expand my Appalachian folk lexicon and coach me on the right way to 'talk country.'"[15] He includes himself in the coterie of foreign physicians who "were completing their training in American urban war zones and moving into these rural havens."[16]

An unexpected note of cognitive dissonance is evident in Verghese's lack of awareness about the possible discomfort his wife may have endured in relocating from India to rural Tennessee after their brief courtship. This is our first indication that there may be deficiencies in Verghese's observations. He writes, "Rajani and I, perhaps because we were of a younger generation, traveled easily between these two worlds: the parochial world of Indians in America, and the secular world of east Tennessee."[17] We are told that Rajani was working as an account executive for an advertising firm in India before coming to the United States. It's hard to imagine how a young professional woman would fit into life in rural Tennessee. One wonders what she was told that her life would be like? Were job opportunities available to her?

We are given one explanation for Verghese's lack of curiosity about Rajani's feelings when, later in this same chapter, he calls himself selfish. This bold and unadorned statement stopped me in my tracks. It is customary for physicians to use the "humble brag" motif, defined in the new Oxford Dictionary as: "An ostensibly modest or self-deprecating statement whose actual purpose is to draw attention to something of which one is proud."[18] As applied to doctors, this could be a statement like, "It's very selfish of me to want to leave early so that I can go home and spend the night reading all of our supervisor's papers in preparation for rounds tomorrow." But when Verghese describes himself as selfish for choosing infectious diseases as his subspecialty interest, he explains that "[c]omparatively few people went into ID," thereby increasing his chances for getting a more prestigious fellowship.[19] He further explains his reason for wanting to be an academic physician:

> If there was glory in medicine, then I was not satisfied with the glory of saving a patient and having the family and a few others know about it. ... The acclaim of the lecture hall, the lead article in the *New England Journal of Medicine*, the invitations to be a keynote speaker at gatherings of my peers—these were the coins I wished to hoard.[20]

He lays bare his honest reasons, at the risk of being considered calculating or even mercenary. This vulnerability is not typical of physician culture.

By being transparent and respectful, Verghese was allowed to explore the spread of AIDS into the population that he cared for. He was able to study the epidemiology of the disease in his rural community for academic journals while simultaneously providing a listening ear for his patients who were burdened by physical and emotional pain that they otherwise had to keep hidden. He acknowledged the toll that the socially unacceptable disorder had on rural families while simultaneously forcing himself to consider the possibility that he, too, may have brought his intrinsic biases and prejudices to the care he offered.

Verghese introduces us to wealthy business owners, Will and Sarah Johnson, referred to as "pillars of [the] community."[21] Will Johnson contracted HIV disease through an intraoperative blood transfusion just before the routine screening of blood products began, and unknowingly passed along the virus to his wife soon after. Verghese recognizes with his first meeting with the Johnsons that he is moved by their situation in a way that he has not felt with his other patients: "I was deeply affected by the story of the Johnsons, very sympathetic to them. Why? Was it easier for me to sympathize ... with this beautiful couple because they were not gay, not intravenous drug users?"[22] He goes on to consider: "I liked to think of myself as nonjudgmental; I thought I didn't discriminate in my services. ... But did I have a blind spot?"[23]

Curiously, while Verghese demonstrates his curiosity and willingness to share his thoughts as they pertain to his patients, a very notable omission is his inability to be as introspective about his relationships with his wife and sons. As he describes the competing pulls of being a husband and being a father with his almost compulsive "need" to understand the full effect that AIDS was having on the community he served, he seems remarkably unaware of the toll that his profession is taking on his wife. For example, after admitting Mr. Johnson, he returns home and attempts to share the patient's story with his wife because "[i]t was a gripping story, one she could obviously relate to. A husband infected 'innocently' who then infects his wife. I was describing our very own nightmare. But she had little to say."[24]

Verghese attributes this to Rajani's ability to "master professional detachment," which he ascribes as a characteristic of doctors' spouses.[25] At the time, he does not consider the possibility that her quietness reflects the depth of her fear, that she might be worried that he could bring home a disease, considered a death sentence, to infect her or the children. Later, Verghese speculates, "I wondered if subconsciously Rajani viewed me the same way ... tainted by the people I took care of."[26] His blindness to his wife's emotional suffering is in stark contrast to his imagined musings about his patients' suffering. Rajani's subsequent comments, sparse as they are, provide foreshadowing for the state of their marriage: "I wish this disease was gone that you were not so close to it. It's kind of become who you are and what you do."[27] It is revealing that, while he seems to have no difficulty asking intimate questions of his patients, much of what he says about his wife lies in the realm of speculation. He rarely writes about actual conversations wherein they discuss these more sensitive aspects of his work and the repercussions pertaining to their family life. The reader is left to wonder whether the conversations happened, but were not included in the memoir, or whether the conversations did not happen, and, if so, why they didn't.

Many of us were trained to believe that medicine is a calling rather than an occupation. In order to be a good physician, conventional and perhaps current thinking is that one has to commit fully to medicine, sacrificing family, personal time, and self-care. For me, this was the first time that I had read of a physician revealing the cost of this commitment. As he later describes his decision to leave Johnson City for an AIDS-only practice in Iowa, Verghese writes:

[My wife] is reluctant about this move; she senses, I think, that this is perhaps our last chance. She has agreed to come because she is trying to make herself believe that once I am removed from the maelstrom, I may become someone she can live with again.[28]

He talks about having a better understanding of what his wife disapproves of, but continues to engage in those acts, only at other people's houses and without mentioning anything to his wife. Likewise, he admits to her that he has had an affair during a time when she returned to India. Verghese's lack of transparency with his wife, when he seems committed to honesty in his interactions with patients, is another discordant note.

Later, he writes, "The minor differences in our two personalities … became more exaggerated every year, as if we were driving each other to the polar extremes," adding that the decision to leave for a sabbatical in Iowa was "an act of self-preservation" so that "in a new landscape, surrounded by strangers, there was no need to put on an act for anyone. And when the pretense was gone, there was nothing left."[29] This could be viewed as a cautionary tale: there can be tangible and long-lasting costs from embracing the tradition of full dedication to medicine to the exclusion of one's self.

One additional point that spans both memoirs is the issue of sexuality. When Verghese and his wife make the decision to settle in Johnson City, Tennessee, after he completes his fellowship, he expresses his satisfaction with the decision by saying, "I felt at peace in this corner of east Tennessee. Finally, this was my own country."[30] By this point in the memoir, Verghese has already explicitly pointed out that the immigrant community in his region primarily consists of other physicians who have relocated as he has, so exactly what he means by "my own country" is not clear. He admits to his curiosity about "the gay lifestyle," and when his wife asks if he is gay, he is slow to respond. While there is, of course, no requirement that an author reveals everything of importance in a memoir, if Verghese had been exploring his sexuality more openly during this time, it could be an explanation for why he chose not to be as introspective about his personal relationships.

As this book is going to press in 2021, the world is still contending with the ongoing coronavirus pandemic. There are similarities between Verghese's introduction to HIV disease and our introduction to COVID-19. In particular, the themes of fear, isolation, and the physician as a hero bear some consideration.

As 2019 drew to a close, a cluster of cases of what would come to be known as SARS-CoV-2 were reported to the World Health Organization.[31] In the months that followed, we watched as the infection spread across the world, leaving death in its wake. In the beginning, the method and extent of COVID-19 transmission was unknown; it seemed that becoming infected might be a death sentence, and how to protect oneself from infection was not well understood. We were told to self-isolate, but the requirements of daily life—getting food or groceries, picking up medications, going to work—were potentially high-risk situations. This was particularly true for frontline workers: emergency personnel, nurses, doctors, and hospital cleaning staff. Verghese describes the fear of passive transmission when he describes the dilemma of what to do about the respirator used for the first AIDS patient in Johnson City:

> Some favored burying the respirator, deep-sixing it in the swampy land at the back of the hospital. Others were for incinerating it. As a compromise, the machine was opened up, its innards gutted and most replaceable parts changed. It was then gas disinfected several times. Even so, it was a long time before it was put back into circulation.[32]

This echoes the measures people took and some still take with conventional inanimate items such as groceries and mail delivery during the COVID-19 pandemic, leaving the items to sit for several days or wiping down the outside of the items with disinfectant wipes. The popular press has been filled with multiple accounts of doctors and nurses choosing to live apart from their families so as to avoid inadvertent contamination, changing clothes several times in going from hospital to home, and following complex routines to ensure proper decontamination and to prevent inadvertent exposure of their families.[33]

The need for months of social distancing coupled with the significant and tremendous fear of infection has led to feelings of isolation, for patients and for frontline workers. With both direct and aerosolized transmission a reality, and challenges associated with vaccine allocation and effectiveness, we are likely to need to continue some version of social distancing for many months to come. Being without a human touch as providers is challenging; who couldn't benefit from a hug after a lengthy day caring for patients in the intensive care unit? From a clinical perspective, Verghese himself wrote eloquently about the value of touch in the patient-doctor relationship, indicating that the touch during physical examination represents "a sacred privilege," helping to "quiet and reassure" patients.[34] What are we then sacrificing during the COVID-19 pandemic when, to prevent doctors and nurses from becoming infected, particularly with limited personal protective equipment, we limit entry to ICU bed spaces, and restrict visitors? Verghese describes this fear of contagion when his patient George is hospitalized with *P. carinii* pneumonia; several nurses refused to care for George, but a few assigned themselves to him over and over again, as if "he was a prize patient."[35]

Throughout the COVID-19 pandemic, countless articles and news stories promote the idea of the doctors and nurses as heroes for being willing to put their lives on the line to treat patients with this disease. While the physician's duty to treat requires that doctors place themselves in harm's way in order to provide patient care, the lack of sufficient personal protective equipment and unclear transmission patterns made doing this particularly risky for doctors and nurses with the onslaught of COVID-19, and, in some communities, there was neither time nor resources available to offer doctors and nurses respite from the huge burden of necessary patient care. That frontline workers continued to show up for work, with some volunteering to travel to places where the contagion was more rampant, gave further strength to the idea of heroism in these acts.

By way of contrast, it was not clear that those doctors and nurses caring for AIDS patients in rural Tennessee were viewed as heroes. Verghese writes about the few infectious disease specialists that existed in the community he served in the mid-1980s, and he describes a "feeling of alienation" due to caring for people with AIDS; this is quite the opposite of the accolades that physicians currently caring for COVID-19 patients are receiving.[36]

One might imagine that reading *My Own Country* might feel dated; so many decades have passed since HIV and AIDS first appeared on the scene. Certainly, the introduction of retroviral therapy and the presence of celebrities such as Earvin "Magic" Johnson and Charlie Sheen who are living their lives with their HIV positivity a matter of public knowledge has changed the public perception of what this disease can do. LGBTQ activism has also shifted some of the homophobia that was inextricably linked with the spread of AIDS. However, to this day, the presence of a dangerous communicable disease, even with a known mechanism of transmission, can continue to propel people into a whirlwind of misinformation and misunderstanding. The nonjudgmental way in which Verghese describes the thinking of the average rural inhabitant of his community, the initial journey of gay men toward the cities, and then their return home if AIDS took its toll allows the reader to feel sympathy for the families caught in the tension between love for their sons and brothers and the concern about what their neighbors and friends may think. This is a relevant learning point for clinicians and trainees alike.

There are other themes that resonate in this memoir that are as applicable today as they were 30 years ago. Recognizing the story behind the illness allows patients to be seen as people first. It is impossible to be a doctor in the Western world, and not feel the intrusion of technology into every aspect of the medical experience. We rely more on scans than on physical diagnosis and on the contents of our computers rather than the history presented by our patients. With the requirement for utilization of an electronic health record, we physicians are being forced to avoid eye contact with our patients in favor of maintaining eye contact with an electronic screen. We are further required to allow for a mechanism for bidirectional electronic communication, generally referred to as a patient portal. Given the challenges patients face when trying to communicate with their harried physicians, many prefer to type out a message and send it into the electronic void to await a reply.

Shorter appointment times mean that there is less time for the social niceties and for the nonmedical information that defines our patients in their entirety. And, finally, the lack of primary care providers creates even more pressure upon overworked clinicians to try to fulfill this enormous need. The profusion of the so-called minute or urgent clinics can further disrupt the traditional doctor–patient relationship.

There is another, less obvious but more important reason why reading—or, in my case, rereading—*My Own Country* can be helpful. A major problem affecting clinical medicine in our current era is burnout, defined by the World Health Organization as a "syndrome conceptualized as resulting from chronic workplace stress that has not been successfully managed."[37] The WHO's International Classification of Diseases manual lists a characteristic symptom as "increased mental distance from one's job or feelings negative towards one's career."[38] Unfortunately, conceptualizing patients as collections of symptoms or signs allows for this type of separation to occur effortlessly.

As someone with a lifelong terrible memory for names and faces, I have taken Verghese's narrative lessons to heart and have developed two changes to my clinical practice to allow me to engage quickly and deeply with patients. I am a clinician specializing in the care of patients with epilepsy. My patients, too, face a cultural stigma because of their disorder. They often try to keep their diagnosis a secret, and because of the infrequent nature of the seizures themselves for most patients, they are able to do so much of the time. In my office practice, however, I encourage my patients to tell me the "story" of their disorder, and I very intentionally use that word: story. This opens the door for patients to tell me what's of greatest concern to them, by weaving the narrative of their condition into the fabric of their lives. Second, when my trainees assess and present patients to me, I request that the trainee identify one, nonpejorative, nonmedical "fun fact" about each patient that will allow me to recall the patient in full Technicolor brilliance. This approach allows me to connect with the patient upon entering the room and demonstrates to the patient my interest in knowing them as whole and complete people. I always hope that after a month of identifying these "fun facts" and seeing how important they are, some of my trainees may choose to incorporate this technique into their own practices.

In the early 1990s, Verghese, Rajani (his first wife), and their five- and seven-year-old sons moved to El Paso, Texas, where the content of his second memoir, *The Tennis Partner*, takes place. The subtitle, as noted, to this volume is *A Doctor's Story of Friendship and Loss*. If we were judging this book by its cover, we would assume that the word "loss" refers to the friendship between Verghese and his tennis partner. There are, however, multiple losses that will be explored: loss of a marriage, loss of the connection between a father and his sons, and loss of self to addiction, to name a few.

The Tennis Partner represents a more focused story of a physician exploring and pushing against traditional boundaries. Much as he led readers through the onslaught of the AIDS epidemic in small town Tennessee, Verghese, then on the faculty of the Texas Tech School of Medicine, was on the leading edge of writing about the havoc that substance use disorders bring to medical care. And as he did with his first memoir, we again meet the person before the condition.

In the prologue, we are introduced to medical intern David Smith as he fails another drug test, and is being sent to the Talbott-Marsh clinic in Atlanta, a residential facility for doctors with substance use disorders. David (as he is referred to in the book) meets clinicians with alcohol, benzodiazepine, and other addictions, and we see him struggle with the ferocious denial described by his colleagues while recognizing that successful passage through the program represents his only hope of continuing on in medicine.

When Verghese meets his new intern, he discovers that David once played tennis professionally. We learn that Verghese also played tennis at a young age, and that he also started keeping journals, containing his observations of professional matches, records of particularly memorable shots, and reminders to himself as a way to improve his game. He later modified this journalistic approach to keep track of his medical knowledge and observations, hoping to improve his performance as a physician.

We move from hearing about the place that tennis had in Verghese's past to watching the senior physician and junior medical resident begin their friendship over a match. In the hospital, Verghese is the teacher, and David is the student; on the tennis court, their roles are reversed, and Verghese resumes his habit of making notes. Anyone who plays tennis can, perhaps, learn much from the detailed descriptions of matches and specific strokes embedded within the memoir. Those of us who are not devoted to the sport may find our thoughts wandering with the pages and pages of matches Verghese describes; we want to ask him, as David ultimately does: "It's like, this ... you're as passionate about tennis as you are about medicine. It seems like ... one of those would be enough."[39] Verghese thinks but does not attempt to explain: "Keep the ball in play. Keep your eye on the ball. Follow through. These were admonitions for both tennis and life, and they spilled over from the one into the other."[40]

Verghese's relationship with David grows stronger, until, one day, David reveals his past: "I'm a recovering cocaine addict. ... I wasn't just snorting it either. I was injecting it. As much as I could, as many times a day as I could."[41] When Verghese admits that he had "tried just about everything else at one time or another," it allows David to reveal the extent of his addiction history, with a causal connection to his tennis career.[42] Later, when David relapses again, Verghese has to decide whether or not to turn him in for violating the terms of his reinstatement into the internship. He decides to remain quiet, justifying his decision by saying that David replied honestly to his query only because they were friends, not because they were mentor and mentee.[43]

While substance use disorder in our modern era represents an expanding epidemic, the reality of physician addicts does not receive as much publicity. Verghese does not shrink from a thorough examination of the condition. His curiosity, eye for detail, and singular voice allow us to appreciate the shared pain, suffering, and humanness of addicted patients, whether members of the medical profession or not.

Throughout the book, he considers not just the medical understanding of substance use disorder, the neurological and biological features that result in certain patients becoming addicted while others don't, but he also discusses the social, environmental, and cultural drivers of substance use disorder. He discusses the loneliness of the medical profession and addresses the culture of medicine preventing the expression of feelings:

> The Citadel quality to medical training, where only the fittest survive, creates the paradox of the humane, empathetic physician, like David, who

shows little humanity to himself. ... It is not individual physicians who are at fault as much as it is the system we have created.[44]

In a perspective piece in the *New England Journal of Medicine*, Verghese reminds the reader that the unremitting stress of being a doctor frequently drives physicians to self-medicate rather than seek help. He acknowledges the general discomfort with confronting other physicians when signs of substance use disorder may be apparent and urges a return to the principles of Alcoholics Anonymous, which underscore the need to uncover the secrecy of substance use disorder.

In this volume, more so than in his first memoir, we see Verghese's clinical acumen at its finest. He provides a three-page exposition on his examination of the human pulse, beginning with reaching for the patient's hand and ending with his personal compulsion: to check for the so-called radio-femoral delay, a specific sign associated with coarctation of the aorta, an extremely rare but life-threatening condition. In between, he describes several potential abnormalities of the pulse, and admits, "I know I linger too long on the pulse, as if wanting my hands to remain submerged in this subterranean river, feel it wash over me."[45] To have a physician who cares as much about every physical finding of the human body sounds like a gift that most patients would crave, particularly as it requires the "laying on of hands," often felt to confer therapeutic benefit as Verghese espouses.

Verghese states that a diagnostic or therapeutic touch can be a "healing ritual or bond."[46] In a particularly prescient scene, Verghese attempts to teach his students the power of the human touch:

> Picture yourself lying on that bed. ... It's a terrifying experience. It's important that you realize that every illness ... comes with a spiritual violation that parallels the physical ailment. A doctor has to be more than just a dispenser of cures, but also ... a minister of healing. That's what that touch is about. Recognize this ability in yourselves, think of it as a potent instrument. Sharpen it and learn how to use it.

Sadly, he acknowledges that

> [they] had the uh-oh look, the concern that we were straying into touchy-feely territory, an area of medicine that was not fashionable, particularly in an ICU where it was as if the high-tech gadgetry stood in for the spiritual, the emotional.[47]

While memoir as a genre represents first-person narrative, there is risk in using the physician voice to describe a patient's experience. One wonders if the ease with which Verghese attributes dialogue to his characters is valid, or whether his literary license allows him to take liberties. For example, in describing a woman presenting with a herpes lesion on her mouth, he says:

> To me, that lesion on the vermillion border of her lip had been a marker for the devastation of her immune system, of how she was approaching the steep part of the inexorable downhill slope of [HIV] disease. To her, it had meant much more than that; it had stigmatized her, hurt her vanity, made her struggle to hold her head up.[48]

Unless Verghese specifically asked the patient how her HIV disease influenced her sense of self, this description could be perceived as offensive or insulting. In his 2014 article, physician-author Abraham Nussbaum suggests that Verghese's work "gives a physician undue authority in assigning meaning to the human experience," and "gives a physician 'full responsibility' for telling the story of his patient."[49]

In an editorial, Verghese explains that he became aware of the presence of physician-writers by reading a pathology textbook, which "made [him] aware of literary voice, the ability of authors to place themselves in the text, let their personality come through, and subtly become a character in the reading experience."[50] Attributing stigma or lost vanity could be construed as originating from bias on the part of the narrator, and biases, disclosures, and other conflicts embedded within the art of narrative writing are not explored as fully by Verghese as one might anticipate.

A significant omission that marks both of Verghese's memoirs is his inability or unwillingness to explore his own relationships with family. In *My Own Country*, Verghese's initial mention of Rajani is so brief that she seems an afterthought in his narrative. He devotes just one paragraph early in the book to their meeting and marriage; later, while describing their first home in Tennessee, he says that Rajani would look forward to decorating it. He spends a single sentence talking about how well she had done and how respected she had been in her professional life. An account executive for an advertising firm when he first meets her, he goes no further in questioning whether Rajani would miss her job when she moves to Tennessee; he does not seem to consider the possibility that she might be bored, or lonely, or homesick.

In a too-late sign of self-awareness, and reflecting on his habits of keeping journals for tennis and for medicine, Verghese writes:

> If I had kept notes on love, if I had tuned my act each time there was a discordant note, a flubbed move, if I had recorded the things that worked, perhaps we could have saved the relationship, moved to a higher level, made it as effortless and automatic as lifting a glass to one's lips.[51]

During an evening of brief reconciliation, Verghese comes to the realization that "[he] had found it necessary to be angry because [he] knew [he] was at fault. It was so much easier to be angry with her than with [himself]."[52]

As Verghese considers the dissolution of his marriage, his interactions with his two sons range from touching to self-centered. When he and his wife are preparing to separate, Verghese says, "What I realized tonight is that when I move, I'm the one the boys will think abandoned them."[53] This conversation, powered by guilt, culminates in his wife's suggestion that they resume counseling; one day later, it is clear that reconciliation is out of the question. When Verghese finds an apartment, he refers to it as the time-out place. The boys visit the apartment and reassure their father: "'It's so great, Dad,' Steven said. 'Don't worry, everything will be all right.'"[54] Verghese finally allows himself to admit the depth of his need for his children:

> The boys were the one constant in my life, my unchanging ritual. If I had thought of myself as needing to be there for them, they were, in fact, much more there for me, secure in their routine, giving me faith.[55]

Finally, *My Own Country* in particular contains multiple descriptions of patients' interactions with partners, parents, siblings, and children. Yet, we are given no information by Verghese about his own siblings and their interactions with each other or with him. His parents are seen marginally more, but his relationship with them is never rendered in three dimensions, as virtually all of his relationships with patients are. Certainly, his friendship with David is explored from multiple angles over time. We see very little linearity or persistence in his descriptions of relationships with his wife or sons.

As doctors, we need to probe and explore the patient's story as readily as we investigate the patient's medical history. We may not always be able to provide a specific, curative treatment, but we can always leave people with hope, comfort, and confirmation that they have been heard. As patients, we need to demand care that is patient-centered and holistic. We must also recognize that families require support from us, particularly when they are struggling with disorders that may be poorly understood, or culturally shunned. The salient message from both memoirs is that listening is a critical skill in medicine.

When people ask me why I became a doctor, I respond that there is no story there. In an opinion piece in the *New England Journal of Medicine*, Verghese wrote about his "call" to medicine.[56] Like many first-generation immigrant children, myself included, his first stated decision to pursue medicine was to make his parents happy. If I am asked why I stay a doctor, I point to *My Own Country*. Reading it was liberating, it broadened my understanding of what was permissible in the patient-doctor relationship and allowed me to be more creative with how I connect with my patients. I am more adherent to boundaries (or more fearful of crossing them) than Verghese, but when using his technique of allowing patients to tell their story directly, I feel better equipped to explore my patients' needs. While I do not expect to achieve the breadth of Verghese's work, in my small way, I flatter myself that I may be able to continue the legacy that he has created by incorporating elements of narrative into my daily practice.

Verghese tears apart the idea that emotions weaken us as clinicians and allows us to reframe emotion as something that allows us to resonate with our patients. This may serve as another outlet for us to cope with the other consequences of burnout. Following his time in El Paso, Verghese became the founding director of the Center for Medical Humanities and Ethics at the University of Texas Health Science Center in San Antonio, where he developed a program using bedside rounding as a way to incorporate empathy into the medical education curriculum. More recently, he was recruited to Stanford University as a full professor; there, he focuses on the theory and practice of medicine. In 2016, he received a National Humanities Medal from President Obama in recognition of his work toward allowing physicians to see patients as individuals. As physicians, we can learn from Verghese to open our eyes and open our hearts to our patients and to each other.

Notes

1 Abraham Verghese, "Culture Shock—Patient as Icon, Icon as Patient," *New England Journal of Medicine* 359, no. 26 (2008): 2748–2751.
2 Andrew Elder, Jeff Chi, Errol Ozdalga, John Kugler, and Abraham Verghese, "The Road Back to the Bedside," *JAMA* 323, no. 17 (2020): 1672–1673.
3 Abraham Verghese, *My Own Country: A Doctor's Story of a Town and Its People in the Age of AIDS* (New York: Simon & Schuster, 1994).
4 Abraham Verghese, *The Tennis Partner: A Doctor's Story of Friendship and Loss* (New York: HarperCollins, 1998).
5 Verghese, *My Own Country*, 16.
6 Ibid., 5.
7 Ibid.
8 Ibid., 13.
9 Ibid., 10.
10 Centers for Disease Control, *MMWR Weekly*, June 5, 1981: https://www.cdc.gov/mmwr/preview/mmwrhtml/june_5.htm, accessed August 20, 2021.
11 Centers for Disease Control, CDC-HIV Surveillance Report, 1985: https://www.cdc.gov/hiv/pdf/library/reports/surveillance/cdc-hiv-surveillance-report-1985.pdf, accessed August 20, 2021.
12 Verghese, *My Own Country*, 18.
13 Ibid., 19.
14 Ibid., 22.
15 Ibid., 21.
16 Ibid., 22.
17 Ibid., 23.
18 *Oxford English Dictionary*: https://www.lexico.com/en/definition/humblebrag, accessed August 20, 2021.
19 Verghese, *My Own Country*, 26.
20 Ibid., 25.
21 Ibid., 233.
22 Ibid., 250.
23 Ibid.
24 Ibid., 253.
25 Ibid.
26 Ibid., 309.
27 Ibid., 254.
28 Ibid., 426.
29 Verghese, *The Tennis Partner*, 41.
30 Verghese, *My Own Country*, 46.
31 World Health Organization, January 12, 2020: https://www.who.int/csr/don/12-january-2020-novel-coronavirus-china/en/, accessed August 20, 2021.

32 Verghese, *My Own Country*, 12.
33 ABC News, April 16, 2020: https://www.abc.net.au/life/couples-living-apart-during -coronavirus-pandemic/12150500, accessed August 20, 2021.
34 Abraham Verghese, "A Touch of Sense," *Health Affairs* 28, no. 4 (2009): 1177–1182.
35 Verghese, *My Own Country*, 84.
36 Ibid., 309.
37 World Health Organization, May 28, 2019: https://www.who.int/mental_health/e vidence/burn-out/en/, accessed August 20, 2021.
38 Ibid.
39 Verghese, *The Tennis Partner*, 91.
40 Ibid., 92.
41 Ibid., 125.
42 Ibid., 126.
43 Ibid., 258.
44 Ibid., 341.
45 Ibid., 132.
46 Verghese, "A Touch of Sense."
47 Ibid.
48 Verghese, *The Tennis Partner*, 254.
49 Abraham Nussbaum, "'I Am the Author and Must Take Full Responsibility': Abraham Verghese, Physicians as the Storytellers of the Body, and the Renewal of Medicine," *Journal of Medical Humanities* 37, no. 4 (2016): 389–399.
50 Abraham Verghese, "Writing Medicine," *JAMA* 323, no. 17 (2020): 1649–1650.
51 Verghese, *The Tennis Partner*, 50.
52 Ibid., 72.
53 Ibid., 71.
54 Ibid., 137.
55 Ibid., 242.
56 Abraham Verghese, "The Calling," *New England Journal of Medicine* 352, no. 18 (2005): 1844–1847.

5 Atul Gawande

Doctoring, dying, and the pursuit of "Better"

Thomas D. Harter

On the one hand, writing a chapter on Atul Gawande should be easy. He has such a wide volume of material covering a vast number of topics, there is no shortage of content to analyze and discuss. Not including his research articles in medical journals, he has published nearly 100 articles in popular media and four books. On the other hand, his writing has resonated so broadly among the American public—each of his four books has been a *New York Times* bestseller; he won the MacArthur Foundation "genius" award in 2006 at age 40 and has been named one of the top 40 important voices by *Becker's Hospital Review* for his work shaping contemporary healthcare practices and policies[1]—that writing a single chapter on a single work or small subset of works seems almost impossible. Indeed, shortly after *The New Yorker* published his article "The Cost Conundrum" in 2009—which compares differences in medical outcomes and costs between two nearly demographically identical Texas locales—the then US president Barack Obama called an emergency meeting of his staff who were working on health reform to discuss the article.[2]

If I had asked Gawande what this chapter should focus on, he probably would have told me to write about what I am curious about. Performing tasks that one is apt at doing and honing one's skills to perform those tasks extraordinarily well is a common theme in Gawande's works. Given that, the bulk of this work will be on death and dying and the ways in which hard conversations about treatment limits can be standardized and made to function routinely as part of good medical care. I am, after all, a clinical ethicist working for Gundersen Health System in La Crosse, Wisconsin, which has been described by some media outlets as the best place in America to die.[3] Still, it is equally important that I highlight and discuss a couple of the general themes found throughout all of Gawande's works, because without understanding those foundational pieces, it is impossible to fully appreciate how Gawande has been able to generate such a broad impact with his works.

Background

To me, Gawande's background is just as interesting and humbling as any piece of writing he has published during his still bourgeoning career. His parents were physicians—his father a urologist, his mother a pediatrician—who met and

DOI: 10.4324/9781003079712-5

married while practicing in New York. After Gawande was born, they moved to Athens, Ohio. It is clear from Gawande's writings the influence growing-up in Athens has on his strong belief in an unfettered, equal right of all people to healthcare. Athens is a small town in the Appalachian foothills whose main economy until the 1950s was coal. As the coal industry declined, so too has the economy and health of Athens. Today, the largest employer in Athens is Ohio University, where the annual student enrollment of approximately 36,000 is larger than the city's population of approximately 25,000. In 2017, while the national US median household income was $63,000, the median household income in Athens was meager $24,000.[4] Opioid addiction and health disparities in that part of the country are well-documented.

From Athens, Gawande studied biology and political science at Stanford University. Given that Gawande's parents were physicians, it should not be surprising that he intended to become a physician too. Immediately after Stanford, though, he attended Oxford University where he studied politics and philosophy as a Rhodes scholar. This is an important detour in Gawande's life for two reasons. First, as Gawande's later writings and works indicate, he is immensely concerned about health disparities and the role of public policy in providing equal access to healthcare. His interest in politics also drove him to be politically active prior to and during medical school.

Gawande took a break from his studies at Oxford to work on Al Gore's 1988 presidential campaign, and then as one of Gore's senate campaign staffers. Shortly thereafter, he returned to Oxford to finish his studies. He then came back to the United States and enrolled in Harvard Medical School but deferred his education to first work on healthcare policy with Congressman Jim Cooper of Tennessee. This work, per Gawande, is some of his proudest since it helped revive the National Health Service Corps loan repayment program that helped bring medical doctors to work in rural areas of the country.[5] Soon after beginning his studies at Harvard, Gawande took another break to work with the 1992 Clinton presidential campaign as the head of Clinton's healthcare and social policy unit. After Clinton was elected, Gawande finally returned to Harvard to complete medical and Master of Public Health degrees.

The second reason his time as a Rhodes scholar in Oxford was important is because of the clear influence studying philosophy has on his thinking and writing about medical practice. Gawande is a surgeon and so it would not be surprising for someone unfamiliar with his work to expect him to write in the way surgeons are known to think and practice: to quickly analyze a problem, devise and execute a plan to approach the problem, and then move on to the next surgery, addressing complications only as they arise. However, Gawande's writings—while well-researched in the way we expect of medical academicians—involve far deeper questioning, analysis, and introspection than many typical researchers or storytellers. He typically asks philosophical questions—questions without easy or obvious answers such as "why do good doctors go bad?," "why does medical care cost more in some places than others?," and "is there a right to healthcare?" He starts from a position of curiosity—looking from the ground-up.

When asked where he gets ideas for his pieces, he states, "I don't know. I'm interested in things that are confusing to me, so I write them down."[6] He is the closest thing to a philosopher in surgeon's clothing I can imagine.

In reviewing Gawande's biography, it may also strike some that becoming both a surgeon and writer was not planned or intended. As Gawande notes, he thought he would be an internal medicine physician with a clinic on the side that would allow him time to work in the realm of public policy. However, upon being exposed to the operating room during medical training, he recognized a similarity between surgeons and politicians. Per Gawande:

> I thought surgeons were like politicians. Surgeons are grappling with having limited information and knowledge, imperfect science, but have a necessity to act in the face of both imperfection in their own abilities and imperfect knowledge in the world. I saw a lot of the same incredible range of characters and people [in politics and the operating room]. ... I wanted to be more like surgeons and more like the politicians I admired who could make decisions, live with the consequences, and learn from the consequences.[7]

Writing, it appears, was similarly accidental for Gawande. One of Gawande's friends, Michael Kinsley, founded the now widely popular Internet magazine, *Slate.com*, in 1996. Looking for writers, he asked Gawande to write something for *Slate* about his life as a doctor. Gawande obliged figuring this was an opportunity to keep his interest in public policy sharp without having to divert much time away from the rigorous demands of surgical training. His first piece, "Gulf War Syndrome," questions the US government response and care of US veterans returning from the first Persian Gulf War with a variety of unexplained illnesses after exposure to sarin gas from a destroyed Iraqi ammunitions depot.[8]

Gawande wrote for *Slate.com* for two years, honing his ability to write good stories while conveying the underlying meaning and ideas driving them. By 1998, his articles on *Slate* generated about 300,000 hits. One reader of his work was an editor at *The New Yorker*, who asked if he would be willing to write something a bit longer for them. He agreed, and after writing three articles for them in 1998, they offered him a staff-writer position.

As a writer

Being a staff-writer required him to write longer articles, and this forced Gawande to become a more creative writer as well. His *New Yorker* articles follow a typical pattern in which he begins with a brief history or story of the topic at hand, intermingled with basic explanations of the topic to help readers better understand the complex medical subject. At some point, he then interludes with one or two anecdotal stories—often from his professional career—that he uses to further iterate and explore the point he is making.

For example, his first *New Yorker* article, "No Mistake," is about the utilization of technology in medical care, specifically machines that read electrocardiograms

(EKGs).[9] The article focuses on two basic questions: (1) can machines perform some medical tasks better than humans?, and (2) to what degree or extent should medical providers rely on machines and other technology to make medical value judgments and perform complex medical tasks? The topic may not be intriguing to some, but herein lies the brilliance of Gawande. The questions he focuses on are intellectually seductive: on the surface they appear empirically bland (the answer to whether machines do a task better than a human is solved via scientific analysis—i.e., observe the two and determine which does a better job), but really, they are deeply rich, philosophical questions. What does it mean, for example, to "do a better job," at reading an EKG or performing a complex medical task? How much is the practice of medicine about technical proficiency versus value-laden assessment and judgment? Gawande does not directly provide answers but instead provides perspectives for readers to think about in cultivating their own answers to these questions. In many ways, while his audience are nonmedical providers, Gawande is really writing for his medical peers, junior colleagues, and medical students.

A philosopher's education

My introduction to Gawande's work was during my first year of graduate school. I was studying philosophy with a concentration in medical ethics at the University of Tennessee. As I progressed through my first year, analyzing the applications of moral and ethical theory to medicine, I longed for a bridge between the two worlds that would help me better understand the medical profession and, more importantly, the medical mind. I wanted to know how doctors think of the situations and dilemmas I was reading about; what sorts of things bother them about being a doctor and providing patient care and are these the same worries I had in thinking about the issues from the classroom and not the clinic? Do physicians put as much weight on ethics principles like respect for patient autonomy, beneficence, and justice that, at the time, solely comprised the nexus of my educational orbit? Or do they value different aspects of patient care than I was being taught?

At a local bookstore, I searched for medical humanities books that would help inform my studies. The title of Gawande's first book stood out to me. *Complications: A Surgeon's Notes on an Imperfect Science*[10] immediately tells readers this is a book of self-reflection. The title implies it is a critical look at a profession often popularly associated with terms like "ego," "arrogance," and "perfection." Perhaps more importantly, though, the title hints that the book is a humbling look at one's role in that profession. As I read through the table of contents, the last chapter of the first section, "When Good Doctors Go Bad," further sparked my interest. Quickly flipping through the chapter, I saw Gawande openly talk about and attempt to understand why surgeons such as himself are reluctant to confront colleagues whose bad practices harm people. Here is Gawande, lifting the shroud on some of the mysteries of the medical profession, writing about what it means to be a practicing doctor caring for individuals during one of their most vulnerable times. It is a confession that the pearly pedestal on which we tend to socially regard physicians is, on closer inspection, covered in some unsightly scuffmarks. This was exactly the kind of insight I needed for my education.

Throughout graduate school, I had made the occasional habit while perusing the isles of bookstores to drift away from the philosophy sections to the medical sections and spend an equal amount of time there looking over the humanities books to see who else, like Gawande, was writing about being a doctor in a way that was not glossy but earnest. I was thrilled when a couple of years after reading *Complications* I saw a second book by Gawande, *[B]etter: A Surgeon's Notes on Performance*.[11] This book would be a game-changer for me.

Complications is a wonderful book for identifying the "what" of some worries and concerns doctors face in medical practice. It tells several stories of what Gawande has seen or been contemplating to that point in his career. But it does not move the conversation about medical, ethical care, much farther than that. *[B]etter* does. It moves the conversation from identifying problems to identifying solutions, with in-depth explanations of what it takes at both micro and macro levels to find implementable, scalable solutions to specific problems. However, I do not see the value of *[B]etter* in the individual frameworks Gawande sets for thinking about and working through specific issues in medical care needing improvement, such as thinking about hand hygiene and appropriate compensation and salary for one's work. Certainly, those are important. For me, though, the value of *[B]etter* is the philosophically existential point Gawande makes— perhaps unwittingly—several times throughout the book.

As Gawande discusses in the chapter "The Bell Curve," to be average is both acceptable and, for most of us, inevitable. For whatever practices people engage in, there are some who are low performers, some who are high performers, and in the middle, a swath of average performers. Even when the average performers adopt the practices and standards of the high performers, the high performers continue to accelerate their performance to higher levels more quickly—high performers, Gawande shows, get better faster. This realization might cause some to experience an existential crisis; what is the value of continuing one's work if one is fated to be average. Gawande's response to this concern is that while the bell curve will continue to exist, to settle for being average is a matter of choice and is neither inevitable nor acceptable. One can make an argument that the reason the title of the book is not capitalized is that Gawande recognizes that pathways to improvement most often only require small, incremental changes, not complete overhauls of medical systems; one ought to work with what they have to improve their performance and that those incremental changes are what likely will have a lasting impact on patient care. This was the lesson I needed to complete my graduate work during the times when I was bogged down with doubts of finishing my dissertation. "[B]etter is possible," writes Gawande, "It does not take genius. It takes diligence. It takes moral clarity. It takes ingenuity. And above all, it takes a willingness to try."[12]

The idea that medical providers are obligated to constantly strive toward improvement and that improvement is possible is the underlying theme—the underlying lesson—that ties together all Gawande's writing and research. His ability to write philosophically from a medical perspective continues to resonate with me and, I suspect, is one reason for his mass popularity. He is a philosopher not only in the sense that he has an unquenchable curiosity about people and the ways medicine affects lives, but he is also a philosopher in his willingness to be self-examining, self-critical, and humble in admitting when he makes mistakes, while not only accepting help to become a better physician but also seeks out those who can help him improve.[13] He neither professes to have the answers to many of the questions he raises; nor does he sit idle and hope the answers simply come to him. He researches. He confronts the bell curve of medical care, challenging himself and readers to strive toward incremental improvements that, over time, have demonstrable effect and can become habitual.

Being Mortal

Being Mortal, Gwande's most recent book, is the culmination of his most ambitious writing to date. Death is an inescapable fact of all biologic life that touches everyone regardless of one's social circumstances, demographic background, or medical history. How people live their lives toward the end and how people die in the United States, however, has changed and, as Gawande finds and writes throughout the book, comes with some qualitative variances that readers see in the stories he tells.

One such story is that of Dr. Felix Silverstone and his wife Bella. Felix was a geriatrician who nearly suffered a cardiac arrest at 79 and finally had to retire at 82—not, as Gawande highlights, because of his own failing health but because of Bella's. She started to experience a rapid decline in her vision, hearing, and neurological functioning, ultimately leaving her totally blind, almost totally deaf, and with poor memory. One day, as Felix was walking with Bella, she fell, breaking both her fibulas. She was immediately taken to the hospital and placed in bilateral casts from her ankles to above her knees. She was discharged to a nursing home where Felix was still able to be with her. Six weeks later, the casts came off, she was able to move back home with Felix and started to walk again. But a mere four days after moving back home with Felix, she collapsed again and during the ambulance transport to the hospital, died.[14]

One reason this story resonates so deeply with me is that while I have never met the Silverstones, I immediately recognize their story as my own. When I was 18, halfway through my senior year in high school, my 83-year-old grandmother, Wilhelmina, slipped on ice while getting her mail and broke her hip. She underwent hip replacement surgery—mostly to mitigate the pain. What was not made clear to her or my family was that, from a medical perspective, there was no expectation that she would ever walk again. Still, shortly after surgery, she was discharged to a skilled nursing facility for rehabilitation. Those with experience in caring for geriatric persons will not be surprised to know this hope and plan for rehabilitation failed. Worse was that at the rehab facility she was alone, miserable, and unable (and my guess, unwilling) to participate in therapy. It was recommended she be transitioned to a nursing home. After touring several facilities, my mother refused all the available options and she and my grandmother decided instead that she would come live with us. The transition was especially hard since my grandmother lived more than 5 hours away, several states over.

Three months later, while still adjusting to our new shared norms of life, my mother was rearranging some pictures on my grandmother's dresser so she could see them better from her bed. My grandmother asked my mother to adjust one of the frames. Within the few seconds it took my mother to get up and move the picture, a tiny blood clot, that doctors suspect had formed during surgery, gradually made its way from her hip to her brain, clotting off a blood vessel, causing a fatal stroke. When my mother turned around, my grandmother had slumped backward and became unresponsive. Emergency medical crews arrived within 10 minutes. My parents sped-off behind the ambulance, leaving me at home to notify my older siblings of what was happening. Two hours later, when my parents returned home, their faces silently telegraphed the news I was expecting that my grandmother had died.

The study and practice of medicine, for all the amazing ways it can cure disease, treat illness, and slow the dying process, has yet to prevent the fatal flaw in all living creatures of being mortal. This is perhaps why, as Gawande notes, medical school training largely neglects this aspect of patient care. Physicians treat and cure illness and disease, and when they cannot, often no longer see their services as needed. Yet, the role of physicians in end-of-life care is not only increasing but also that dying has become a medicalized endeavor. As Gawande points about, prior to 1945, most deaths occurred in the home. But, as medicine allowed for aging persons to live longer, healthier, independent lives, and as economic opportunities widened, leading to changes in traditional family systems, how the elderly die has also changed. It is no longer the case that older persons can expect or rely on their children to care for them as they age. A recent study found that approximately 45% of Medicare beneficiaries in 2015 died either in an acute care hospital or nursing home, while approximately 45% and 27% were, respectively, cared for in a hospital or intensive care unit (ICU) in the 30 days prior to death.[15]

Two decades later, as I reflect on my grandmother's life and death, I realize that in one sense, her end is all too common, while in another sense, it is not common at all. That she fell, broke her hip, and was immediately treated in a hospital where she was given a new hip, and then ultimately developed a blood clot months later and whisked away again to a hospital where she died, is not surprising to me or anyone in the medical profession. That she came to live and be cared for by my family over her last few months of life is now, however, atypical.

Being Mortal is a unique—but unsurprising—book in Gawande's catalog. It is unique in that the majority of his writings prior to *Being Mortal* tend to focus on improving medical performance or on interesting medical oddities such as why people itch or blush, while the majority of his writings since *Being Mortal* focus on innovative health policies and reform to ensure wide and fair access to needed healthcare goods and services. It is not surprising, though, given what we know of what inspires Gawande to write, that he set out to closely examine human mortality and the process of dying. Death and dying is one of the greatest mysteries about biologic life, and clearly there has been a notable culture shift in how that process occurs in the United States, with the majority of persons now commonly receiving high-level, invasive medical care within the last 90 days of life.[16] Moreover, many will remember that during the Obama administration, death and dying in America became a divisive political issue when a provision was included in the Affordable Care Act to reimburse physicians for talking with their patients about end-of-life treatment preferences.

Given this take on *Being Mortal*, one could argue that it is a transition piece of sorts for Gawande. It is an exploration of death and dying and medicine's evolving role in helping persons facilitate that process that not only allows Gawande an opportunity to examine best practices that medicine can and should adopt for managing this new responsibility but to also explore the politics and policies of dying in the United States. This, however, is not how I read *Being Mortal*. At its core, *Being Mortal* reads more as an homage and eulogy to Gawande's father.

Hard conversations and letting go

On March 22, 2011, Gawande gave a talk at Cleveland Clinic based on his work detailed in his third book *A Checklist Manifesto*. I was in Cleveland at the time completing a bioethics fellowship and so was able to attend. After introducing Gawande, then Cleveland Clinic CEO, Dr. Toby Cosgrove, sat next to a pair of older people in the front row who were not wearing the standard physician coats all Cleveland Clinic practitioners were expected to don. Toward the end of his talk, Gawande introduced the pair as his parents and thanked them for attending. I recall him saying that it was the first time that they had seen him give a professional talk. It was not until I read *Being Mortal* that I realized during this special talk that his father was entering the terminal phase of his long battle with spinal cancer. Approximately six months after this event, Gawande's father passed away. It was shortly after this that Gawande began to formally write *Being Mortal*.

One reason I find this event notable is from what Gawande writes in *Being Mortal* about letting go and having hard conversations with those who we love. Gawande details the painstaking and sometimes uncomfortable conversations he felt compelled to have with his father and mother about his father's end-of-life preferences; namely, what his father's treatment limits were, what his worries were, and what trade-offs he was and was not willing to accept regarding attempts to prolong his life. As Gawande writes, these are not natural conversations people have—whether with their physicians or loved ones—and, in referencing palliative care specialist, Dr. Susan Block notes that having these types of conversations is really a procedure that requires developing skills akin to surgery.[17] One of the most common mistakes that occurs during these types of conversations—especially treatment discussions between physicians and patients—is that they typically begin with a brief survey of the treatment options and *then* turn the focus to asking people what treatment goals they have that can be molded to fit the available options. The problem with having treatment conversations this way is that it assumes peoples' treatment goals are what should change to fit the treatment options and not the other way around. Instead, as Block recommends—and as I've come to experience in my own work—these types of conversations should start with asking people what treatment goals they have, then molding the treatment options to fit the goals.

Another reason this event is notable is because of my current position. As previously stated, much of Gawande's writing and research focuses on how certain practices are or can be standardized to improve areas of noted deficiency in medical practice. It seems natural, therefore, that Gawande's research for *Being Mortal* would eventually bring him to La Crosse, WI, where I took a position post fellowship and where, for the past 30 years, we have been pioneering efforts to standardize advance care planning and help patients and physicians adapt to the new norms in how people die.

The development and rise of advance care planning in La Crosse stem from ethics consultation. Not long after being hired to lead Gundersen's ethics education and consultation service in the mid-1980s, my predecessor, Dr. Bernard "Bud" Hammes, received three consults in our dialysis unit involving patients who lacked treatment decision-making capacity. These patients all had other chronic medical problems that were beginning to rapidly advance, resulting in diminishing benefits from continuing dialysis. Yet, despite the overall health decline of these patients, stopping dialysis predictably would cause these patients to die within days. None of the loved ones for each of these three patients knew what the patients' preferences were; they had never talked—either with the patients or the patients' physicians—about if or when to stop dialysis. These cases were distressing to the families because they did not want to make a "bad" choice for their loved ones; they were distressing to the staff because they did not want to continue with the treatment they believed might be harming the patients rather than benefiting them; and it was distressing to Bud because he could easily see the ethical and moral tensions in each case but could not easily resolve them and he understood that had the patients had better conversations with their loved ones and providers before becoming uncommunicative, they possibly could have prevented the distress the patients' loved ones and providers were now experiencing.

Bud therefore worked to develop a standardized method to talk with persons about their treatment preferences before chronic or acute illness would strike and leave persons unable to clearly communicate. Over the next several years, he engaged in a collaborative effort with the leadership of La Crosse's local hospitals, clinics, and nursing facilities to create a process for asking people during clinic checkups whether a person had completed an advance care plan and, if not, whether they would be willing to schedule an appointment with a trained facilitator. These facilitations—which take about 60-90 minutes—are in-depth conversations aimed at answering three basic questions: (1) who would the person trust to make decisions for them if they lost decisional capacity, (2) what goals are important to the person in making treatment decisions, (3) what would the person want in the event they suffered an irreversible condition that prevented them from being able to meaningfully interact with the environment around them?

As Gawande details in *Being Mortal*, these are hard conversations for many people. As this new process for talking about and attempting to understanding and document persons treatment preferences began to flourish throughout the La Crosse community, it was clear that for many persons, this was the first time they were being asked to think about medical care in a way that forced them to confront their own mortality. It was also clear that for many, they had never thought about their life goals and how illness and medical treatment could impact their lives in ways that may thwart—or potentially help them meet—those goals. When Gawande writes about the failure of treatment conversations in which medical providers lay out treatment options and ask patients to tell them what option they want, the fact that many persons have never truly considered their treatment goals is the primary reason that this conversational style fails. Persons who have never been asked to think about and reflect on their life and treatment goals and have not had the opportunity to talk about goals and values with their loved ones or medical providers are not in a position to answer questions about their treatment preferences at the moment when chronic or acute illness takes hold.

Two initial studies show the impact of this work toward standardizing advance care planning conversations. The first study—known as the La Crosse Advance Directive Study (LADS I)—was conducted in 1996, five years after the implementation of this new process. It showed that of 540 decedents in La Crosse county over 11 months, 85% had an advance directive or healthcare power of attorney and that of those with an advance directive or health-care power of attorney, 95% had copies of their documents in the medical records at the time of death.[18] Twelve years later, in 2008, the study was repeated and showed an increase in the numbers of people who died in La Crosse county over a seven-month period with an advance directive and power of attorney for healthcare on file. Of the 400 decedents included in the second study, 90% had an advance directive or healthcare power of attorney at the time of death, with 99.5% of these documents found in the medical records.[19] If you were to ask those of us working in La Crosse's hospitals and clinics what the true value of this advance care planning system has had on the local community, it is not only that people are talking about and documenting their preferences and that the preferences are available to care providers at the places where they receive care but also that when surrogate decision-makers are utilized, they have a much clearer sense of what choices the patient would make and that medical providers strive to honor patients' preferences.

For Bud and myself, the takeaway from the advance care planning work in La Crosse has less to do with the logistics and legalities of getting people to complete advance directives and naming surrogate decisions and more to do with the relationships people have with their loved ones and care providers. There has been a clear culture shift here—a shift that we admittedly have not been able to accurately study and quantify—that is obvious during many patient care encounters.

Gawande touches on this in *Being Mortal* when he talks about visiting La Crosse and speaking to one of our critical care specialists, Dr. Greg Thompson. Gawande observed that none of the patients populating the ICU were entering the final stages of a terminal disease or imminently dying from some chronic medical condition. I have been rounding in our ICU every week since I started at Gundersen, and I can confirm this is still the case. Moreover, for many of the patients who we treat in the ICU who have experienced an acute trauma, such as devasting stroke or cardiac failure, who may not have completed an advanced care plan, in talking with their loved ones, it is still evident that conversations occurred between the patients and their loved ones about treatment goals and upper-treatment limits. Having hard conversations remains our community norm because there is a recognition that the value of advance care planning is not about end-of-life care or treatment preferences *per se*. It is about how people care for one another. As noted by Bud in a 2014 interview with CBS about the La Crosse advance care planning program:

> I think the ultimate topic that's being discussed is how people care for each other. And so what comes out at the end of the conversation is, 'I love you, and now I know how to take good care of you.'[20]

Toward "Better"

As a bioethicist and philosopher, I would be remiss in writing a chapter on Gawande—or any doctor-writer—filled with introspection and praise but not addressing criticisms or problems with his writing. There are two criticisms I address here: the existential and the issue of simplicity. Neither criticism is necessarily about the form or content of the writing; it is about something more foundational that, like the bell curve, is unlikely to be overcome, but in which there is must be a continued striving toward improvement.

The existential criticism

All doctor-writers, when they move from scientific to narrative writing, from the epistemological to the personal and anecdotal, from an objective to subjective voice, place their readers at risk. What is at risk is trust toward both the general public and their colleagues and profession. Narrative writings are valuable exercises—like journaling—that help physicians reflect on their practices and develop a better understanding of their changing identities from not being a medical student to becoming a medical student to becoming a practicing physician. They can help uncover biases and they can help identify and solidify virtues to be emulated. When these writings are made public, and doctor-writers shift from writing for themselves to a broader audience, they provide glimpses behind the curtain, into the inner working of medical practice, and perhaps most fascinating, into their psyches—how *they* as individuals see the world of medical care. Obviously, when doctor-writers make this shift, there is no shortage of interest from the general public; recall my *hope* in reading Gawande was to identify a bridge into the world of the medical mind. But what is most fascinating about these writers is the very thing that puts us all—readers and the writers alike—at risk.

Storytellers, as the creators and sculptors of the stories they tell, have great power over their audiences. They are the mapmakers and the guides who take the audience across the landscape of the story. Doctor-writers have even greater power by virtue of their social positions outside of being a storyteller. Physicians hold special places in every society as those entrusted to care for people at their weakest, most vulnerable moments. As such, society at large expects physicians to behave according to varieties of ethical codes, values, and virtues of the societies in which they practice. Yet most doctor-writers—Gawande included—detail personal failings or problems in medical practices. When they do this, they not only risk sensationalizing those practices, problems, and errors as the norm as opposed to the exception (or as a surgeon friend of mine says, confusing the numerator for the denominator), but they also risk exploiting audiences (as actual or future patients whom these stories are about) and, perhaps the most damning problem, potentially undermining public trust in medical practices and institutions (including the trust of their colleagues who might question their intentions in writing [is it for the sake of patient care or personal profit from book sales?] or the competency of the doctor-writer as a practicing physician).[21]

Among doctor-writers, Gawande is unique regarding the "existential" criticism. Any one of his writings engages in several types of narrative style and structure, and because of this, his writings have different meanings to different readers depending on the individual reader's focus. In many ways this is what we hope for and expect of successful doctor-writers: appeal to broad audiences. But because of how Gawande writes, he never fully engages in any one style, making it seem as though his writings are at best, incomplete, and at worst, irresponsible.

Many doctor-writers engage in a form of reflective and confessional writing, lamenting their personal failings in patient care. Some use a journalistic and descriptive approach—or what I call the 15,000-foot view of writing—to report, rather than reflect on, a practice failing. Others will engage in manifesto-esq writing—the 30,000-foot view—to identify, via personal narrative, structural problems in medical practices at large. Gawande's use of all these styles in a single narrative can be analytically troubling. Whereas confessional writing typically ends with a reflection or moral that speaks to the individual's growth and identity as a physician, Gawande often makes an impersonal reflection—see, for example, the epilogue of *Being Mortal*, where he talks about his worries of developing an infection from drinking from the Ganges River—or he will make an appeal to policy-making.[22] When Gawande provides analysis or impersonal reflection, it can detract from the richness of the overall narrative, perhaps causing audiences to question whether he has crafted a narrative story or argument. For those who see Gawande as attempting to formulate an argument by use of the impersonal reflections and inclusion of data toward grounding a normative claim about policy changes, they note that either narrative writing is not the most effective means to makes these points or that engaging in narrative writing that makes normative claims based on a limited selection of remarkable stories is essentially irresponsible storytelling and an invalid use of the narrative ethics writing style.[23]

One reason I call this the "existential" criticism is that no matter how hard Gawande—or any doctor-writer—works to avoid placing him or his audience at risk of undermining trust, it is Gawande's willingness to risk trust that makes the writing so valuable. He exposes his failings, the failings of colleagues, the failings of the general public to understand or appreciate the complexity of medical care, and the failings of the medical profession in a way that seemingly jeopardizes the sanctity of medical practice and the position and license bestowed on medical providers to treat the ill—i.e., he risks violating the social contract that exists between medicine and society.[24] Yet, to change the style of writing would deplete it of the very thing that makes it valuable to audiences—that of a physician telling real-life stories about the trials and tribulations of being a physician and how it might be possible to make medical practice better in a way that benefits all.

The simplicity criticism

What sparks Gawande's curiosity to write on a particular topic is tantamount to either a problem in current medical practice or a lack of justification for variances in medical care with demonstrable negative impact. After identifying and closely examining the problems, he provides exemplars that demonstrate the possibilities for correction. Gawande is a big-picture thinker whose writings are like home remodeling projects; there is dissatisfaction with the current layout, clearing of the room and demolition of the walls, and finally a rebuilding. Where Gawande's writings are sometimes lacking is in the description of the rebuild and unclear use or explanation of the materials used in the project.

For example, Gawande touts La Crosse as a paradigm of advance care planning, making it seem as though we've got advance care planning totally figured out and that we know how to correct problems quickly as they occur. Neither of those is true. As laws change, providers change, institutional and other local priorities change, new problems arise while the integrity of the program develops cracks that requiring fixing. This aspect of advance care planning is not addressed in *Being Mortal* or any of Gawande's other writing on advance care planning and end-of-life care.

The concern is that some may read Gawande's works and consider his suggestions for correcting problems as equivalent to offering hope. While this is not Gawande's intention, it is understandable how one could read Gawande's writings on improving healthcare and say, "This is easy. Why aren't we doing this?" Gawande does not always make his rebuttal of this view obvious.

This is not to say that Gawande thinks answers to complex issues or systematic concerns are simple. It is to say that there is the potential to misrepresent solutions to these issues or concerns as broadly applicable without giving due consideration to the logistical and cultural obstacles that can hinder the implementation of big ideas. To this end, Gawande's writing would benefit, at the very least, from an acknowledgment that the issues, as he discusses and addresses them in his narrative writings, are both from a privileged position and are incomplete (this is perhaps true of all doctor-writers). For example, in *Being Mortal*, the idea of a "good death" is one that follows from autonomously chosen or identified goals, values, and preferences; absent—almost categorically—is how or whether the conception of a "good death" could apply to children, those suffering from substance addictions, mental illnesses, neurological diseases, such as dementia, or those who are socioeconomically oppressed or disenfranchised and lack access to social or medical supports.[25]

Conclusion

Gawande's writings are engaging. He deftly balances the shifting focus from a patient-based story to the broader medical issue he is wanting to address and back to the story. He takes complex issues such as death and dying, medical error, and insurance and health policy, and makes them more understandable in the stories he tells. He relates to his audience by providing just enough engagement with the personal "I" to entice readers but enough third-person discussion to keep readers focused on the questions he is asking. The questions he asks are difficult to answer and teeter between the need for empirical and philosophical assessment. Perhaps most importantly, he reminds us that medicine is not inherently a science but rather an artform that progresses via the scientific method. His writings are the embodied observation of renowned ethicist Edmund Pellegrino's quote, "Medicine is the most humane of sciences, the most empiric of arts, and the most scientific of humanities."[26]

Notes

1 Becker's Hospital Review, "40 of the Smartest People in Healthcare," *Becker's Hospital Review*, March 4, 2014: https://www.beckershospitalreview.com/lists/40-of-the-smarte st-people-in-healthcare.html, accessed August 20, 2021.
2 Atul Gawande, "Atul Gawande on the Secrets of a Puzzle-Filled Career: Interview with Eric J. Topel, MD," *Medscape*, December 6, 2013: https://www.medscape.com/viewarticle/815241.
3 Joseph Shapiro, "Why This Wisconsin City Is the Best Place to Die," *National Public Radio*, November 16, 2009: https://www.npr.org/templates/story/story.php?storyId=1 20346411.
4 Data USA, "Athens, OH," *Data USA*, 2014: https://datausa.io/profile/geo/athens-oh, accessed August 20, 2021.
5 Tony Kirby, "Atul Gawande: Making Surgery Safer Worldwide," *The Lancet* 376 (2010): 1045; Gawande, "Atul Gawande on the Secrets of a Puzzle-Filled Career."
6 Gawande, "Atul Gawande on the Secrets of a Puzzle-Filled Career."
7 Ibid.
8 Tony Kirby, "Atul Gawande: Making Surgery Safer Worldwide," *The Lancet* 376 (2010): 1045; Atul Gawande, "Gulf War Syndrome," *Slate*, October 26, 1996: https://slate.com/news-and-politics/1996/10/gulf-war-syndrome.html.
9 Atul Gawande, "No Mistake," *The New Yorker*, March 23, 1998: https://www.new yorker.com/magazine/1998/03/30/no-mistake.

10 Atul Gawande, *Complications: A Surgeon's Notes on an Imperfect Science* (New York: Picador, 2002).

11 Atul Gawande, *Better: A Surgeon's Notes on Performance* (New York: Henry Holt and Company, LLC., 2007).

12 Ibid., 246.

13 Atul Gawande, "Personal Best," *The New Yorker*, September 26, 2011: https://www.newyorker.com/magazine/2011/10/03/personal-best.

14 Atul Gawande, *Being Mortal: Medicine and What Matters in the End* (New York: Henry Holt and Company, LLC., 2014), 46–59.

15 Teno, Joan M., Pedro Gozalo, Amal N. Trivedi, Jennifer Bunker, Julie Lima, Jessica Ogarek, and Vincent Mor, "Site of Death, Place of Care, and Health Care Transitions among US Medicare Beneficiaries, 2000–2015," *JAMA* 320, no. 3 (2018): 264–271.

16 Ibid.

17 Gawande, *Being Mortal*, 181.

18 Bernard J. Hammes and Brenda L. Rooney, "Death and End-of-Life Planning in One Midwestern Community," *Archives of Internal Medicine* 158 (1998): 383–390.

19 Bernard J. Hammes, Brenda L. Rooney, and Jacob D. Gundrum, "A Comprehensive, Retrospective, Observational Study of the Prevalence, Availability, and Specificity of Advance Care Plans in a County that Implemented an Advance Care Planning Microsystem," *Journal of the American Geriatrics Society* 58, no. 7 (2010): 1249–1255.

20 CBS News, "Being Prepared for the Final Days," *CBS News*, Aired April 27, 2014, on CBS Television: https://www.cbsnews.com/news/being-prepared-for-the-final-days/.

21 See, e.g., Terrence E. Holt, "Narrative Medicine and Negative Capability," *Literature and Medicine* 23, no. 2 (2004): 320–333; Delese Wear and Therese Jones, "Bless Me Reader For I Have Sinned: Physicians and Confessional Writing," *Perspectives in Biology and Medicine* 53, no. 2 (2010): 215–230; Ruth Cigman, "How Not to Think: Medical Ethics as Negative Education," *Medical Health Care and Philosophy* 16 (2013): 13–18; and Abraham M. Nussbaum, "When the Doctor Is a Gardner: Victoria Sweet, Hildegard of Bingen, and the Genres of Physician-Writers," *Literature and Medicine* 32, no. 2 (2014): 325–347, 494.

22 Gawande, *Being Mortal*, 259–263.

23 Wear and Jones, "Bless Me Reader for I Have Sinned," 215–230; Anne H. Jones, "Narrative Ethics, Narrative Structure," *The Hastings Center Report* 44, no. 1 (2014): S32–S35; and Abraham M. Nussbaum, "Trains Departing from Different Stations: Being Mortal and Dying in the 21st Century," *Perspectives in Biology and Medicine* 59, no. 3 (2016): 425–436.

24 Jonathan Oberlander, Larry R. Churchill, Sue E. Estroff, Gail E. Henderson, Nancy M. P. King, and Ronald P. Strauss, eds., *The Social Medicine Reader: Health Policy, Markets, and Medicine*, 2nd ed. (Durham, NC: Duke University Press, 2005).

25 Karen Kopelson, "Dying Virtues: Medical Doctors' Epidemic Rhetoric of How to Die," *Rhetoric of Health & Medicine* 2, no. 3 (2019): 259–290.

26 Edmund D. Pellegrino, *The Philosophy of Medicine Reborn: A Pellegrino Reader* (Notre Dame, IN: University of Notre Dame Press, 2008).

Part III
Medicine, meaning, and identity

6 Danielle Ofri

Offering lessons for all

Susan Stagno

Biographical information

It was never her intent to become a writer. Nor does she regard herself as a humanities or literary scholar. After ten years of intense educational and training experiences in science and medicine, the stories inside her simply came pouring out onto the pages. She needed to decompress, process, and make sense of the dizzying world of medicine in which she had been immersed, embedded, maybe even at times, imprisoned.

Danielle Ofri was born and raised in New York City, the daughter of parents who were both teachers. As a high school student who was smart and excelled in the sciences, there seemed to be only one logical option—becoming a doctor. Having had a dog as a child, she considered veterinary school but thankfully ended up in human medicine. She enjoyed writing as a young person, but she didn't get back to this form of self-expression until after the long, arduous (and sometimes wonderful) journey of medical school, graduate school, and residency training.

She left high school a year early, matriculated college at McGill University in Montréal, majoring in physiology, and was "full steam ahead" on her choice to go to medical school. The educational system at McGill in her field was "100% science"—no humanities. But she met a departing senior during her freshman year who told her that if she didn't take advantage of classes taught by Professor Wisse, she would be wasting her education at McGill. Interestingly, this professor taught Yiddish Literature. Ofri, who is Jewish, enrolled and loved it! This opened a door for her and she continued to take classes outside of her science studies, including Russian Literature and Russian History.

"The zeitgeist [at McGill] was that if you love science, you become a scientist. Medicine was for technicians! … So I couldn't decide what to do. Then someone told me about an MD/PhD program, and that was perfect."[1] So she began her seven-year journey of the combined medicine and science education at New York University, focusing on the neuroscience of opioid receptors. Influenced by this work, neurology seemed a good fit, so she started her training doing the required preliminary year at Bellevue Hospital. During that time, she "fell in love" with the patients, their stories, and the opportunity to provide care to underserved and

DOI: 10.4324/9781003079712-6

vulnerable patients at Bellevue, which is her "medical home." She decided to stay with internal medicine and put her heart and soul into becoming a primary care physician.

Something that had a powerful influence on Ofri was the death of her good friend, Josh, who died during her first year of residency training from a genetic heart condition. He was 27 years old, the same age that she was. This was a huge loss and also something of an existential crisis. Up until that point, she had been barreling through, from early departure from high school to college, and then an intense MD/PhD program. "This was the first time I sort of stopped," she remarked to me. She needed a break.

For 18 months, she traveled widely, and when she needed money, she worked as a locum tenens doctor (meaning she served short stints of filling in for medical practices, often in remote areas). This peripatetic and (sometimes) less stressful approach to medical practice allowed her the time to process the many experiences she had during her medical training. Having not written creatively since college, and with no formal training in writing, she began putting down on paper the tales of herself, patients, and the world of medicine she had encountered. She wasn't planning to publish these stories, but after writing and refining them, she did submit stories to literary journals. And they got noticed. Although she had prepared a collection of stories and sent them to various publishers, a publisher actually contacted her after seeing one of her pieces. And so *Singular Intimacies*[2] was born.

She is now an attending physician at Bellevue Hospital, the oldest public hospital in the United States. She holds a clinical faculty appointment at New York University School of Medicine, where she teaches in an outpatient environment. She is cofounder and Editor-in-Chief of the *Bellevue Literary Review*, the first literary journal to arise from a medical setting. She sees her professional life as equal measures of writing, editing, and medical practice—one informing the other. After the publication of her first book, her publisher suggested that the success of the book might afford her the opportunity to move out of patient care and be a full-time author. This idea was frankly abhorrent to her—she couldn't imagine her life without providing patient care, and her experiences with patients, of course, are the source of her inspiration.

She is a frequent contributor to various publications, including *The New York Times*, the *New England Journal of Medicine*, *Lancet*, and she has appeared on CNN and National Public Radio. Her lectures are renowned for her use of dramatic stories (and avoidance of PowerPoint). Ofri also served as Associate Chief Editor of *The Bellevue Guide to Outpatient Medicine*, which was awarded Best Medical Textbook of 2001 by the American Medical Writers Association.

Her awards and accolades are many: her essays have been selected for inclusion in *Best American Essays* (twice) and *Best American Science Writing*. She is the recipient of the John P. McGovern Award from the American Medical Writers Association for "preeminent contributions to medical communication," was awarded an honorary Doctorate of Humane Letters from Curry College, and the Editor's Prize for Nonfiction by *The Missouri Review*.

She grapples with the ethical concerns of writing about patients. Many of her stories are fictionalized, based on real experiences but with details changed; for those that are about the actual patients, she gets their permission and spends time with them outside of the medical encounter. She considers how the patient might react if they were to read the stories about them, avoiding topics that could be hurtful. She points out that most of her patients don't know that she has published books (and many, frankly, don't read English), and only one patient has sought her care because of having read her work.

Ofri lives in New York with her husband and three children. She enjoys mastering the cello in what little free time remains after doctoring, parenting, writing, and editing. With such a busy professional and personal life, finding balance is a challenge. She is good at setting limits: "I say no an awful lot," she told me. She prioritizes those things that have value to her: family, work, writing, and editing. She also told me, "I haven't watched TV since 1980, and I do all my shopping online. I don't care what my kids wear, don't care what I wear. I pare down my life to its most basic."[3] One thing she carves out time for is practicing her cello an hour a day. She regards her greatest accomplishment as "crafting a life that I am happy with" and allowing serendipity to have its influence.

A unique "doctor voice"

Unlike other doctor-writers, Ofri has evolved in her writing from telling compelling, dramatic medical stories to books that help both healthcare practitioners and the people they serve have a better relationship and a better medical experience. She helps all readers appreciate the humanity of doctors while also emphasizing the issues and barriers that people face as they enter the medical system, particularly the underserved, immigrants, and people of color.

She strives for authenticity both as a writer and as a physician. She says, "It is about being honest about being human. We need to be honest about our shortcomings too, or we have no credibility out there." She regards listening as the greatest skill that doctors have, "and if we just listen hard, we will get there."[4]

She also provides readers with a "female voice" in medicine, which is one of her goals. While women in medicine are growing in numbers and many medical schools' rosters are about 50% female, this was less common in the time that Ofri was a student, and so there are far fewer women doctor-writers. Because women tend to bear more of the responsibility in child-rearing, and may also choose part-time work, especially when their children are young, coupled with working in what is still a male-dominated culture, this voice is important to hear. Ofri's writing weaves her womanhood and motherhood into the texts beautifully, particularly her stories about her sabbatical year in Costa Rica where she could fully focus on parenting.

What we all can learn

Ofri's *Singular Intimacies* traces her experiences in training, beginning with medical school and progressing into residency. The prologue and epilogue of this volume are told from her vantage point as an attending physician, flanking the stories of "becoming" that lie between.

Ofri was trained in the early days of the AIDS epidemic, and this had a profound influence on her. An early piece in this volume, entitled "Stuck,"[5] is a gut-wrenching story in which she gets stuck with a suture needle during an operation. She fears the worst. Did she get stuck with a needle contaminated by HIV? Hepatitis? Some other dread disease that would change the course of her life? But there is much more to this story. The actual event of the needle stick is preceded by a rich description of the experience of being a medical trainee: the unpleasant quarters known as the "call room" for students and residents who are on duty overnight. She writes: "Every fourth night I slept on a mattress on the floor of that freezing, grimy, windowless room. I didn't dare contemplate how old those mattresses were or what creatures live inside."[6] She also reflects on the overwhelming work load; the sense of uselessness a student has and the humiliation they often experience, when, for example, the attending physician says, "You the medical student? ... Keep your hands where I can see them. I don't want anything contaminated."[7] This and more lead up to the needle stick. When it happens, Ofri tries to determine if others noticed and whether someone would help. But no one did. She thinks, "Was I allowed to speak? Did third-year medical students have that right?"[8] This was followed by the sense of panic and vulnerability of not knowing what to do, and this is the tragedy. What one is *supposed* to do in this situation is quite clear: you report the stick and get tested. But the culture of medicine is such that you don't ask for help and you don't admit to a "mistake." Still, she has to know whether she is at risk, so she reads the patient's chart that reveals that this patient had been a nurse at an inner-city hospital for 34 years. This strikes fear in Ofri's heart, assuming that not only had this patient been exposed to a wide variety of dread diseases, but that "[s]he'd probably gotten a million needle sticks."[9] So instead of asking someone or reporting to infection control, she decides to ask the patient directly. But in the asking, she becomes quite emotional, and the patient, who tells Ofri that she is, thankfully, free of any infectious diseases, embraces and comforts her. So much about this story speaks to what is so wrong with the culture of medicine. To not report the stick, to burden a patient with her own worries are serious problems. Because this book is a series of medical vignettes, readers do not get the benefit (unlike in her later books) to process and better understand what went awry here.

Another notable story in this volume is "Merced."[10] In this story, named in part for the patient (Mercedes) and, also in part, one assumes, from the root of the Spanish meaning "mercy," Ofri is near the end of her residency. With only weeks to go, she feels confident in her diagnostic skills, proud of her ability to apply her intellect to patients' symptoms. A woman is admitted to the hospital when Ofri is on duty with a headache and a vague history suggesting "bizarre behavior"— "classic aseptic meningitis," she thinks, wondering why the emergency doctors had chosen to admit and, in her opinion, overtreat her. Ofri does a careful history and physical exam and orders the "million-dollar workup" looking for "zebras" (medical jargon for the rare diagnoses). A bout of witnessed odd behavior leads her neurology colleagues to believe Mercedes has herpes encephalitis and she is transferred to their service. However, when the litany of lab results come back, the test for Lyme disease was positive. She had been the one to think of it and, once again, felt quite proud of herself. Treatment was started and Mercedes was discharged, only to return several days later. Turns out the Lyme result was a false positive. It was unclear what she had, but whatever it was, caused her death. Standing at the bedside with Mercedes's family surrounding this beautiful young woman who looked quite lifelike but was brain dead, Ofri's world came crashing down. It brought back all the deaths that had remained unprocessed, not the least of which was her dear friend who died young, unexpectedly. She began to weep and was comforted first by the chaplain who was present to help the patient's family and then by the patient's sister who later thanked her for her care of Mercedes. She finally came to terms with the limitations of medicine: despite the high technology and sophisticated testing, not everything has an answer. And she found that sharing her grief at the loss of Mercedes was

> perhaps my most authentic experience as a doctor. Something was sad. And I cried. ... Standing in the ICU, the chaplain's arms around me, surrounded by Mercedes's family, I felt like a person. Not like a physician or a scientist or an emissary from the world of rational logic, but just a person.[11]

The story of Mercedes highlights the kinds of experiences that are common in medicine but often are unprocessed. The culture of medicine expects that this is all in a day's work, that we should shore ourselves up and move on. That Ofri chose to be at the bedside, to comfort and to be allowed to be comforted, to accept the appreciation of the patient's family for her care even though the outcome was not good—these are the elements of connection that are so vitally important but so woefully lacking in medical encounters. This story stands as an important lesson that doctors are human, too. They have feelings. And they care about the patients in a profound and unique way. To pretend that they do not harms everyone.

Ofri's *Incidental Findings: Lessons from My Patients in the Art of Medicine*[12] chronicles her professional life following residency. She relates stories that shaped her thinking about medicine and patient care, keeping true to the subtitle. These experiences became profound events that caused her to reflect on herself, her values as a physician, and the way medicine is practiced outside a large teaching hospital. She also writes about her own experience being a patient while she is pregnant, allowing her insights into the patient-physician relationship that inform her own way of practicing.

In "Living Will"[13] she confronts the notion of "rational suicide." This story, which takes place during one of her locum tenens jobs in rural Florida, involves a man with a long list of diagnoses coupled with an equally long list of medications that are intended to keep his symptoms at bay. However, his life has been reduced to being a "shut in" who can no longer even walk to his mailbox. His wife has essentially abandoned him for her own activities, and many of the important people in his life have died, as has his dog. The patient, Mr. Reston, chooses to stop taking his medications which results in his lungs filling with fluid. He comes to the emergency room and, despite having a Living Will in which he directs that he does not want any life-sustaining procedures, agrees to be intubated. Once he is stabilized and the breathing tube removed, Ofri is able to have a conversation with him during which he describes his limited life, his losses, and his despair, including nearly life-long depression. Having made what is deemed a suicide attempt, she feels the obligation to send him for psychiatric care against his wishes but grapples with forcing him to get a treatment that has already been tried without success and with the patient facing a dismal future. She questions whether this is ethical. She then has an "ah-ha" moment when she realizes that, when given the option of "life-sustaining treatment" in the emergency room, he chose to be intubated. She seizes on this ambivalence and decides that, underneath it all, he probably still does want to live. It appears that this patient was not provided with any other options, nor was there a conversation about how his discomfort could be eased if he did wish to stop taking his medications. Although her "ah-ha" moment allows her to feel that she is off the hook for forcing more treatment (and, presumably, more misery), this story raises many issues about patient autonomy, end-of-life choices, and limits of a doctor's obligations. The patient's decision to discontinue his medication could have been understood in a variety of ways—possibly a suicide attempt, but it could have been a "call for help" or a true expression of a desire to discontinue treatment and die (a choice that, with proper discussion and options presented, is an ethically justifiable one). When one is drowning in one's own fluid is not the time for in-depth discussions about medical choices, and most people opt to do whatever it takes to breathe again. This story also speaks to appreciating the patient's context, their narrative, and their values.

In "Common Ground,"[14] Ofri is serving in a locum tenens job in a small-town Catholic hospital with restrictions on birth control and abortion. She is faced with a patient who finds herself unexpectedly pregnant after a sexual encounter with an old friend and who, after carefully considering her options, wishes to terminate the pregnancy. Ofri struggles with this situation on many levels, including the obvious restriction that is being placed on her by the confines of practicing in a religious institution with values different from her own but, more poignantly, the reminder of her own choice to have an abortion when she was 17 years old. She maintains close phone contact with this patient both leading up to and immediately following the abortion, and desperately wants to tell the patient about her own experience, but recognizes the professional boundary that needs to be maintained and refrains from sharing that information. She closes this story with the reflection that "we are all made of the same stuff."[15] This story highlights the need for all medical practitioners to be reflective, and to work on resolving their own issues so that they do not interfere with patients' care and well-being.

Medicine in Translation: Journeys with My Patients[16] takes up issues related to immigration and healthcare—two topics that were a prominent part of public discourse in 2010, the year this book was published and the year that the

Affordable Care Act (ACA) was passed. While the ACA provided the opportunity for immigrants to obtain health insurance, it was available only to those who were in the country legally. It is interesting to note that while Ofri's earlier books were reviewed in high-profile medical journals, this one received more attention in the business world and the lay press. A review[17] in *Inside Business* suggests that before readers make up their minds about the debate regarding using taxpayer's money to insure the uninsured, they should read this book. Once again, the subtitle of this book shouldn't be overlooked. She *is* journeying with her patients both literally (by going to Costa Rica for sabbatical) and figuratively as she accompanies her patients on their paths of illness—sometimes recovering and flourishing, sometimes dying, but always by their side.

Herself the child of an immigrant (her father having come from Israel to America), she has a more acute awareness of the issues of those who have come to America seeking a better life for themselves and their children. Spending every clinical day caring for patients whose primary language is not English, and many who are unable to communicate in English at all, she finds herself surprised when having a conversation with her father who has a rather undisputable Israeli accent that she hadn't really noticed before. Her sensitivity to languages and the nuances that they hold in relating in the clinical encounter are palpable throughout this book.

The first patient that we meet is Samuel, a young man from Africa with a harrowing tale of having been assaulted because of his evangelical Christian faith, his assailants cutting off an ear, beating him severely, and then pouring sulfuric acid down his throat, leaving him for dead. Samuel is in the Survivors of Torture program at Bellevue, and when he first meets Ofri, having waited a very long time for the appointment, his chief complaint is that he needs career training and an ophthalmologist to repair the holes in his retina sustained as a result of his attack. Samuel eventually is one of the patients who overcomes, with Ofri's help and guidance along with her willingness to hear his story and support his goals.

Because of Ofri's conviction that the communication between the doctor and the patient is the key to care, and that careful listening is the doctor's best tool, having so many patients with whom she is unable to freely communicate due to the language barrier is a frequent theme in this book. Most interpretation is done over the telephone, which Ofri finds disconcerting. She muses over language, and although she speaks some Spanish, she is not fluent. This spurs her to take a sabbatical, living in Costa Rica with her husband and two children, immersing herself in the language and culture. She learns just before her departure that she is pregnant and will deliver her child in Costa Rica, thereby becoming a patient in a foreign land as well. She found an obstetrician who speaks English, Hebrew, and Spanish, and she felt very well cared for throughout her pregnancy in a significantly more child- and family-friendly culture than New York. She witnessed her children's quick acquisition of the language, somewhat envious as she continues her private Spanish lessons and still carries on many of her conversations in English. She was also surprised at how much she enjoyed attending to family, cello lessons, and her writing, and how little she missed practicing medicine. But she knew that was only temporary.

The story that threads its way through this volume is that of Julia Barquero, an undocumented immigrant from Guatemala who, despite her young age and otherwise good health, has a failing heart and needs a heart transplant but is not eligible for it due to her immigration status. Ofri identifies with Julia in many ways; they are the same age, and they have children who are of similar ages, "[b]ut chance had thrown us on opposite sides of the border and with the opposite genetics and there was nothing I could do about it."[18] Ofri is deeply troubled by the injustice of Julia's situation and, at the same time, unable to tell her that she will die because a procedure that could cure her condition is not available to her. We hear more about Julia in a future book.

Intensive Care: A Doctor's Journey[19] contains stories that are published in other volumes, and so it won't be discussed here.

What Doctors Feel: How Emotions Affect the Practice of Medicine[20] takes a decided turn from her other books. Her prior work tells doctor and patient stories, while this book examines the emotional side of medicine: the shame, fear, anger, anxiety, empathy, and even love that doctors experience, which impacts patient care. This book helps the readers, whether they be health professionals or patients, to have a better understanding of the consequences that emotions have on doctors. She draws on the medical literature related to these issues as well as other doctors' stories.

She begins by taking up the issue of empathy, whether it can be taught, why medical students who seem to have an abundance of it when they start medical school appear to lose it during their training, and what might help doctors to "walk a mile in their patients' shoes." She uses examples from her own experience, but also cites studies and commentaries that discuss factors contributing to the erosion of empathy in medicine.

She describes, sometimes in graphic detail, the realities of what doctors encounter with some patients who may have illnesses or symptoms that are extremely unpleasant, such as an elderly, cachectic man with advanced dementia who had bed sores that were so severe that amputation was necessary. Ofri states: "We were so deeply unsettled by Mr. Easton's body, by seeing someone whose physical condition appeared incompatible with life, that we reacted by shutting him out of our moral vision."[21] Seeing this patient as human was nearly impossible—until his family arrived. Suddenly he was a person with a life, a story, and connections, allowing Ofri and her colleagues to see him as the person who has the disease rather than the disease the person has (borrowing on a phrase from Sir William Osler).

Fear is a ubiquitous emotion for healthcare professionals: the fear that a patient will die on their watch, that they will not know what to do in an emergency, that a mistake will be made. Ofri examines this in the chapter "Scared Witless."[22] Equally encountered is sadness and grief. Death and untoward outcomes are part and parcel of providing care for sick persons, and it is not surprising, then, that doctors encounter their own sense of loss and sorrow as they get to know and care for their patients. In one gripping story, a pediatrics resident, Eva, is asked to be present at the delivery of a baby with Potter syndrome, a diagnosis incompatible with life. Her role was to remove the baby from the room, ensure that the parents did not see the infant (by their request), and allow it to die. Once the baby was delivered and handed off to Eva, she was at a loss as to what to do. She searched, in vain, for a room she could use to hold the baby until it died, but every room was occupied. She ended up in a cramped supply closet watching this dysmorphic infant breathe its last. But even after the baby's breathing stopped, its umbilical cord was still pulsating, indicating that the baby's heart was still beating. Eva felt stupid for not knowing when the baby was dead, guilt for not resuscitating the dying child followed by "a wave of immense sadness" for a baby who had never been held by her parents or anyone else but Eva. She rocked her, saying "I love you," while awaiting the umbilical cord to cease its pulsations. With no time or opportunity to process this horrible event, she pushed through the night, the next day, and the remainder of her residency, having "stuffed the whole thing way down in [her] consciousness."[23]

This was not the only traumatic experience that Eva had. They piled up over time, and she decided to leave pediatrics to pursue child psychiatry. With no chance to rebound, and her reserve of empathy empty, she chose to quit psychiatry training mid-way through. By this time, she had full-blown post-traumatic stress disorder. Ofri points out that the culture of medicine doesn't typically provide opportunities to process these painful experiences and emotions.

Unresolved grief not only can adversely affect doctors but can also have reverberations in the way they approach patient care. Ofri cites a study[24] that looked at the effect of grief on doctors providing care to patients with cancer. Findings showed that grief was pervasive and affected doctors' professional and personal lives. Some of the fallout from these unresolved feelings include overaggressive treatment of other patients after caring for a patient who died because the doctor felt like a failure; emotionally withdrawing from a patient after witnessing unnecessary suffering; and providing less aggressive (possibly inadequate) treatment when it may have been warranted.

Another important example of her examination of emotions is the anger, shame, and humiliation that arise when a doctor is being sued for malpractice. She says, "If there is a sucker-punch for a doctor, the word *lawyer* is it."[25] In the chapter "Under the Microscope,"[26] she returns to Mercedes, the young woman who died mysteriously in *Singular Intimacies*. Ofri is contacted by the hospital's lawyer to review the chart in an effort to "be prepared." Although a law suit was not filed, the experience shook her to the core.

Ofri's next brush with malpractice involved a woman whom she followed as a primary care doctor through her treatment for metastatic breast cancer. This was a patient with whom she had a great professional relationship. The patient had clearly indicated that she did not want any heroics at the end of life. However, once a patient dies, family members who may have had different opinions about how the care should have proceeded are left behind. In this case, she was required to give a deposition and experienced the difficult questioning by lawyers who demanded yes or no answers to questions that needed a more nuanced explanation. And, of course, they can frame those questions in a way that makes the doctor appear negligent. She observes that

> [b]eing judged stirs up a powerful and distinctive blend of emotions that can unsettle even the most stable, confident doctor ... having my medical care parsed and scrutinized by these lawyers—even the ones who were there to defend me—was an incomparably awful feeling.[27]

While the suit was dropped, she notes that "emotions cannot be dropped with similar briskness. I still retain the sting of those examinations."[28] That retention, especially for doctors who have been subject to the full process of a malpractice suit, regardless of the outcome, parlays itself into a change in the way a doctor is likely to practice, such as "defensive medicine" in which more tests get ordered in order to cover any potential diagnoses, no matter how unlikely. Exposure to more tests can easily lead to more adverse effects and overtreatment. Law suits may also lead to doctors leaving medicine, or doing work that takes them out of patient care.

Woven throughout this book is a re-visitation of the story of Julia Barquero, the Guatemalan immigrant from *Medicine in Translation*, who needed a heart transplant. With Ofri's advocacy, Julia miraculously does get the transplant only to have two strokes afterward, at a time when Ofri was away. Swelling in her brain caused devastating damage and the decision was made to withdraw life support. Ofri was crushed by this news. She made it back to Julia's bedside after the ventilator had been removed, but with Julia barely alive. The way Ofri felt she could best honor Julia was to read the section of her book, *Medicine in Translation*, in which Julia's story is told. She then listened, for one last time, to Julia's weakly beating heart.

This book reveals Ofri at her most vulnerable, and perhaps her best. It is in the vulnerability that doctors truly face humanity, their own limitations, and the fact that we can't possibly know everything. But it is exactly that humanity that allows meaningful connections that are healing.

What Patients Say, What Doctors Hear[29] examines the issue of doctor–patient communication. It is an extension of her previous book in that it incorporates how emotions might interfere with what the doctor is able to hear. Her opening story is a classic example—a patient who is persistent, a bit pushy, shows up when he doesn't have an appointment, and won't "listen" to her when she recommends that he see a doctor in the urgent care clinic on a day she is not in the office. Then he arrives in her doorway with no appointment, saying he must see her, and collapses on the floor with a rapid heartbeat and undetectable oxygen saturation. Apparently, he was trying to tell her something.

She reviews the literature on doctor–patient communication, including the study that demonstrates that, on average, a doctor interrupts a patient within 12 seconds of the start of the encounter. Ofri runs her own experiment during one of her clinic days and decides that she will "shut up" and let the patient tell her why they are there for as long as they need. One patient on her schedule, she is quite certain, will take up her entire day and wonders if she should rethink this plan. But she sticks to her commitment and finds that even the patient she feared would take an inordinate amount of time takes only 4 minutes and 7 seconds. Several take less than a minute, and on average just under 2 minutes. And in those two minutes the patient feels heard, the doctor has a better understanding of what is going on (medically, socially, psychologically) for the patient, and this allows medical care to proceed in the context of the person's life.

She briefly examines the issue of self-disclosure in a discussion about efforts to provide more humanistic care. She provides a lovely example of why having appropriate boundaries is important, and she provides research that supports this, demonstrating that primary care encounters in which the doctor talks about themselves are associated with lower patient satisfaction. Patients aren't interested in hearing about the doctors' experiences, nor are they interested in having someone tell them, "I know just how you feel." Healthcare professionals need to deal with their own "stuff" and mostly keep it to themselves.

Prejudice, implicit bias, and the judgments that doctors have about patients is the subject of the chapter "Rushing to Judgment." She describes an obese patient in her practice:

> I had to be honest—I was uncomfortable with my new patient … [she] was petite in stature but massive enough in width to meet the medical criteria for morbid obesity. Her pendulous belly hung like a third appendage between her legs and impeded her gait. A lovely-featured face was entirely swallowed up in layers of neck and jowl. Her arms could not hang straight down at her sides because of her girth.[30]

The thing that Ofri wants to convey is to be authentic. She can admit, examine, and reflect on her own uncomfortable feelings—and then do something useful with it. Saying these things out loud or writing them on paper can allow other doctors or healthcare professionals to realize that we all have our biases, weaknesses, vulnerabilities, but having awareness of them and being reflective allows us to modify our responses and behaviors.

What Ofri finds is that the more a doctor is able to hear the individual patient's narrative—in this patient's case, the stresses of raising children while trying to tend to her medical problems, her challenges in controlling her eating, and her depression which contributed to her craving of sweets—the less likely these biases interfere with appropriate care. She also cites studies demonstrating how communication and patient education can positively impact issues of adherence with recommended medical care as well as pain management, two major issues in medicine.

In addition to her books, she has contributed significantly to the medical literature through thought pieces that have been published in high-profile medical journals as well as in the lay press. One particularly interesting article entitled "The Covenant"[31] was an invited commentary on the robust discourse occurring about the problem of burnout in healthcare professionals. Ofri suggests that the medical system is taking advantage of physicians because of the covenant of professionalism that defines them, but the business-focused medical system takes advantage of the goodwill and intent that physicians bring to the table. She admits that not every doctor is a saint but that "the vast majority of doctors put in a good faith effort to place their patients' needs front and center. The commitment to do the right thing for our patients remains the guiding—and treasured—principle for most doctors."[32] She refers to the healthcare system as "an assembly line-style factory" and concludes that "doctors and nurses are not burned out by patient care but rather by their inability to give patient care the way they know it should be done."[33]

Ofri writes eloquently about the progress and the pitfalls of the electronic medical record (EMR), which plagues doctors and is regarded as the biggest contributor to physician burnout. She acknowledges the benefits but points out the ways in which the EMR literally gets between the doctor and the patient. Due to expectations of documentation and time efficiency, doctors find themselves interfacing more with the computer than the patient during a clinical visit. In an essay from *The Lancet* she states:

> The connection between doctor and patient is the foundation of empathy. How can we even begin to sense our patients' world if we are hardly glancing in their direction, listening with only half an ear, or cutting them off every time they try to talk because we ourselves are drowning in the EMR?[34]

Although she doesn't have any easy answers, she has developed strategies that include devoting the first part of the patient's encounter to direct eye contact, listening, and inviting the patient's input into the medical record. She adds that this electronic intrusion makes doctors decide whether they are taking care of patients or the EMR.

Her most recent book, *When We Do Harm: A Doctor Confronts Medical Error*,[35] again uses compelling stories to make her points. Chapters toggle between the accounts of two patients and their families who were the subject of medical errors, leading to their deaths, and providing insight into how errors occur due to systems issues, overwhelming situations in which clinicians are expected to work, technologic problems (where she again finds a lot of fault with the EMR), cognitive errors, and bias. This would be a pretty frightening book for patients to read. The litany of the ways things can (and do) go wrong in a hospital is staggering, and you really have to push through to the end of the book where she describes things being done to try to address these problems in order to feel that there is much hope that you will actually survive a hospital stay.

The story of Jay, a previously healthy young man who develops leukemia, is gut-wrenching. It is told largely from the vantage point of his wife, who is a nurse and who tried repeatedly to draw the attention of the various members of the healthcare team to her husband's multiple signs heralding his steady decline. Having significant clinical knowledge herself, she points out the way in which multiple organ systems are shutting down. It seems that each person—whether a nurse or a doctor—minimizes, ignores, or writes off her concerns, whether from hubris, tunnel vision ("It's just a side effect of the chemo"), or because the staff felt threatened by her pointing out these failures. He continues to decline and goes into cardiopulmonary arrest. A code is called, which she painfully witnesses, but he dies. Not only do we hear about multiple errors, but we also witness what it is like for Jay's wife, Tara, and her family in the aftermath of this horrendous situation. Tara brings suit against the hospital, and Ofri chronicles the way in which the legal system inflicts its own trauma. Tara suffers from post-traumatic stress disorder and complicated grief as a result of witnessing her husband's suffering, decline, and his final moments, and presumably also from the legal system. She attempts to return to her work as an emergency room nurse, but cannot. This narrative points out that our American way of redress (malpractice suits) for medical errors is no walk in the park, and frankly is not accessible to many individuals. And it is, of course, adversarial, and that alone is traumatic for the plaintiff. While the case eventually settled and she received some compensation, money cannot, of course, compensate for the loss of life, pain, and suffering by the patient who died and the family who suffers in the wake of the disaster.

The second narrative is that of Glenn, who suffered significant burns while volunteering to help rebuild a dam in his community. Living in a small town in Nebraska, his local hospital—although trying to be quite sophisticated—did not have the resources or personnel to properly address the severity of Glenn's situation. He was eventually transferred to a burn unit but the damage had already been done with inadequate care, mismanagement of his fluids (a critical aspect of the care of a burn patient), and a system that apparently didn't want to lose business.

Ofri examines causes of errors quite extensively and concludes that people with medical complexity and individual variations simply cannot be reduced to a checklist in the way that airplanes can. While checklists are helpful, they don't always apply, and they can give a false sense of security to a complex situation. She emphasizes again that communication is often the key:

> When it comes to minimizing diagnostic error, the focus should be on the conversation. The conversation between the patient and the medical team is the single most critical diagnostic tool, so you want to make sure it does not get short shrift.[36,38]

She also includes a chapter entitled "What's a Patient to Do?" providing practical advice to ways in which patients can advocate for themselves, encourage the doctor to think broadly and critically, share their thinking process, and assertively get answers to important questions about their care. These strategies provide some solace, but the book is still pretty frightening.

What's missing?

Ofri is, without question, a truly gifted writer and storyteller with very important messages to bring not only to doctors but to patients as well. She has received accolades from a wide variety of sources and individuals, including Oliver Sacks. It is frankly difficult to be critical of her work—work that comes from the heart, tells thoughtful, caring, and compelling stories that hopefully can and will benefit both health professionals and the people they serve. Besides all of that, she is "gutsy" and tells it like it is—both from the side of vulnerabilities, problems, and weaknesses in the medical system (and sometimes with individual doctors), and also from the strengths. She speaks passionately and brilliantly to the altruism, resilience, care, and dedication that the vast majority of doctors have. She "calls a spade a spade" when it's needed, as she did recently in *The New York Times*. Commenting, as a frontline worker in the midst of the coronavirus pandemic, she states:

> We [referring to health care workers] watch the news with just as much anxiety as the general public. We're relieved that one of our trusted own is up there, though we wish Dr. Fauci had the authority to quarantine the less evidence-based politicians. The way in which this public health crisis is continuously being refracted through a political lens—playing down risks for the sake of ratings, worrying more about the stock market than about lives—leaves medical professionals steaming with anger. We want rational policy, not meaningless fluff. We don't have time for this. ... There's a point at which those without relevant knowledge simply need to stand down. From the perspective of the medical community today, we've long since passed it.[37]

While she doesn't invoke Trump's name, it seems pretty clear to whom she is referring.

If there is a criticism, it is perhaps that she doesn't go quite far enough. In an overall very positive review of her book *What Doctors Feel*, Robert Arnold says:

> Sadly, Ofri does not talk about two topics that also are important for building a more emotionally resilient physician. First, how physicians view their role as physicians (what are sometimes called identity issues) shape their emotional reactions to patient care. ... I would have liked a longer discussion about how our societal norms regarding the role of physicians impact our emotional reactions. In addition, I think she missed an opportunity to talk about how individuals can build emotional resiliency. ... Finally, this is a book that is more descriptive than normative. The degree to which emotion should influence our ethical decisions, and the role of emotions in making ethical decisions is not discussed.[38]

Arnold adds: "Pre-medical and medical students should read it so that they have a better idea of what they are getting into. It is the most honest and clear picture of doctoring that I have read."[39]

These are excellent points about what this book, if taken a step or two further, could have done. In addition, Ofri assiduously avoids using the terms most often used in psychiatry but are present in every doctor–patient interaction: transference and countertransference. In a personal communication,[40] she indicates that this was because she wants her work to appeal to a broader audience, and also, it occurs to me, because doctors tend to cringe when these terms are used. The problem is that not acknowledging the dynamics that occur in a medical encounter, no matter who the provider is or what the context, leaves one rife for problems that can profoundly influence both the care of the patient and the well-being of the doctor. Her book on error also seems a missed opportunity to talk about the effects of burnout and its impact on medical error, a problem that is well documented.

One could also criticize Ofri for writing about some of her patients without their consent. However, she is not insensitive to this issue, and even takes it up in an article written in *The Lancet:*

> [F]or whom do I write? Was my writing simply cathartic, an unloading of pent-up frustration, pain, occasional exhilaration? Or was this part of a nobler cause, something that would fall under the purview of healing, something with ultimate benefit for my patients?[41]

She concludes that as long as two conditions are met (being honest about the motivation for writing about patients and treating patient stories with the same respect we have for them as persons) that writing about them is not wrong. She says:

> We must probe the patient's story as gently as we palpate their abdomen, never going beyond the point of wincing, never causing pain for pain's sake. We must listen for the human underpinnings as delicately as we listen for diastolic murmur. We must examine the tender edges of despair as gingerly as we would explore the ragged edges of a wound. And then we must look the patient—and their story—directly in the eye at the end of the encounter and ask ourselves if we have made a connection that is healing. Then, and only then, can we put the pen to rest. Then, and only then, have we become part of the patient's story.[42]

Conclusion

Ofri brings a fresh and unique voice both to readers who provide care for patients and for those receiving care. She is willing to be vulnerable and to acknowledge her emotions, things that most doctors don't admit out loud. These all serve to uphold her desire to be authentic and to convey lessons that can help doctors and patients better understand one another and lead to better care while also providing a more satisfying and meaningful experience for both doctors and patients.

Acknowledgment

I would like to thank Dr. Ofri for her generous gift of a personal interview and the time she gave in talking with me.

Notes

1   Danielle Ofri, Personal communication, July 30, 2019.
2   Danielle Ofri, *Singular Intimacies: Becoming a Doctor at Bellevue* (Boston, MA: Beacon Press, 2003).
3   Ofri, Personal communication, July 30, 2019.
4   Ibid.
5   Ofri, *Singular Intimacies*, 33–52.
6   Ibid., 36.
7   Ibid., 40.
8   Ibid., 44.
9   Ibid., 47.
10 Ibid., 222–236.
11 Ibid., 236.
12 Danielle Ofri, *Incidental Findings: Lessons from My Patients in the Art of Medicine* (Boston, MA: Beacon Press, 2005).
13 Ibid., 11–24.
14 Ibid., 25–37.
15 Ibid., 37.
16 Danielle Ofri, *Medicine in Translation: Journeys with My Patients* (Boston, MA: Beacon Press, 2010).
17 Terri Schlichenmeyer, review of *Medicine in Translation: Journeys with My Patients*, by Danielle Ofri, *Inside Business*, January 22, 2010.
18 Ofri, *Medicine in Translation*, 243–244.
19 Danielle Ofri, *Intensive Care: A Doctor's Journey* (Boston, MA: Beacon Press, 2013) Kindle.
20 Danielle Ofri, *What Doctors Feel: How Emotions Affect the Practice of Medicine* (Boston, MA: Beacon Press, 2013).
21 Ibid., 58.
22 Ibid., 64–94.
23 Ibid., 102.
24 Leeat Granek, Richard Tozer, Paola Mazzotta, et al., "Nature and Impact of Grief over Patient Loss on Oncologists' Personal and Professional Lives," *Archives of Internal Medicine* 172, no. 12 (2012): 946–966.
25 Ofri, *What Doctors Feel*, 174.
26 Ibid., 173–201.
27 Ibid., 185.
28 Ibid., 186.
29 Danielle Ofri, *What Patients Say: What Doctors Hear* (Boston, MA: Beacon Press, 2017).
30 Ibid., 179.
31 Danielle Ofri, "The Covenant," *Academic Medicine* 94, no. 11 (November 2019): 1646–1648.
32 Ibid., 1646.
33 Ibid., 1647.
34 Danielle Ofri, "Empathy in the Age of the Electronic Medical Record," *Lancet* 394, no. 10201 (September 7, 2019): 823.
35 Danielle Ofri, *When We Do Harm: A Doctor Confronts Medical Error* (Boston, MA: Beacon Press, 2020).
36 Ibid., 222.
37 Danielle Ofri, "Why Doctors and Nurses Are Anxious and Angry," OpEd in *The New York Times*, March 20, 2020.
38 Robert Arnold review of the book *What Doctors Feel: How Emotions Affect the Practice of Medicine*, by Danielle Ofri, *Kennedy Institute of Ethics Journal* 25, no. 1 (2015): E1–E4.

39 Ibid.
40 Ofri, Personal communication, July 30, 2019.
41 Danielle Ofri, "Dissecting Room," *The Lancet* 361, no. 9386 (May 3, 2003): 1572.
42 Ibid.

7 Paul Kalanithi

Sometimes, they break—craft as a window

Lise Saffran

Paul Kalanithi understood how human brains were put together. By the time he wrote his memoir *When Breath Becomes Air*, he had completed a postdoctoral fellowship in neuroscience and a residency in neurosurgery at Stanford University.

He also knew how stories were put together. Before choosing a career in medicine, Kalanithi had studied English literature and completed an MPhil in History and Philosophy of Science and Medicine at the University of Cambridge. He imagined that someday he would enter into the tradition of physician-writers, a community well represented in this volume. He had, he wrote, "mapped out this whole forty-year career for myself—the first twenty as a surgeon-scientist, the last twenty as a writer."[1]

Kalanithi's view of his future, based on his conception of himself as a clinician and a scholar, conformed to what psychologist Dan McAdams describes as "the internalized and evolving story of the self that a person constructs to make sense and meaning out of his or her life."[2] The disruption of this story, or narrative identity, is a central theme of memoirs that involve serious illness and in writing about the end of life.[3] The act of writing can be a powerful tool for integrating and exploring the disorder of illness. Discussing the autobiography of an author with a terminal illness, Deborah de Muijnck offers, "the occasion for telling ... can be expected to lie in the need to process what one is going through."[4] The act of reconstructing a narrative contains within it the possibility of forging a new identity, one that is transformed through rigorous reflection and self-examination. Identities borne out of serious illnesses, writes Arthur Frank, are those that, "no one wants but which are nonetheless affirmed as honorable in their consequences for self-discovery and service."[5]

Kalanithi was widely read, and he was deeply interested in literature and philosophy, and so it is perhaps unsurprising that the sudden pressure exerted on him to create a new, internalized narrative would inspire an externalized narrative, as well. The prologue to *When Breath Becomes Air* describes how Kalanithi detects cancer while reading his own slides in the hospital. Part I, called "In Perfect Health I Begin," dives into his early family life and training, his love of literature and his initial resistance to, and then the ultimate embrace of, medicine. Part II, "Cease Not Until Death," circles back to the moment of diagnosis and documents his declining health and the decision that he and his

DOI: 10.4324/9781003079712-7

wife undertake to have a baby. The epilogue was then written by his wife, Lucy, after his death.

Kalanithi's book touches on a number of themes that arise in memoir generally, including perspective and point of view, the subjectivity of truth, the unreliability of memory, and the inclusion and representation of secondary characters, including family members. Some of the themes common in end-of-life memoirs noted by Jeffrey Berman that arise here include the lack of time—both to process and potentially complete the story—and the drive to question previous fundamental assumptions about the world.[6] *When Breath Becomes Air* further belongs to a smaller subset of illness and end-of-life memoirs: those written by physicians. Physicians writing about illness must contend with the particular tension of being both doctor and patient.[7] For Kalanithi, as a neurosurgeon, this is particularly acute; he describes his clinical role as being concerned with protecting, "not merely life, but another's identity; it is perhaps not too much to say another's soul."[8] He is presumed to be doubly cognizant then of what is at risk when he himself becomes ill. If it is true, as Margaret Morgenroth Gullette observes, that "in the American milieu … dying has emerged as something to be learned,"[9] Kalanithi positions himself as both teacher and student. "Death may be a one-time event," he tells us, "but living with a terminal illness is a process."[10]

Kalanithi's process included, almost necessarily, reading and writing. "The most sacrosanct regions of the cortex," he writes, describing the areas of the brain that surgeons consider near inviolable "are those that control language. … What kind of life exists without language?"[11] Kalanithi respected the craft of writing, noting, "Great literary works provided their own set of tools, compelling the reader to use that vocabulary."[12]

In this chapter, I will attempt to use the vocabulary of a creative writer to examine the ways in which Kalanithi used those tools and I will attempt to highlight some ethical and narrative questions that his literary choices illuminate. The choices that Kalanithi made as a writer, I will argue, are not arbitrary or merely aesthetic; they are meaningful and consequential. For example, with a few exceptions (a story he recounts in which another doctor-turned-patient ties the quality of his care to the quality of the socks he wears to his appointments), Kalanithi does not focus, as Jonathon Tomlinson describes other doctor-writers doing, on how "medical education and clinical practice have prepared them so poorly."[13] He attaches lapses in empathy and humility to the individual failures of clinicians (see the discussion of the character Emma Hayward below) rather than to training or institutional pressures.

In *When Breath Becomes Air*, Kalanithi raises about his own life and prognosis questions that preoccupy the narrator of any story worth telling: where do I stand in relation to the chronology of this narrative? Where does it begin? How close am I to the end? What is crucial to include and what, though true, is unnecessary? Perhaps most important, what is the story about? What does it all mean? Behind these big questions and aims lie a series of smaller choices a writer makes, including how much of the story is looking backward and how much forward, the selection of scenes and dialogue, tone and language, and the artful use of metaphor. Even the tense in which a story is told has much more significance than a casual reader might suppose and Paul Kalanithi was neither a casual reader nor a casual writer. When he was diagnosed with lung cancer in his 36th year, he understood that not just his life but also the *story* of his life was changing. Stories mattered to Kalanithi as *stories*—more than just a series of events or facts strung together, they were artifacts crafted and interpreted through a singular human consciousness.

At almost exactly the mid-point in *When Breath Becomes Air*, Kalanithi describes an encounter with a close mentor and friend, the head of a neuroscience lab at Stanford in which he has been working, a man he calls "V." Having been diagnosed with pancreatic cancer, V asks Dr. Kalanithi for his medical advice. Kalanthi's response is: *tell me the story*. The story he is asking his friend for is a biomedical one; it involves his friend's weight loss and the results of his CT scan. This was the information that V wanted to present when he had asked Kalanithi to "wear your doctor hat." Yet, as useful as it might be, it was not enough: "Paul," he said, "do you think my life has meaning? Did I make the right choices?"[14]

Kalanithi was a storyteller, but he was also a scientist, immersed in the world of evidence and data. I teach storytelling to public health students and early on I always ask them: does data have meaning? Often they think it is a trick question. Public health is an evidence-based field. Data drives priorities, the development and continuation of interventions, surveillance and emergency response systems, and the understanding of health disparities. Being aware of the mountains of misinformation on the internet, my students are leery of anecdotes and narratives. They believe that the data can, and should, speak for themselves. I remind them that data speaks only when arranged in a way that makes sense, and that requires the ordering, selection, and omission of other data. A single data point, V's weight loss, for example, means something different when it is combined with the results of his CT scan. Kalanithi observes that even those data points, facing toward a conclusion of cancer, do not provide all the meaning that is required. He notes that "the problem" (of knowing you will die) wasn't "really a scientific one. The fact of death is unsettling. Yet there is no other way to live." He writes:

> What patients seek is not scientific knowledge that doctors hide but existential authenticity each person must find on her own. Getting too deeply into statistics is like trying to quench a thirst with salty water. The angst of facing mortality has no remedy in probability.[15]

In writing *When Breath Becomes Air*, Kalanithi wasn't asking someone else to tell him the story of his life; he took the job into his own capable hands. He understood that the ways of knowing that the humanities offered—contemplation, interpretation, imagination and critical analysis to name just a few—were at least as, if not more, central to understanding the experience of being a human alive on this planet as anatomy, diagnostic imaging, and biopsies. He viewed literature not just as entertainment, or consolation, but instead as "a powerful reflecting tool for thinking about life."[16]

Though medicine, the natural world, literature, philosophy, spirituality, and an attention to domestic life were all crucial to Kalanithi's identity both pre and post diagnosis, this chapter will argue not just *what* he writes—the content—but *how* he writes—the form—reveals a reshuffling of those elements in his evolving search for meaning.

At an important turning point in his career, Kalanithi judges medicine, as opposed to literature, as offering a more "direct experience of life and death questions." He recalls that "Words began to feel as weightless as the breath that carried them."[17] Closer to the end of the book, in contrast, he recounts himself to be "[l]ost in a featureless wasteland of my own mortality and finding no traction in the reams of scientific studies, intracellular molecular pathways, and endless curves of survival statistics."[18] It is at this point that he writes, "I began reading literature again." It may also be, I presume, when he began to write. Solving the mystery of where the book began in the writing process, however, does not answer the question for Kalanithi of where to begin the *story*.

Where to begin

In *When Breath Becomes Air*, Kalanithi places the growing suspicion of his illness and his ultimate diagnosis in the prologue. Introducing his diagnosis immediately makes sense both from a human point of view—a significant thing had happened; it might, in the end, be the most significant thing—and a narrative point of view.

Ordering events on a timeline is key to crafting a tale with the power to engage, move, and even transform. Too much background information too soon can bore readers. Beginning too far back in a narrative is a common first draft mistake. I've been in many writing workshops where the leader, sometimes it's me, identifies a spot near the middle of the story and suggests that the story begins *here*.

When I teach creative writing, I employ a tool of chronology that relies on the ABCs—action, background, and character, in that order. Action captures a reader's interest and pulls them into the story. It casts a shadow of significance over details that might otherwise be easily dismissed. A novel that begins with a scene of a child having an ordinary breakfast with his parents is not likely to hold the attention of a reader. But if that scene comes after an opening in which the child has disappeared, it becomes riveting, containing even in its ordinariness potential clues to understand the extraordinary thing that has happened.

Most important about the story of *When Breath Becomes Air* is, of course, is that the diagnosis coaxed it from its writer in the first place. Though he notes that he intended to write eventually in his career, Kalanithi clearly was not intending to write this story at this time. The drive to leave a thoughtful and fully examined record of his life translates to the page with an urgency that is compelling and moving. In narrative terms, the diagnosis is a powerful hook, both dramatic and surprising: a young man, a surgeon, threatened by cancer. It is almost impossible not to read on, to find out who this man is, and how he faces death. Having set that hook, the structure that he chooses provides Kalanithi time to develop the character of who he was before tragedy struck—the passions, the curiosities, the failings. It allows him to capture our attention with his diagnosis, but then to create a picture in our minds of a person who is not defined by illness, who is, in fact, *in perfect health*. In so doing he also sets the stage for the transformation of the central character—of himself—which contributes to a compelling narrative. There is a clear demarcation in the book, the second section of which is entitled, *Cease Not Until Death*. There is a before and there is an after—both in terms of the state of Kalanithi's health, but also of his character.

Time

As described in the forward to the book by another doctor-writer, Abraham Verghese, the story of Kalanithi "turned time on its head."[19] All pieces of serious writing are put under pressure by time. The sense of urgency—narrative drive—is what keeps a reader turning pages. In embarking on the story of his life even as his life might be ending, the stakes were that much higher for Kalanithi. Time, this central feature of all narratives, was not on his side. In the epilogue, his widow, Lucy Kalanithi, describes the book as carrying "the urgency of racing against time, of having important things to say."[20]

A dilemma for Kalanithi, indeed for anyone writing a memoir under the pressure of a potentially terminal illness, is that nuanced, complicated narratives require time to cohere in the mind of the writer. In the midst of cohering, they require time to come apart and reform and change. The meaning of things is often muddled and unclear when they are happening. To a young man facing death and hoping to write something that communicated the essence of his life, however, this was time Kalanithi didn't have. The moments he chooses, describes, orders, and reflects upon *have* to mean something. The force of that pressure—the desire for certainty in the midst of inherent uncertainty—is a central theme of health humanities, an area of study for which *When Breath Becomes Air* is an important text. It is also one that Kalanithi bears with grace throughout the book. The instances where, in my view, he delivers moments to the reader that have not been allowed sufficient space to evolve into other meanings in either the text or the reader's mind are important not because they are frequent but because they are instructive of that tension. The way that Kalanithi's marriage is addressed in the book is particularly illustrative, in my view, of a moment when a conflict is resolved prematurely, before it might be allowed to disrupt the narrative.

In a description of himself as a younger man he writes:

> Throughout college, my monastic, scholarly study of human meaning would conflict with my urge to forge and strengthen the human relationships that formed that meaning.[21]

Coming as it does in the first section of the book, this passage seems to reflect an aspect of Kalanithi's character that he has reflected upon and understood and that has perhaps changed through his subsequent struggles by the time—later in his life—when the book is begun. But what reads to me as a fairly neat summary of a complicated situation begs a number of questions that seem almost as unre-solved in the book's present moment as in this memory from the past. Conflict in what way, the reader is left to wonder? Might that struggle be connected to the conflict with his wife Lucy that is hinted at in the prologue? It is there that she glimpses the history of a search for the "frequency of cancers in thirty- to forty-year olds" on his cell phone and confronts him. He writes:

> She was upset because she had been worried about it, too. She was upset because I wasn't talking to her about it. She was upset because I'd promised her one life, and given her another.[22]

The couple is drawn closer together through the ordeal of Kalanithi's illness, and he even goes so far to write that "[i]n truth, cancer had saved our marriage."[23] After periods of hope and treatment—a brief return to work—the book ends with them having had a baby, in spite of Kalanithi's understanding that he may not live to see the child grow. At that point, I felt like I understood the centrality of their marriage to his life while nonetheless understanding relatively little about that relationship or the nature of the conflicts that were in many ways swept away by this unexpected tragedy. And exactly because it was so central, this gap felt unexplained.

Certainly, this cannot mean that a memoirist is obligated to reveal everything on the page. In her interview with Karin Babine, author of *All the Wild Hungers*,[24] a memoir about her mother's cancer, memoirist and teacher Julija Sukys argues that it does not:

> Beginning memoirists and essayists often struggle, on the one hand, with fears of betrayal and, on the other, with the notion that they must strip themselves bare in the name of honesty and vulnerability. I remind my stu-dents that they control which secrets they reveal and which ones they keep. *They* get to decide what to divulge and what to keep to themselves.[25]

As a reader, I'm not looking for the details of the messy fights that Paul and Lucy Kalanithi must have had. My point is that if it is true what Kalanithi writes, that relationships form the meaning that literature only seeks to illuminate, this par-ticular relationship at the center of his life, arguably the most important of his life, arrives on the page somewhat too neatly packaged.

The former director of the Iowa Writers' Workshop, Frank Conroy, used to tell his students when they began a story to hold the destination only lightly in their minds. You can buy a ticket to England, he would say, but you have to be prepared to get off the plane in France. This was a reminder that stories must be allowed to change as you are writing them. It can be frightening when that begins to happen in a story you care about deeply. As a former student of Conroy's, I encourage my students in the health professions to become alert for data that doesn't fit their narrative. How do they do that? By turning in the direction of complexity. In this case, it might have involved Kalanithi looking more deeply into what still seems mysterious in these relationships—and resisting the impulse to protest: *but it's not about that*. It would have been a risky approach. He might have worried that he'd end up in a city where he didn't speak the language.

This reminds me of another thing Frank would tell his students. When speaking of the writing life he would warn, "[t]his is a dangerous way to live."

What I think he meant is that you could pour everything you had into the work and it still might not lead anywhere. It might not be good. Or even if it was good, people might not read it. To a young man with a story to tell, and the skills to tell it well, to a young man facing death who has a family whom he loves, how could that be an allowable outcome? My argument is not that *When Breath Becomes Air* should have been the story of a marriage. As it is, it is a remarkably self-reflective, beautiful, and thoughtful account of an examined life at its end. And yet, in those few instances where he touches upon the tension between his mind and his heart, his intellect and his relationships, and then steps away, I hear the ping of buried treasure, the echo of some central questions about who he was that he might yet have explored had there been more time.

What to include

The ubiquitous admonition among writers to *show* and not *tell* is not without its critics. Pulitzer-Prize-winning novelist Viet Thanh Nguyen notes that it can sometimes silence marginalized voices with stories that require more directness, more telling, lest they be ignored by the majority.[26] As moments that happen in real time, scenes are perhaps the most vivid example of *showing*. Scenes offer readers the sense of being in the action without mediation. They feel like they are unfolding without the writer's hand, though they are as much the product of selection and omission as any other part of the story. They direct the reader's attention where the writer wants them to look. Indeed, the inclusion of some moments as scenes and others as a summary is an important way in which the writer guides the reader's focus. This can be problematic in the context described by Nguyen, in which readers may be approaching certain stories already carried along by meta-narratives that are not easily challenged. Kalanithi's inclusion of detailed hospital scenes reflect, in my view, an emphasis that is both practical in a storytelling sense (it is interesting) and significant in a philosophical sense (it reflects what Kalanithi viewed as important).

While the first pages include vivid descriptions from Kalanithi's boyhood, such as when he encounters some black widow spiders,[27] the most emotional and resonant scene in the early pages, involves his visit to a home for brain-injured patients. He contrasts this visit with previous attempts to find meaning in analytic philosophy. He worries that the products of the human brain—philosophy, literature—seem inadequate in conveying the experience of living with that brain, and with a body, in the world. He senses a way to understand the messiness of life among the injured. "Brains give rise to our ability to form relationships and make life meaningful," he writes. "Sometimes, they break."[28]

Subsequently, Kalanithi "trained for years to actively engage with death, to grapple with it, like Jacob with the angel, and, in so doing, to confront the meaning of a life." He moved toward the mystery, toward the brokenness, as he had moved toward the spiders, though they frightened him. "I had started in this career, in part, to pursue death: to grasp it, uncloak it, and see it eye-to-eye, unblinking."[29] If the brain was "the crucible of identity,"[30] then becoming a doctor who studied and healed the brain was a source of identity conferred by few vocations.

Eventually, the physical reality of Kalanithi's illness made the continued practice of medicine impossible. Even before he became ill, however, his confidence in medicine as the key to understanding life and death began to falter. He began to suspect that the undeniable presence of death unfolding all around him might paradoxically render him *less* able to discern what he actually sought, which was meaning in life. He writes:

> But in residency, something else was gradually unfolding. In the midst of this endless barrage of head injuries, I began to suspect that being so close to the fiery light of such moments only blinded me to their nature, like trying to learn astronomy by staring directly at the sun.[31]

A shift that began in residency is accelerated by his experience of illness. He continues:

> Coming in such close contact with my own mortality had changed both nothing and everything. Before my cancer was diagnosed, I knew that someday I would die but I didn't know when. After the diagnosis, I knew that someday I would die but I didn't know when. But now I knew it acutely. The problem wasn't really a scientific one.[32]

The idea that deeper meaning might be found just alongside but not in those moments in a story that *seem* most likely to promise meaning makes sense to a teacher of creative writing or to anyone who begins a story about *an unbelievable true thing that really happened*. The unbelievable thing is, in one sense, just the pitch. Though Kalanithi's book is about a 36-year-old neurosurgeon who gets terminal cancer, it is also—perhaps more importantly—a profoundly representative story of mortality and grief and love in all its ordinariness and poignancy.

Though the details about the residents' lives (they drink energy drinks at 2:00 am), the variety of tragedies they address (cancers, head traumas, stillbirths), the description of the procedure called a Whipple (a nine-hour operation that involves the re-arranging of organs) are all compelling, they are not, in the end, the heart of the story. The heart lies underneath. It can be found as much, if not more, in the ordinary moments as in the dramatic ones. For example, in this early description of sunrise at Sierra Camp, where Kalanithi spent a summer working in college:

> And then we would sit and watch as the first hint of sunlight, a light tinge of day blue, would leak out of the eastern horizon, slowly erasing the stars ...

craning your head back you could see the day's blue darken halfway across the sky, and to the west, the night remained yet unconquered—pitch-black, stars in full glimmer, the full moon still pinned to the sky ... you could not help but feel your speck-like existence against the immensity of the mountain, the earth, the universe.[33]

One might argue that shifts in the narrative focus from medicine to philosophy and literature toward the end of the book merely reflect the physical reality of Kalanithi's illness. He grew too sick to work as a physician. Elsewhere, however, Kalanithi resists a purely chronological structure. Further, all experience, when written about, lies in the past. All of it is available to the writer to interpret, emphasize, or omit in the construction of a story. I believe that the structure of the book reflects a growing awareness that the meaning of life lies in a focus on *life*, rather than the battle against death, however interestingly that unfolds in the skilled hands of a neurosurgeon.

What to leave out

The job of a memoirist, of any kind of writer, is as much to decide what to omit as what to include. In his introduction, Verghese notes that Kalanithi decided not to use the names of any of the people (aside from family) who appeared in the book, with the exception of one person, who is not identified. What to make of Kalanithi's decision not to use the names of all but one of the secondary characters besides his family, including the physician who treats him and, presumably, could be identified with some sleuthing? What might that decision tell us about where he placed his story on a continuum of health-related stories that stretch from, on the one hand, patients who tell stories about their own experiences with illness and healthcare and, on the other, doctors who write? How might those decisions echo the deliberations of memoirists in other fields, who also write about friends, family, and colleagues?

In the interview with Julija Sukys referenced earlier, memoirist Karen Babine discusses the question of whom to identify by name in her memoir, a matter much considered by writers of creative nonfiction. She says:

> The easy answer is based in my ethics of nonfiction: the first is not to violate the contract with the reader to tell the truth, and the second is to Do No Harm.[34]

Easy, perhaps, until it becomes clear that the first ethical imperative can present itself to be in conflict with the second. Whose truth? One might ask. What if the story one is telling *includes* a description of harm done—can it still be told? The decision of whether or not to identify secondary characters by name is one that often features in the trade-off between truth and harm, but even that decision is rarely as straightforward as it may seem at first.

As stated above, questions of privacy and consent are central to the considerations of memoirists of all kinds, but there are particular issues when it comes to memoirs written by physicians. Jack Coulihan notes the risks to patient privacy with even de-identified patients if they have not given their consent.[35] Even when patients do consent, physician memoirs are open to charges of exploitation considering the power imbalance between the clinician and the patient, the possible release of private medical data, and the potential for implicit bias, among other things.[36] But if the patient is also a doctor, the rules about confidentiality and consent—at least in a legal sense—do not apply in the same way.

Kalanithi could not have known that his book would reach the large audience that it did but he was clearly writing for publication. The decision of whom to name, or not, must have been a considered one and reveals, I believe, Kalanithi's particular approach to the tensions that exist when a doctor becomes a patient. How much of their authority do they retain, in this case? How might their presumption of credibility contrast with those patients who, having always been medical outsiders, may struggle to be believed?

Though many characters are given a first name only, one important character, his treating physician, is given both a first and a last name: "Emma Hayward." She is described as a caring and competent doctor in the book and her willingness to take charge is mostly presented a source of comfort to Kalanithi. When describing how she kept his identity as a surgeon in her mind, he writes:

> She had done what I had challenged myself to do as a doctor years earlier: accepted mortal responsibility for my soul and returned me to a point where I could return to myself.[37]

At the same time, there are scenes where her vulnerability is on display. In a medical system that prizes objectivity and professionalism, that is a portrayal that carries risks. The most poignant of these moments is shortly before Kalanithi's death when she tells him that he has, "Five good years left."[38] Kalanithi understands that she is speaking to him as a fellow human being as much as a physician and that her statement is more likely anchored in hope, rather than evidence:

> She pronounced it, but without the authoritative tone of an oracle, without the confidence of a true believer. She said it, instead, like a plea." ... There we were, doctor and patient, in a relationship that sometimes carries a magisterial air and other times, like now, was no more, and no less, than two people huddled together, as one faces the abyss. Doctors, it turns out, need hope too.[39]

In the opinion of Seamus O'Mahoney, it is a "generous" portrayal.[40] While Amy Caruso and Rebecca Garden observe that Kalanithi "creates a space for patients who do not believe that fighting until the end (with the hope of a miraculous cure) and hoping for a peaceful death are mutually exclusive,"[41] O'Mahoney describes Emma Hayward's reassurance and hope-seeking as "fudging and fibbing, this hesitation to be brave."[42]

Kalanithi does not appear to share O'Mahoney's negative view of his oncologist's behavior ("Emma hadn't given me back my old identity. She'd protected my ability to forge a new one."[43]), but he is less generous in his portrayal of Brad, a medical resident who argues with him about the medicine that he should be taking while hospitalized. While it is true that masking these characters in the narrative might serve to spare them from some of the consequences of a negative portrayal, they are no doubt recognizable to themselves and potentially to others. Further, I would argue that the decision to de-identify or mask characters can influence how those characters take shape in the writer's mind during composition.

Given the potential downsides of identifying characters such as Emma Hayward or Brad by their real names, I would suggest there are nonetheless arguments in favor. Jack Coulehan's case study, which involves a fictional memoir of an urban doctor named Cushman, might be instructive here. Coulehan imagines that readers, among them medical colleagues, might object to the negative portrayal of a doctor. He argues that Dr. Cushman has the right to include it, nonetheless:

> If, in fact, Dr. Cushman's anger over his attending physician's attitudes contributed significantly to his decision to dedicate his life to caring for the poor, the portrayal represents a crucial feature of his life experience and should be included in the memoir, even though it reflects negatively on his teacher.[44]

In addition, while it seems like a small trade-off with what Karen Babine identifies previously as the "contract with the reader to tell the truth," changing names is not without consequence, in part because it is rarely just the names that are changed, it is often also identifying details. Details that might at first glance seem trivial can, upon further reflection, prove to be important. The fact that Emma Hayward is a woman, for example, might seem inconsequential in some respects but could become more noteworthy in a narrative that included more consideration of systemic problems within the American healthcare system. A discussion of structural issues in healthcare and how those might color his or others' experiences is largely absent from Kalanithi's book. Physician Paul D'Alton observes:

> At times the boyish unquestioning enthusiasm for the adrenalin of the hospital emergency department or the 100-hour weeks is challenging. Failing to address these and almost any of the other systemic problems of medicine, such as the inherent inequality of a privatised healthcare, is unfortunate but understandable. Time was not on Kalanithi's side.[45]

Even outside of health settings, I find it useful when working with students to examine the pressure on the storyteller that *not* choosing to mask or de-identify characters puts on the writer. A scene you are writing that portrays the actions of another person in a negative light is a prime opportunity for reflection. What are your feelings about writing it? Are you angry? If so, how might that emotion color the representation of the character in the work? Writing about the therapeutic power of creating an autobiographic work that displays a "unitary, organizing, masterful consciousness," Arthur Frank notes that "[t]he limitation of this story is that it imagines the storyteller becoming *alone*."[46] He suggests there is ethical merit to a dialogical approach, in which the perspective of others is allowed to disrupt the narrative. Using real names for people in your narrative requires you to consider, even more deeply than you might otherwise, their perspective on the events you describe. It puts more pressure on the internal conversations that an ethical memoirist has with him- or herself, in which they imagine secondary characters speaking up in their own defense. These are conversations in which the writer asks him- or herself: How would this person I'm writing about explain this moment from their perspective? How would they characterize their behavior or, perhaps, even my own? How might external factors be at play? The burden that memoir places on a writer is not just a technical burden (did it happen this way?) but one that requires us to enter into these conversations with the others in our stories—sometimes in person as many memoirists do, at other times in our imaginations. Rather than merely assuming the power to tell or not tell, to reveal or not reveal, we embrace the subjectivity inherent in our own point of view.

The issue of subjectivity versus objectivity raises another interesting question related to the use of pseudonyms in *When Breath Becomes Air* that is specific to the context of health and illness. Much health and medical humanities scholarship involves the examination of patient narratives: their value in amplifying marginalized voices, as critiques of the healthcare system, as well as how they should be viewed in terms of their believability.[47] Angela Woods explores this tension in the following way:

> To what extent can we trust that people's stories of illness faithfully describe, "what it was really like?" As Mark Freeman has noted in relation to qualitative research more broadly, there is "widespread concern that narratives are untrue to 'life itself.' Whether this is cause for alarm (the data are distorted!) or celebration (a toast to the imagination!) depends on who is offering the critique." The issue of whether narratives are "true" of course immediately prompts us to ask "for whom, and in what situation?"[48]

Narratives written by doctors—particularly when writing about patients—are put under ethical scrutiny in great part because of the authority they carry, the risk that they might reveal not just private things about patients but private things that are also assumed to be true. Patient narratives rarely carry the same authority, even when, or perhaps most especially, the patient is describing their own experiences.[49] The anguish that Kalanithi experiences in his shifting role from doctor to patient is one that he explores elegantly throughout the book:

Eighteen months earlier, I'd been in the hospital with appendicitis. Then I'd be treated not as a patient but as a colleague, almost like a consultant on my own case. I expected the same here.[50]

Verghese's tantalizing "all but one" implies that Kalanithi's deliberations about whether or not to include names and identifying details were the result of a thoughtful process, rather than a blanket decision. It is not clear which of the considerations explored above were foremost in his mind. Nonetheless, it seems to me that in a significant respect Kalanithi believed that he carried one aspect of the power that he held as a physician into the part of his story where he became a patient: the power to be believed.

Where to end

When Breath Becomes Air ends in an embrace of uncertainty that is active. In my view, it is not just *where* and *when* the story ends that is significant, it is *how*. The wisdom of the final pages of the book lies not in resolution but in the suspension of it, as represented, most vividly, by a shift in the final few pages to the present tense. "Yet there is dynamism in our house," writes Kalanithi.[51] In these passages, Kalanithi notes a feeling of languor associated with this focus on the present, a feeling of openness. Tying the ambiguity and uncertainty in which he finds himself explicitly to tense, he writes: "So what tense am I living in now? ... Have I proceeded beyond the present tense and into the past perfect?"[52] *When Breath Becomes Air* includes a series of events, reflections, and encounters at the end of Kalanithi's life but it is not a mere recording of those things. It is, as underscored earlier in this chapter, the *story* of those things. This might seem like an inconsequential distinction until you consider this difference: a story has many possible endings. A life has only one.

"Death always wins," writes Kalanithi.[53] This is a sentence I think of often while drafting this reflection on his work. It is a sentence I return to when sitting at the kitchen table with my son who, at the time of my writing, is graduating from high school in the middle of a pandemic. He's excited and worried about his future in discreet chunks: Will he go away to college? What will he become? As his mother, my worries are more amorphous and far ranging. In addition to the pandemic, my home state of California is burning in increasing swaths each year. It is all but certain that the world will be a very different place when my sons are as old as I am now. What, I worry, will become of them? Of us? I find myself wishing I could jump to the end of the story to see how it turns out. But how far ahead would I want to leap? As Kalanithi observed, if you look far enough ahead there is no end but one.

The idea of a resolution to a story is particularly confusing to my storytelling students who are mostly concerned with telling true stories about public health issues. The work of public health is complicated and nuanced and rarely offers neat endings of the kind they are looking for. I remind them that the end of a story isn't necessarily the end of the action. It certainly isn't always a happy ending, which my storytelling students often take a long time to understand. They want to write a story about addiction that ends in sobriety, or with an effective, affordable policy solution to a seemingly intractable public health problem. Sometimes there is one. More often, the resolution they land on is like a clearing at the top of the mountain you have climbed, where you can look back and understand something more about how you arrived where you are.

And yet, even if we give up the fantasy of a happy ending, our urge toward narrative is a powerful impulse. It is, as described by the communication scholar Walter Fisher, the "paradigmatic mode of human decision making and communication."[54] It propels us toward at least the illusion of answers and sometimes, as I touched on earlier in this chapter, toward premature sense-making. Writing about *When Breath Becomes Air* during these particularly troubled times, I feel a palpable pressure to mine it for wisdom, a pressure to find a way to translate that wisdom into something meaningful on the page. I experience confusion approaching despair when I think I might miss the mark. I believe in those moments that I might understand something of Kalanithi's urge toward narrative under the pressure of time. I believe he might have understood mine.

The urge to make sense of events through narrative may be innate, as Fisher argues, but it is not without its own risks. The world is full of false narratives: stories that reinforce stereotypes and oppression and that revise history to flatter those in power. As Angela Woods observes, "narrative is not, and never has been, innocent; it is not, and never has been, inherently oriented towards the good."[55]

What's more, the power of events to undermine our narratives can overwhelm even our strongest attempts at making sense of them. Arguing against a preoccupation with narrative, philosopher Crispin Sartwell notes that it "comes apart at the extremes … it comes apart in ecstasy, in writhing pain, at death."[56] Indeed, Kalanithi describes how his illness precipitates just this kind of narrative coming apart. Shortly before his diagnosis, he believed he had arrived at a place where "[i]t felt to me as if the individual strands of biology, morality, life, and death were finally beginning to weave themselves into, if not a perfect moral system, a coherent worldview, and a sense of my place in it."[57] He notes that "[s]evere illness wasn't life-altering, it was life shattering. It felt less like an epiphany-a piercing burst of light illuminating What Really Matters-and more like someone had just firebombed the path forward."[58]

For most of us it is near-impossible to live in that nonnarrative space, to walk that firebombed path where all meaning has been blown to pieces. An oft-stated goal of health humanities training is to inculcate in health professionals a tolerance of ambiguity. I would argue that one of the things that *When Breath Becomes Air* shows us in its final section is that *tolerance* is too passive a word. Kalanithi was no fan of passivity. When he writes about feeling like the illness has robbed him of his agency, he notes that the word patient comes from fourteenth-century philosophy to mean "the object of an action."[59] He reiterates the desire for agency when he writes: "Most lives are lived with a passivity towards death—it's something that happens to you and those around you."[60]

One of the things that this book illustrates, I believe, is that living with ambiguity is much more about embracing it than tolerating it. It is an approach in which each moment is open to active questioning. A narrative forms, is blown apart, and reforms, changed. Wisdom, in my view, lies neither in the narrative moment nor the nonnarrative moment. Rather, it can be found in the moving back and forth between narrative and nonnarrative, in making sense of things without allowing them to solidify. It can be found in the way Kalanithi no longer asks himself: Who am I? What do I want? But rather: Who am I *now*?

The answer keeps changing. As it must. What's more, as observed by Elise Smith, the answer to these questions becomes increasingly relational and less individualistic as Kalanithi advances in his journey toward death.[61] She notes the passage where he writes: "Human knowledge is never contained in one person. It grows from the relationships we create between each other and the world, and still it is never complete."[62]

As his energy wanes, Kalanithi burrows further into language. Whereas he had once worried that "words were as weightless as the breath that carried them,"[63] he judges them, finally, useful in their way in grappling with the angel. Though he finds himself unable to think into the future, he writes toward it. "Words have a longevity I do not,"[64] he writes, and, indeed, Kalanithi's text at the end moves with languor between moments that are static and those that are dynamic. It contracts. And expands. And then contracts again.

Notes

1 Paul Kalanithi, *When Breath Becomes Air* (New York: Random House, 2016), 136.
2 Dan McAdams, "Narrative Identity," in *Handbook of Identity Theory and Research*, edited by S. Schwartz, K. Luyckx, and V. Vignoles (New York: Springer, 2011): doi: 10.1007/978-1-4419-7988-9_5.
3 Lars-Christer Hydén, "Illness and Narrative," *Sociology of Health & Illness* 19, no. 1 (1997): 48–69.
4 Deborah de Muijnck, "'When Breath Becomes Air': Constructing Stable Narrative Identity during Terminal Illness," *Colloquy* 38 (2019): 44.
5 Arthur Frank, "Illness and Autobiographical Work: Dialogue as Narrative Destabilization," *Qualitative Sociology* 23, no. 1 (2000): 137.
6 Jeffrey Berman, *Dying in Character: Memoirs on the End of Life* (Boston, MA: University of Massachusetts Press, 2013).
7 Jonathon Tomlinson, "Lessons from 'The Other Side': Teaching and Learning from Doctors' Illness Narratives," *BMJ* 348 (2014): g3600. https://www.jstor.org/stable/10 .2307/26515125. Accessed August 20, 2021.
8 Kalanithi, *When Breath Becomes Air*, 98.
9 Margaret Morganroth Gullette, "How We Imagine Living with Dying," *Embodied Narration: Illness, Death and Dying in Modern Culture* 15 (2018): 67, 68.
10 Kalanithi, *When Breath Becomes Air*, 161.
11 Ibid., 108.
12 Ibid., 40.
13 Tomlinson, "Lessons," 1.
14 Kalanithi, *When Breath Becomes Air*, 101.
15 Ibid., 132.

16 Stanford Medicine, 2015, "A Strange Relativity: Altered Time for Surgeon Turned Patient," https://www.youtube.com/watch?v=d5u753wQeyM. Accessed August 20, 2021.
17 Kalanithi, *When Breath Becomes Air*, 43.
18 Ibid., 148.
19 Ibid., xi.
20 Ibid., 213.
21 Ibid., 31.
22 Ibid., 8.
23 Ibid., 138.
24 Karen Babine, *All the Wild Hungers: A Season of Cooking and Cancer* (Minneapolis, MN: Milkweed Press, 2019).
25 Julija Šukys and Karen Babine, "A Season of Cooking and Cancer," *Fourth Genre: Explorations in Nonfiction* 21, no. 2 (2019): 183.
26 Viet Thanh Nguyen, "Book Review: Viet Thanh Nguyen Reveals How Writers' Workshops Can Be Hostile," *The New York Times*, April 26, 2017: https://www.nytimes.com/2017/04/26/books/review/viet-thanh-nguyen-writers-workshops.html. Accessed August 20, 2021.
27 Kalanithi, *When Breath Becomes Air*, 22.
28 Ibid., 38.
29 Ibid., 80.
30 Ibid., 71.
31 Ibid., 81.
32 Ibid., 131.
33 Ibid., 34.
34 Šukys and Babine, "A Season of Cooking and Cancer," 183.
35 Jack Coulehan, "Ethics, Memoir, and Medicine," *AMA Journal of Ethics* 13, no. 7 (2011): 435–439.
36 Rimma Osipov, "Healing Narrative: Ethics and Writing about Patients," *AMA Journal of Ethics* 13, no. 7 (2011): 420–424. Also see: Danielle Ofri, "Doctor-Writers: What Are the Ethics?" *Huffington Post*, July 5, 2010.
37 Kalanithi, *When Breath Becomes Air*, 163.
38 Ibid., 193.
39 Ibid., 193–194.
40 Seamus O'Mahony, "Hope, Oncology and Death," *BMJ Blog: The Reading Room*, May 9, 2016: http://stg-blogs.bmj.com/medical-humanities/2016/05/09/the-reading-room-when-breath-becomes-air/.
41 Amy Caruso Brown and Rebecca Garden, "From Silence into Language: Questioning the Power of Physician Illness Narratives," *AMA Journal of Ethics* 19, no. 5 (2017): 501–507.
42 O'Mahony, "Hope, Oncology and Death."
43 Kalanithi, *When Breath Becomes Air*, 166.
44 Coulehan, "Ethics, Memoir, and Medicine."
45 Paul D'Alton, "When Breath Becomes Air Review: A Neurosurgeon's Story of Terminal Illness," *Irish Times*, January 21, 2017.
46 Frank, "Illness and Autobiographical Work: Dialogue as Narrative Destabilization," 138.
47 Johanna Shapiro, "Illness Narratives: Reliability, Authenticity and the Empathic Witness," *Medical Humanities* (2011): 68–72.
48 Angela Woods, "The Limits of Narrative: Provocations for the Medical Humanities," *Medical Humanities* 37, no. 2 (2011): 74.
49 Shapiro, "Illness Narratives." Also see Rebecca Garden, "Telling Stories about Illness and Disability: The Limits and Lessons of Narrative," *Perspectives in Biology and Medicine* 53, no. 1 (2010): 121–135.
50 Kalanithi, *When Breath Becomes Air*, 122.

51 Ibid., 196.
52 Ibid., 198.
53 Ibid., 114.
54 Walter Fisher, "The Narrative Paradigm: In the Beginning," *Journal of Communication* 35, no. 4 (1985): 74–89.
55 Angela Woods, "The Limits of Narrative: Provocations for the Medical Humanities," *Medical Humanities* 37, no. 2 (2011): 75.
56 Crispin Sartwell, *End of Story: Toward an Annihilation of Language and History* (Albany, NY: State University of New York Press, 2000), 65.
57 Kalanithi, *When Breath Becomes Air*, 113.
58 Ibid., 120.
59 Ibid., 141.
60 Ibid., 114.
61 Elise Smith, "Review of Paul Kalanithi, *When Breath Becomes Air*," *The American Journal of Bioethics* 16, no. 10 (2016): W6–W7.
62 Kalanithi, *When Breath Becomes Air*, 172.
63 Ibid., 43.
64 Ibid., 199.

8 Joanna Cannon

Leaving medicine to pursue a physician's calling

Abraham M. Nussbaum

Physicians once wrote war stories about battling against disease, love stories about falling for science, and conversion stories about realizing how hard it is to be ill. Today, physicians write burnout stories about how the practice of medicine has worn them down and run them out.

Burnout is the most common word to describe the contemporary practice of medicine. A recent systematic review estimated the prevalence of burnout among surveyed American physicians at 67%. That two of three physicians report burnout has been associated with increased errors in patient care, reduced satisfaction among patients, and with physicians reducing their clinical practice or leaving practice entirely.[1] Healthcare leaders have responded by naming physician burnout an epidemic[2] and prescribing treatments.[3]

These prescriptions are necessarily targeted at symptoms rather than the cause of physician burnout, because it remains unclear if burnout is another word for depression, for generational change, for declining professional autonomy, for the introduction of electronic health records, or for the experience of moral distress—or if there is some other explanation.

The work of Joanna Cannon, a British psychiatrist turned writer, dramatizes these possibilities while suggesting a further possible explanation for physician burnout. In her writing so far—two best-selling novels and a memoir—physicians still tell war stories, but one of the casualties is themselves. Physicians still tell love stories, but they fall for an avocation outside of clinical practice. Physicians still tell conversion stories, but they become a physician who pursues the doctor's calling without a clinical practice. In Cannon's work, burnout becomes an international phenomenon that occurs even in a single-payer system distinct from the American system where most burnout research occurs. Burnout also becomes an existential phenomenon: physicians, Cannon suggests, are so disenchanted with the institutions of medicine that a physician must leave institutional medicine to practice a physician's calling.

The Trouble with Goats and Sheep

Cannon's first novel, *The Trouble with Goats and Sheep*, is, at least explicitly, a mystery. The novel follows two English ten-year-olds, Grace and Tilly, as they

DOI: 10.4324/9781003079712-8

seek a missing person. Their neighbor, Mrs. Creasy, has vanished. Grace and Tilly set out to find her and God, whom they believe can secure Mrs. Creasy's safety. The children's double pursuit occurs in double time. The novel's present moment, 1976, reveals the secrets of their neighbors from a past moment, 1967. As the novel shifts between chapters set in the transposed years of 1976 and 1967, the dual narratives reinforce a core psychiatric belief: the past affects the present. As the novel's narrator says: "It was strange how often the past broke into the present like an intruder, dangerous and unwanted."[4]

In this line, the double nature of Cannon's narrative voice is fully developed: she writes with a physician's knowledge from a patient's point of view. Unlike physician books that luxuriate over the technical details of illness and care, Cannon compassionately narrates the experience of being ill, especially mentally ill, in a world which mistrusts the ill.

Grace and Tilly live in such a world. Many of their neighbors fear Walter Bishop, a man who often stands alone in his council flat, silently watching the happenings of the neighborhood. Walter's hair is too long, his skin too milky; some call him "Strange Walter" and suspect he is the one who disappeared Mrs. Creasy. But the narrator's sympathy is with the Walters of the neighborhood, the feared outcasts, instead of its conventional inhabitants who fear the odd. A close-minded neighbor tells Tilly: "The point is, these people don't think like the rest of us. They're misfits, oddballs. They're the ones the police should be talking to, not people like us."[5] The neighbor assures the child she too will learn to cross the street when she encounters the odd.

A psychiatrist like Cannon cannot cross the street to avoid the odd; a psychiatrist encounters the odd, the strange, the people who are not the people like us, daily. Grace and Tilly are not psychiatrists, but their interest in the odd and their nascent observational skills are steps toward becoming a psychiatrist. And their story resembles Cannon's own story, because Grace and Tilly make their pursuit during the years of Cannon's own childhood and in a provincial setting similar to her own childhood in Derbyshire.

But Grace and Tilly do not speak like shrinks; they use the language to which they have access as children. They talk of candy, of pop culture. After an initial meeting with the neighborhood vicar, they take up a biblical language of seeking Mrs. Creasy as a lost sheep. The children's search is suggested by the novel's title, which alludes to the Christian parable of the goats and the sheep. The parable promises that when Jesus returns in glory, "he shall separate them one from another, as a shepherd divideth his sheep from the goats: And he shall set the sheep on his right hand, but the goats on the left."[6] The scripture describes Jesus as a shepherd who gathers, classifies, and separates his flock. Grace and Tilly seize upon the parable's divine sorting out who is a sheep and who is a goat as a way to find the two missing persons sought in the novel, Mrs. Creasy and God.

Despite its title, the suggestive names of characters like Grace and Bishop, and the scriptural language of the children, the novel is no doctrinaire Christian allegory. The vicar tells Grace and Tilly that God is everywhere. The children imagine God as a divine parent who keeps people safe. The children attend church primarily for the sweets. And when Jesus is found by the children, He appears not in celestial glory, but within a creosote stain in a drainpipe.

God is, as the vicar promised the children at the beginning, everywhere.

And nowhere. The novel makes it clear that when we classify, we often mistake sheep and goats. Tilly asks Grace: "How does God know which people are goats and which people are sheep?" Grace replies: "I think that's the trouble … it's not always that easy to tell the difference."[7] As the novel progresses, the children realize that Walter Bishop is not the goat their neighbors fear him to be.

Late in the novel, the children encounter Bishop directly. He says: "It is a wise man who make his own decisions. It's very important to remember that, especially if you're looking for God."[8] With Bishop's assistance, the children realize that the security of being a sheep comes at the cost of blind faith. The wise chart their own course.

Doctoring and writing

Cannon's first novel, and its reception, created an additional double narrative. Just as the children gave up a child-like belief in God as the omniscient guarantor of safety, Cannon gave up an early belief in the doctor as the invulnerable guarantor of health. After all, sorting sheep from goats is a diagnostic process undertaken every day while doctoring.

Diagnosis, in the classic Platonic formulation, is a carving of nature at its joints, a sorting of metaphysically different disease entities from each other.[9] As the violence of the Platonic image makes it clear, there can be no ambiguity in the work of the ideal physician as she divides the healthy from the diseased, the normal from the pathological. The kind of physician who carves nature at its joints is akin to the kind of God who divides the sheep from the goats.

However possible that may or may not be in the rest of medicine, psychiatry readily admits that its diagnostic system is incapable of making metaphysically distinct diagnoses. To become a psychiatrist means giving up the diagnostic certainty that other kinds of physicians can more readily enjoy.

Cannon enjoyed the life of a physician only after years of pursuing other labors. In the press reports celebrating her first novel, journalists often told a romantic origin story about the debut novelist. A girl from the Midlands, Cannon's father was a plumber and her mother owned a giftshop. Cannon attended a provincial school and left at the age of 15. She worked—delivering pizza, tending bar, cleaning kennels—before entering university in her 30s. In these publicity materials, Cannon described herself as a tea drinker who rose early to walk her dog each morning and had struggled along the way to becoming a best-selling physician-writer.

Cannon told journalists that she has long preferred reading to socializing but wrote only when she entered medicine.

> As an adult, the first time I wrote with any seriousness, was when I first became a doctor. The medical wards can be quite distressing at times, and

> I found it really helped if I wrote about how I was feeling. It's amazing how things begin to make sense if you write them down.[10]

In these publicity materials, Cannon described herself as becoming an author only when she became a physician and began making sense of the strange worlds of medicine. She described herself as a shy child who found her voice as an adult physician. She became a writer over lunch breaks, writing her debut novel in her car as her colleagues supped in the physician lounge; a physician apart from other physicians. She entered a portion of the resulting manuscript in a writing contest. A bidding auction broke out - Cannon earned a book publishing deal, and she became an author. All from the novel Cannon wrote in response to becoming invested with a physician's authority and responsibility.

So it seems telling that her debut was about diagnostic processes that have gone awry. Characters mistake sheep for goats, the well for the ill, the past for the present. The mistaken diagnoses are corrected only when characters move from judgment to understanding.

It is also a novel about how a person gradually finds herself on the wrong path. Toward the end, the narrator observes:

> When she looks back, the journeys she takes do not seem like journeys at all. They seem like a series of small decisions, one placed thoughtlessly upon the next. It's only when she stops and turns, and realizes she has reached a destination, that the importance of the decisions becomes clear. They stack behind her, the perhaps and the another-times, and the one-day-soons, and they hold her in a place she never meant to be held. The choices she has made are not a part of her. They have stitched themselves into the person she has become, and when she stops to see who that is, she finds that the cloth from which she is cut has begun to suffocate her.[11]

Cannon will eventually write that her own small choices, the choices that made her a physician, that held her in medicalized places, began to suffocate her.

Three Things About Elsie

The Trouble with Goats and Sheep was about the pursuit of missing persons, but it embodied disease with the authority of diagnosing. In Cannon's second novel, *Three Things About Elsie*, a person goes missing because of her disease. The protagonist, Florence, has been removed from the world by dementia, relegated to an institutional facility with the cheery, but placeless name, of Cherry Tree. There are, Florence notes, no cherry trees at the facility; its name is a euphemism obscuring what the place actually is.

Florence repeatedly calls attention to the way medical euphemisms obscure the ill from the view of the healthy. Cherry Tree, Florence says,

> was called sheltered accommodation, but I'd never quite been able to work out what it was we were being sheltered from. The world was still out there.

... We were the ones hidden away, collected up and ushered out of sight, and I often wondered if it was actually the world that was being sheltered from us.[12]

Florence describes the staff at Cherry Tree as competent but distant; the staff makes sure she is "fed and watered."[13] Florence mounts a small resistance by calling the attendants "uniforms," signaling an awareness that the staff is just as depersonalized by institutionalized places as the patients are. Today's institutional places, Florence notes, are all given misleading names that, despite themselves, reveal their truth: "Woodlands, Oak Court, Pine Lodge. They're often named after trees, for some reason. It's the same with mental health units. Forests full of forgotten people, waiting to be found again."[14] Cherry Tree is filled with people like Florence, whose diseases are measured and charted; as Florences are abstracted into patients, they disappear from the world's awareness.

In these institutional spaces, Florence experiences physicians as complicit in the disappearing acts perpetuated upon the ill. When Florence is examined by a physician, her friend Elsie says the purpose of the examination is "to make sure everyone knows who they're supposed to be."[15] The physician performs a minimental status examination, a bedside test of cognition, attention, and executive functioning. Florence says:

He told us there were thirty questions, which didn't sound very mini to me. The world of medicine appears to be littered with understatements—small scratch, slight discomfort, minor abrasion. ... It's strange how easily you can become flustered when someone is watching you.[16]

The physician watches Florence, but his language and examination prevent Florence from feeling seen. Cannon wants readers to see Florence and people like her.

Although the novel is written from a patient's perspective, it evinces sympathy for physicians. The description of one medical encounter reads:

She will sit with me in a cubicle that smells of hand sanitizer and other people's despair. When the doctor finally arrives, he will be unshaven and exhausted, and his eyes will be filled with all the other lives who have sat in front of him that day. But he will still care. He will still listen to what I have to say.[17]

By Cannon's second novel, both the patient and the physician are described sympathetically, but they encounter each other within an institutional setting, which wears them both out.

Cannon writes with a therapeutic compassion for characters traumatized by their experiences and *Elsie* shares, with her first novel, the theme that small decisions can affect a large change. Florence approvingly recalls a friend's counsel: "you can't tell how big a moment is until you turn back and look at it."[18] Only in time, Cannon implies, do we understand the stories of our lives. So, just as in her first novel, Cannon writes in a therapeutic mode, giving neglected characters a healing chance to tell their story. In a fashion, Cannon extends what Florence calls the singular "moment of sympathy," the small obit in a community newspaper with a vanishingly small circulation, typically extended to an elderly person with a dementia.[19] Instead of a few lines of agate type, Florence gets a novel and a character often missing from society's view, an elderly woman with dementia, is compassionately seen.

After the formal conclusion of the novel, Cannon includes an acknowledgments section. Just like in her first novel, she thanks her patients.

> I honestly believe that every person we meet alters us in some ways. ... This book would never have been written without the patients. ... My life was definitely changed by meeting you. My writing and thinking will always be guided by the short time we walked together.[20]

Breaking and Mending

Cannon implicitly suggests that her time walking together with patients as a clinical physician has come to an end. The patients changed her and she will never forget them, but Cannon has shifted from being a physician who writes on her lunch break in the car park to being a novelist who was a psychiatrist.

By the time she fulfilled her three-book deal with a memoir, Cannon was no longer practicing but insisted that she remained a physician. The subtitle of her memoir, *Breaking and Mending: A Junior Doctor's Stories of Compassion and Burnout*, implies that she, like so many physicians today, burned out. Yet, within its pages, Cannon never quite settles on "burnout," offering a variety of descriptions like breaking, exhausting, and suffocating. So she writes:

> I had arrived on the wards filled with joy and enthusiasm, and a desire to be the best doctor I could possibly be. The inadequacies of the system, the lack of funding, the absence of people to provide the necessary care, and the misery and the death and the dying had all whittled away at me until there was nothing of that doctor left.[21]

Joy, enthusiasm, and desire are "whittled" away by her experiences in contemporary healthcare, so Cannon leaves clinical practice but it is unclear if she was whittled away or burned-out or if something else occurred.

Burnout is in the subtitle of Cannon's memoir, but even the book's title provides a different explanation. Burnout is a metaphor for a machine, a running out of a finite supply of energy. Breaking is a metaphor for solid matter, a violent division into parts or fragments of what belongs together. Mending is also a metaphor for matter, a repairing or a reparation of what belongs together. Both breaking and mending are nontechnical, nonmechanical, nonmedical metaphors. They are also words from the language belonging to patients, rather than the language belonging to physicians. Many physicians who become writers struggle to translate medical experiences into popular narratives. Not Cannon. Cannon so consistently chooses the language preferred by patients to describe even medical experiences, that it is unclear she ever adopted the language of physicians as her authorial voice.

Cannon herself raises the possibility that she never fully shifted to a physician's voice by writing that on the first lecture of the first day of medical school:

> We were told that there are two kinds of doctor: white coats and cardigans. Those who love the science and those who love the people. Those who order tests for the patients and those who talk to them. Using those (debatable) parameters, I was so much of a cardigan, I was off the scale.[22]

Cannon imagines a scale, an instrument for weighing, between white coat and cardigan, between physicians who identify with science and those who identify with patients and describes herself as outside its parameters. Throughout the memoir, Cannon describes her reluctance to fully adopt the physician's perspective, repeatedly drawing attention to the ways medical training requires a physician to become a different person with a different emotional state, a kind of invincible calm and confidence that masks the physician's humanity.

Ill-fitting equanimity

Cannon describes becoming a physician as becoming complicit in the work of the institutions that patients like her fictional protagonist Florence resist. Like Florence, Cannon describes herself as unable to directly affect change within the system, but able through re-narration to resist its hold upon her.

So, in her memoir, Cannon repeatedly observes that medical training was a dream that became a nightmare: "This was my dream, my ultimate goal, and yet it had turned into a nightmare so vivid and so brutal that I could hardly bear to look any more."[23] The very tools of a physician are malign instruments because of the unbearable emotional weight of wielding them: "For some, though, a stethoscope is less of a protective talisman, and more of a risk factor, because it carries with it an unimaginable burden."[24] To become a physician, a person has to give up emotional needs, but also material needs. "Sacrifice and the surrender of the self are woven into the job, and going without food and water and sleep are also vows every junior doctor seems to be expected to uphold. *Look after yourself*, we are told."[25] Cannon resists sacrificing herself to medicine's institutions and its admonitions that each individual must pursue her own calling.

Cannon writes as a disappointed idealist. She admires the body and the science which increases our understandings of it. She writes lovingly of wise teachers. She writes compassionately of patients who endure both illness and alienating institutions. But she writes with deep bitterness about those institutions.

> Having time for your patients, being able to explain a treatment to someone in a way they can understand, helping someone's journey to be a little

more bearable. It's only when you arrive on the wards, when you are spat out into an NHS that bends and breaks under the strain of the endless demands placed upon it, it's only then that you realise you will never be able to be the doctor you want to become. The system simply won't allow it.[26]

The problem, for an idealist, is that the system will not allow you to be the doctor you want to become. Systems want to make you into the doctor they need. Some trainees are broken by the system and then rebuilt into the doctor the system needs.

Those doctors become the white coats, their identities subsumed into the professional garment which becomes their public self. Cannon is no white coat; the joy she finds in medicine remains the joy of a cardigan, of participating in the stories of the people she meets as patients.

This participation is, both figuratively and literally, a narrative work for Cannon. When she meets a new patient, she experiences them as a new story. "Someone else was in her place—another story, another set of words."[27] Indeed, Cannon writes that lives are saved by stories.

> Lives can be saved by building up so much trust with a patient, they will still take a medication even if they don't believe they need it. Lives can be saved by listening to someone who has spent their entire life never being heard.[28]

Cannon becomes the storyteller. She carries each story, each patient with her, and it eventually burdens her. "As each day passed, I collected more and more people, and it was inevitable that the weight of those people would prove too much to bear."[29] Our words burden others. Becoming a doctor means hearing and carrying untold stories, a cargo whose weight can cause a physician-storyteller to falter under the unbearable burden.

For Cannon, being both a physician and a writer depends upon stories. Both are also, for Cannon, not jobs, but ways of being in the world. On the opening page of her memoir, Cannon writes: "My eyes swam with too much seeing."[30] As a way of being, becoming a physician means learning to see too much, adopting a seemingly omniscient view. Cannon later returns to the metaphor, writing:

> My hands shook and my eyes swam with too much seeing, and I wondered how someone could walk through a landscape and be at the very lowest point of their life and yet no one who passed by them even noticed.[31]

The physician carries too many stories and sees too much.

The language of seeing too much echoes an aphorism from the first truly contemporary physician-writer, William Osler. Addressing a graduating group of Army surgeons, Osler advised the graduates that "[t]he value of experience is not in seeing much, but in seeing wisely."[32] Osler delivered the speech in 1894, and it was later disseminated in a collection of his writings, *Aequanimitas*, whose very title is one of the professional virtues Cannon describes as ill-fitting. Osler is the physician most responsible for celebrating the equanimity among medical trainees and practitioners that Cannon finds suffocating; he was also the physician most responsible for creating today's training programs.

And yet, Cannon concludes *Breaking & Mending* by writing that she remains grateful she pursued that training because it made her a physician

> I look back and I can't imagine having done anything else. I can't imagine not meeting the incredible people I have had the privilege to meet, and I am amazed at the fragile decisions I made that allowed our paths to cross, even if it was only for the briefest of times.[33]

Cannon expresses gratitude that she became a physician because of the people she met, but an inability to stand with patients if it means standing within the complicit institutions where they seek care. Cannon retains the physician's relationship with patients, but not the relationship with medicine's institutions. Cannon gives up clinical practice, her relationship with institutions, but insists she is still a physician. A physician is a way of being in the world, of relating to ill people, which endures even if you leave its practice.

Practicing outside of medicine

And physicians are leaving the practice either for a time or for good. In its most recent annual report on the state of medical education and practice, the United Kingdom's General Medical Council reported that it has become so common for physicians to interrupt their career, reduce their clinical hours, or even leave clinical practice "that young doctors are pursuing different career paths from their older colleagues," which is now "the new reality" of medical practice.[34] According to the report, 12% of surveyed physicians had taken a leave of absence because of stress in the past year, 52% were planning to reduce their time spent in clinical practice over the coming year, and the only way to secure the National Health Service's future workforce will be to import physicians.[35]

Some of those imported physicians will need to provide mental health services to physicians themselves. The clinical psychologist Caroline Elton, who has spent a career working with British physicians, describes today's National Health Service as requiring physicians to live double narratives. Physicians must reassure their patients while maintaining low specialty referral rates, they must attend to the patient before them while multitasking, they must collect emotionally challenging information from patients while maintaining equanimity, and they must embody the profession's calling while serving the system's priorities. Elton writes that these burdens are most acute on trainees and junior physicians. Trainees, Elton observes, are educated in a system essentially unchanged from a century ago when Osler formulated it, while healthcare systems like the National Health Service have changed dramatically—ever-increasing regulatory and documentation requirements, escalating productivity requirements, and the erosion of clinical agency, all while keeping alive patients who would have surely died a century ago. Medical education no longer matches the needs of the systems into which physicians graduate.[36]

In Cannon's memoir, she writes that the medical school and the hospital teach different institutional lessons. "I was no longer in the safe embrace of the medical school; I was in a job now and this was not a job in which you spoke out."[37] The medical school embraced trainees; the hospital silenced physicians. Describing her first day working in the hospital, Cannon wrote of feeling abandoned by her supervisor, the consulting physician:

> At the end of the ward round, the consultant disappeared to theatre and the rest of us were left in the wake of a tornado, with a jobs list to divide up between us. There were notes to write, discharge letters to type, medications to change and blood tests to chase. Everything in medicine is chased.[38]

Through contemporary training processes experienced as constant chases, Elton writes that physicians like Cannon are enculturated to categorically distinguish between themselves and their patients. Doing so, Elton writes, serves a defensive psychological function.

> On a daily basis, doctors encounter distress, disease, and death. Doctors are mortal, as are the people they love. So any of the difficult things they see in their patients could happen in the future to them, their families, or their friends. … Positioning themselves as 'other' than their patients happens unconsciously, and assists doctors in going about their work without being psychologically overwhelmed by anxiety.[39]

The distinction is a fantasy. Physicians are human, will suffer loss, and will eventually be patients themselves. Yet the fantasy that a physician is different is reinforced by the institutions of medicine throughout medical training.

Medical training especially stigmatizes physicians who experience mental illness, so some psychiatrists have expressed public concern that signs of burnout are actually signs of depression. Leading psychiatrists have observed that the prevalent use of burnout provides a destigmatized way to conceptualize distress within medicine, but worry that it comes at the cost of continued silence about depression among physicians and trainees.[40] At times, Cannon's memoir raises the possibility, as when she writes:

> I barely ate. I hardly slept. I lost vast amounts of weight. My hair was matted and stuck to my skull. I would crawl into bed each night and lie in the darkness, unpicking the day, and each morning I would crawl out of bed, dress in the clothes closest to my hands, and I would walk back into a life I had begun to think of as the worst possible living hell.[41]

Physicians, especially trainees, often find it especially difficult to discuss mental health problems, the possibility of losing one's very mind, in the transition between training and practice.

Even words can lose their meaning.

Cannon writes that she swore humane oaths with her fellow trainees, but later found it impossible to keep a humane oath in an inhuman space.

> We repeated our oath and made our pledges with the utmost sincerity. Each sentence was meant, each vow considered, but words are always defined by their landscape, and words said in a grand auditorium with red velvet seats are very different to words remembered in the rush of a crash call or at the bedside of a dying patient. We thought we knew what those words meant, but their meaning would evolve with every step we took as doctors.[42]

Words, Cannon writes, are defined, not where they are spoken but by the places in which they are lived out.

The National Healthcare Service, Cannon writes, is a place which has weaponized the humane and noble language that physicians use to describe their labors.

> Medicine is a vocation, not a job, we are often told. The reality is, it is both, but when the conditions of the job become unbearable, when the demands made of us are likely to put our own lives at risk, not to mention the lives of the patients in our care, we are expected to continue to bear it because of a deep-rooted sense of purpose.[43]

The stories physicians have long told about their labors, that it is a vocation, now binds physicians to institutions that use a physician's calling against themselves. The job impedes the calling. "You quickly find that you can never be the doctor you wanted to become, because the doctor you wanted to become would not be able to survive."[44] The system, in Cannon's telling, entices a physician with a calling and then prevents a physician from living out her calling, from becoming the doctor she desired which she entered the hospital to become.

This lament is the language of a lost calling, but the subtitle of Cannon's memoir points to burnout, whose history is mechanical. The word entered the profession through the work of George Beard, a nineteenth-century neurologist. In 1869, he coined the term "neurasthenia" to describe a symptom constellation—anxiety, depression, headaches, impotence, insomnia, irritability, lethargy, muscle pain, weight loss—resulting from overwork in newly urbanized areas. Beard's neurasthenia was a diagnosis for the industrial revolution, and it borrowed the era's metaphors, imagining the person as a machine running on nervous energy and breaking down through overwork.[45] In 1974, the psychologist Herbert Freudenberger updated Beard's diagnostic portmanteau, calling it "burnout." In the early 1980s, Christina Maslach refined and operationalized burnout to describe a tripartite pathology of emotional exhaustion, depersonalization, and diminished personal accomplishment. Maslach conceptualized burnout as affecting all professions, but in particular health professions, because of the intimate encounters with the ill, especially the ill whose health could not be improved.[46]

Today, the Maslach Burnout Inventory is the most commonly used measure of physician distress, but physicians are beginning to resist its conceptualization. Contemporary psychiatrist commentators have observed that burnout, and the related concept of resiliency, makes well-being the responsibility of individuals while removing the responsibility for well-being from the institutions in which they labor. These commentators observe that calling burnout an epidemic and prescribing resilience strategies distract physicians from structural problems:

> The issue thus may not be long hours, increased workloads, and excessive charting alone. The larger problem may be that medicine is no longer in the hands of medical personnel, but of those who manage providers. It is to the institutions' and hospitals' benefit if we not only perform better, but also take the onus upon ourselves to make sure that we do.[47]

Burnout is becoming a diagnosis imposed upon physicians by institutional medicine to explain their distress while distracting them from the distress of others.

Perhaps physicians should seek treatments beyond those prescribed by institutional medicine. And diagnoses: Cannon's work suggests that burnout may actually be what Max Weber called disenchantment, the realization that our rationalized callings serve only impersonal, technical gods who make each individual responsible for her own calling.[48]

Cannon, for one, narrates individual solutions as impossible means for reenchanting medicine. Mental healthcare services are the most neglected among the NHS's many neglected services, and they can rapidly disenchant even the most committed psychiatrist if she stands alone against the system. The patients, Cannon observes, also stood alone; they were more isolated and disconnected than other patients in the NHS. Cannon says patients told her that no one knows them and no one would mourn them if, like Miss Creasy or Florence, they disappeared.

Cannon writes that the psychiatric patients were also, despite their disconnection, compassionate.

> It is a true saying that those who have the least give the most. I have seen patients share their very few possessions and clothes with someone who has been admitted with nothing. There are some people who never have visitors or anyone to care about them, and during visiting hours, I have witnessed one patient invite another to join their family instead of sitting with no one. I have seen those who have been on the wards a long time make a cup of tea for someone who had just been admitted, afraid and alone. When you are world-weary, or ward-weary, when you have had your fill of unkindness and cruelty and suffering, to witness small and quiet acts of compassion restores your faith in the world like nothing else.[49]

The acts of kindness and community by the least among us are restorative.

Cannon mercifully recalls these kindnesses from her psychiatric practice. She expresses and embodies real affection for psychiatry and for persons with mental illness, but concludes, for now, that she can best be a psychiatrist by being a writer outside of clinical practice. As she says, the psychiatrist still believes lives can be saved by stories.

Cannon's own stories finally raise more questions than it answers. What comes after you can no longer be the doctor you dreamed of being? What happens when the ending is unexpected and unhappy? What comes after a physician's war story, love story, and conversion story have all become burnout stories? For Cannon, it is becoming a writer who still exhibits the physician's stance in relationship to a patient: she is the someone you can tell.

But while the ranks of physician-writers have swelled, there are surely not enough publishing houses for every physician to practice medicine as a writer.

Burnout is only half of her memoir's subtitle. What if the solution to the disenchantment of medicine is the other half of the subtitle, compassion? Throughout her memoir and her novels, Cannon repeatedly narrates moments of compassion with language which bring her novels and memoir together into a larger project. Might medicine be reenchanted by shifting its institutions toward the compassionate giving away that Cannon found in the presence of persons with mental illness? What if medicine, say, reclaimed Matthew 25, from which Cannon borrowed the title of *The Trouble with Goats and Sheep*, but for an image of the physician as something more than a divine diagnostician? After all, the second half of the parable promises that after dividing goats and sheep, the judgment is meted out based on who fed the hungry, watered the thirsty, welcomed the stranger, clothed the naked, visited the sick and the imprisoned. Such judgment, the parable tells us, will be based in what was done for the least of all. What if the institutions of medicine measured a physician's practice that way: what you do for the indigent, the vulnerable? Is the real solution to burnout changing institutions to serve the least and those who, like Cannon, see them for themselves? Reading Cannon, where two children can find God in a creosote stain in a drainpipe, physicians are left to ask: what will it take for physicians to find their patients and their calling in an equivalently damaged, but redeemable, corner of today's institutions?

Notes

1 Lisa S. Rotenstein, Matthew Torre, Marco A. Ramos, Rachael C. Rosales, Constance Guille, Srijan Sen, and Douglas A. Mata. "Prevalence of Burnout among Physicians: A Systemic Review," *JAMA* 320, no. 11 (2018): 1131–1150.
2 National Academies of Sciences, Engineering, and Medicine, *Taking Action against Clinician Burnout: A Systems Approach to Professional Well-Being* (Washington, DC: The National Academic Press, 2019).
3 Tait D. Shanafelt and John H. Noseworthy, "Executive Leadership and Physician Well-Being: Nine Organizational Strategies to Promote Engagement and Reduce Burnout," *Mayo Clinic Proceedings* 92, no. 1 (2017): 129–146.
4 Joanna Cannon, *The Trouble with Goats and Sheep: A Novel* (New York: Scribner, 2016), 293.
5 Ibid., 113.
6 Matthew 25:33, King James Version.

7   Cannon, *The Trouble with Goats and Sheep*, 89.

8   Ibid., 202.

9   E.g., Joseph K. Campbell, Michael O'Rourke, and Matthew H. Slater, *Carving Nature at Its Joints: Natural Kinds in Metaphysics and Science* (Cambridge, MA: MIT Press, 2011).

10   "Author interview—Joanna Cannon," January 26, 2016. Accessed from https://www.vanessarobertson.co.uk/author-interview-joanna-cannon/ on August 20, 2021.

11   Cannon, *The Trouble with Goats and Sheep*, 338.

12   Joanna Cannon, *Three Things about Elsie: A Novel* (London: The Borough Press, 2018), 16.

13   Ibid., 14.

14   Ibid., 107.

15   Ibid., 323.

16   Ibid., 324.

17   Ibid., 165–166.

18   Ibid., 368.

19   Ibid., 238.

20   Ibid., 371–372.

21   Joanna Cannon, *Breaking and Mending: A Junior Doctor's Stories of Compassion and Burnout* (London: The Borough Press, 2019), 114.

22   Ibid., 149.

23   Ibid., 3.

24   Ibid., 2.

25   Ibid., 77–78.

26   Ibid., 103.

27   Ibid., 39.

28   Ibid., 14.

29   Ibid., 111–112.

30   Ibid., 1.

31   Ibid., 126.

32   William Osler, *Aequanimitas*, 2nd ed. (Philadelphia, PA: P. Blakinson's Son, 1914), 111.

33   Cannon, *Breaking and Mending*, 155–156.

34   "The State of Medical Education and Practice in the UK: The Workforce Report," General Medical Council, p. 9, published December 2019, Accessed from https://www. gmc-uk.org/-/media/documents/the-stateof-medical-education-and-practice-in-theuk---workforce-report_pdf-80449007.pdf on August 20, 2021.

35   Ibid., 22.

36   Caroline Elton, *Also Human: The Inner Lives of Doctors* (New York: Basic Books, 2018).

37   Cannon, *Breaking and Mending*, 102.

38   Ibid., 84.

39   Elton, *Also Human*, 129.

40   Maria A. Oquendo, Carol A. Bernstein, and Laurel E. S. Mayer, "A Key Differential Diagnosis for Physicians-Major Depression or Burnout?" *JAMA Psychiatry* 76, no. 11 (2019): 1111–1112.

41   Cannon, *Breaking and Mending*, 113.

42   Ibid., 77.

43   Ibid., 79–80.

44   Ibid., 104.

45   Tom Lutz, *American Nervousness, 1903: An Anecdotal History* (Ithaca, NY: Cornell University Press, 1991) and David G. Schuster, *Neurasthenic Nation: America's Search for Health, Happiness, and Comfort, 1869–1920* (New Brunswick, NJ: Rutgers University Press, 2011).

46 Christina Maslach, Susan E. Jackson, and Michael P. Leiter, *Maslach Burnout Inventory*, 3rd ed. (Palo Alto, CA: Consulting Psychologists Press, 1996).
47 Helena Winston and Bruce Fage, "Resilience, Resistance: A Commentary on the Historical Origins of Resilience and Wellness Initiatives," *Psychiatric Services* 70, no. 8 (2019): 739.
48 Max Weber, David S. Owen, Tracey B. Strong, and Rodney Livingstone, *The Vocation Lectures* (Indianapolis, IN: Hackett Publishing, 2004); for a further exploration of disenchantment in contemporary medicine, see Abraham M. Nussbaum, "The Worthless Remains of a Physician's Calling: Max Weber, William Osler, and the Last Virtue of Physicians," *Theoretical Medicine and Bioethics* 39, no. 6 (2018): 419–429.
49 Cannon, *Breaking and Mending*, 140–141.

9   Damon Tweedy

Stories on being Black, sick, and marginalized

Keisha Ray

Introduction

Given Black people's overall poor health outcomes, a person might conclude that being Black is bad for your health. In *Black Man in a White Coat: A Doctor's Reflections on Race and Medicine*, Damon Tweedy, a Black male psychiatrist examines how different social inequities map onto the Black race, demonstrating that it's not so much that being Black is bad for your health, but lacking certain social determinants of health is bad for your health.[1] Throughout the text Tweedy recounts some of the interactions he had with Black patients during medical school, residency, internships, and during his time as an attending psychiatrist. As Tweedy tells these stories, it becomes clear that the patients are not the only subject of the story, but that social determinants of health also have a starring role in these stories. For instance, he frequently notes that his Black patients' experiences of illness were almost always complicated by a lack of income, health insurance, transportation, or safe housing. Additionally, racism from healthcare providers also made it harder for them to secure proper health.

Social determinants of health are the social, cultural, and economic goods that we need to ensure our health.[2] Social determinants of health include access to safe housing, recreation areas, and clean drinking water and air, as well as access to transportation, technology, and other social goods. No matter how well our bodies and minds are functioning, a lack of access to such social determinants of health can make us unhealthy and have less well-being. Differential access to social determinants of health is one contributing factor to racial disparities in health because social determinants of health often map onto race. In particular, people of color, on average, have less access to many social determinants of health. Tweedy highlights these inequities in his patients' stories. And it is through their experiences with hypertension, diabetes, uterine fibroids, and other illnesses that Tweedy reveals the ways in which a patient's very identity as a Black person also complicates their experiences with illness and their experiences of seeking care. As race—or, rather, racism—is also a social determinant of health, in Tweedy's stories it becomes clear that his Black patients have this additional barrier to proper health.

DOI: 10.4324/9781003079712-9

What makes Tweedy's story-telling compelling and unique is that in each patient story he uses the patient to represent many other Black patients who are in the same position. For example, Tweedy uses the story of a woman named Pearl and her experiences with untreated hypertension while seeking care in a rural community as the face, as it were, of Black people's overall higher rates of hypertension[3] and rural people's lack of access to quality and affordable healthcare.[4] Pearl is but one of the many patients we meet in Tweedy's text whose experiences of poor health were coupled with inadequate access to social determinants of health.

As much as this text is a compilation of stories about mostly Black patients, it is also a tale of a Black man's experiences in medicine. From a professor in medical school mistaking him for maintenance staff to racism from colleagues and patients to his own experiences with illness, this text also tells Tweedy's story. That is to say, it tells the story of a Black man navigating a racially inequitable healthcare system yet recognizing the class privileges bestowed on him by his position as a physician, which his patients don't have. *Black Man in a White Coat* is Tweedy's reflections on race, social determinants of health, and his own growth as a Black man, who is also a caregiver. In this chapter, I offer a critical, while sympathetic, engagement of Tweedy's story of what it means to be Black, marginalized, and ill in America.

Biography

In *Black Man in a White Coat*, Tweedy gives us a look at some of the experiences that shaped his views of medicine and his perception of what it means to be a Black man who is also a physician. One of Tweedy's more significant and relatable experiences occurred during a lecture at Duke University School of Medicine, where Tweedy was a student. After studying very hard during his first year of medical school, Tweedy received his midterm scores; they were high enough to put him in the top half of the class. After reeling from his high scores, Tweedy chatted with some fellow students during a break in a lecture. He then exited the classroom, and, upon his return, his professor, Dr. Gale, approached him and asked, "Are you here to fix the lights?" Tweedy examined his polo shirt and khaki pants, his clean-shaven face, looking to see if his appearance had given his professor any reason to believe that he was not a Duke student. After telling Dr. Gale that he was not there to repair the lights, the professor asked, "Then what are you doing here in my class?" to which Tweedy replied that he was a student in the course. With Dr. Gale's reply of "Oh," the confidence his high midterm scores gave him were shattered. He had a difficult time focusing on his other courses that day because he could not stop thinking about the meaning of this encounter. Seemingly, in an attempt to prove his worthiness, Tweedy even vowed to study harder than ever before.[5] This experience is significant to Tweedy's story because it is an example of how race and racial biases would continue to be an inescapable and prominent fixture in his career in medicine. Dr. Gale's case of mistaken identity told Tweedy that he did not belong at an elite medical school like Duke. Dr. Gale exacerbated Tweedy's insecurities and feelings of not belonging in medical school. Like Tweedy, many Black professionals have a "mistaken identity" story, including myself.

One of my first experiences with mistaken identity occurred while I was a postdoctoral fellow preparing to teach my morning course. Another university employee entered my classroom and asked me to clean a spill for him. Like Tweedy, I looked at my attire to see if my clothing gave him the impression that I was a member of the janitorial staff. I examined my professional-looking floral dress and dress shoes and wondered what about me said that I am the house-keeper and not the instructor leading this class. When I told him he was inter-rupting my class and that he should seek a member of the janitorial staff, the surprised look on his face told me all that I needed to know about his perception of me. I knew that it was my race (and perhaps also gender and age) that told this person that I did not belong in front of the classroom but, rather, clean-ing the classroom. Like Tweedy, this experience was significant in my career because it was not the first time, nor the last time, that a student or university employee made it clear to me that they did not believe I belonged leading a university class.

When Tweedy started seeing patients as a second-year medical student, he began to see how the intersection of race and social determinants of health played out in Black patients' lives. His observations continued during his third year of medical school when he chose to work at a clinic in rural North Carolina that did not have a doctor's office. The people who came to the clinic were mostly Black and mostly uninsured, which made it difficult for them to get proper care. And by the time Tweedy graduated from medical school in 2000, he continued to witness Black patients' wide-ranging levels of poor health.

In 2003, Tweedy graduated from Yale Law School and then returned to Duke for further medical training. As Tweedy went on to complete his internship at Duke, he encountered both Black and White patients who openly requested to not be treated by a Black doctor. Tweedy also encountered colleagues whose racial biases hindered proper patient care. In these cases, Tweedy was faced with the dilemma of making sure that the patients received proper care but also mak-ing sure that he kept his professional relationships intact and did not become known as "a racially sensitive" person.

During his psychiatry residency, in Duke's emergency department Tweedy treated patients with mental illnesses, some of whom doubted his abilities to treat them because of his race. He contemplated the value of race-matching, a process in which doctors and patients are matched because of their shared race, a practice he ultimately deemed unnecessary. He continued to work for Duke, including working at an outpatient mental health clinic, for seven years. By 2013, Tweedy was a faculty member at Duke. As of 2020, Duke's website lists Tweedy as an associate professor of psychiatry and behavioral sciences and employed by the Durham VA Health Care System where he leads a team of mental healthcare providers.

Tweedy as a patient

As Tweedy tells the stories of his patients and their experience of illness, he also tells his own. For example, as he retells his patients' experiences with hypertension, he also tells the story of when he learned he had hypertension. During his first year of medical school, he and a classmate were practicing taking blood pressure readings on each other. When both the classmate and the instructor got a very high reading, he went to see a doctor. The doctor confirmed that he had hypertension; he also was in the early stages of kidney failure.

Throughout his life Tweedy staved off disease by changing his lifestyle, including his eating and exercise habits. Though there were times when he fell off the path of proper diet and fitness, and his blood pressure would rise enough for him to start the medication to treat it, he would eventually get back on a healthier track. To do this, though, Tweedy had to overcome cultural beliefs and racial biases about a healthy lifestyle. For instance, he associated yoga and eating salads with insecure White women, and eating organic food and running in the woods with White men who wanted to return to nature, which did not interest him. To maintain his health, he had to give up gendered and racialized beliefs that were preventing him from lowering his blood pressure. Though he would overcome these thoughts, it was a struggle for him to consistently eat well and exercise. He referred to himself as a "close cousin to the yo-yo dieter who loses twenty or thirty pounds only to gain it all back each time."[6] But, in time, he was able to make consistent lifestyle changes to maintain his health.

Tweedy also tells the story of his experience with seeking treatment for knee pain. After years of playing basketball in high school and college, and then playing in local leagues and local pickup games after college, in his 30s Tweedy experienced great knee pain. While seeing Dr. Parker for his troubles, Dr. Parker dismissed his pain without a physical examination of his knee. With just a visual examination, he attributed his pain to a bruise or sprain and told him to rest his knee for a while. After Tweedy made a comment about a previous surgery, Dr. Parker recognized that he must be in the medical profession based on the language Tweedy used. After asking if Tweedy was an X-ray tech, Tweedy informed him that he was a physician. Dr. Parker's demeanor changed. He then began to treat Tweedy with more regard. After chatting, Dr. Parker suggested that he take a deeper look at his knee. He then performed an actual exam and ordered X-rays. Dr. Parker offered him pain medication, a knee brace, and crutches. He even personally called Tweedy the next day with the radiologist's reading of the X-ray. Dr. Parker also had acquired a better brace than the one Tweedy had been given, free of charge, although Tweedy told him it wasn't necessary. Tweedy's visit with Dr. Parker and his experience with medical racism parallels the stories that he tells of his own patients and their experiences with medical staff whose racial biases influenced their level of treatment. (Of note, Tweedy's story is a lot like the story Gary in the text, a patient who was diagnosed with a psychiatric disorder because the White physician treating him thought he was exaggerating his complaints of chest pain.[7])

What makes Tweedy's analysis of his own health journey fascinating is that he recounts how his determination to get healthy coincided and was inspired by his own patients' struggles with health and maintaining a healthy weight. By showing these parallel experiences, Tweedy is saying that as a Black man he experiences some of the same health and social ailments that are rampant in the Black community. His status as a physician in many ways does not protect him from poor health. He even experiences racial biases from caregivers like when Dr. Parker who assumed that he must be an X-ray technician and not a physician.

Similar to Tweedy, physicians have also assumed that I am a teaching assistant and were very shocked when I told them I was a professor. As the latter half of his interaction with Dr. Parker shows, however, being a physician gives Tweedy some advantages in the healthcare system when he is seeking care just like being a college professor gives me certain advantages, advantages that Tweedy's patients and many other Black patients do not have. In the next section, I will continue to explore Tweedy's reflections on the ways his patients' Black race disadvantaged them in the healthcare system.

Tina and Pearl: Black, poor, and rural

During Tweedy's third year of medical school, he volunteered to work at a pop-up clinic in a rural area of North Carolina, where no physician had an office. The clinic opened one Saturday each month and was staffed by Duke students, one senior resident, and one faculty member. The patients were all Black, uninsured, and poor. Here is where he met Pearl and Tina.

Pearl, a Black woman in her 50s, came to the clinic to be screened for diabetes and hypertension. Her visit began with an interest in Tweedy. Pearl was happy to see a Black man in the role of the physician, noting, "It's so good to see a young brother in a white coat. That don't happen much 'round here.'"[8] When the focus of the visit returned to Pearl, she told Tweedy that one or two years ago she was told that she was borderline diabetic and hypertensive. She came to the clinic because her brother started dialysis and his situation encouraged her to get a checkup herself. After taking Pearl's vital signs, Tweedy determined that her blood sugar levels and blood pressure were both higher than they should be, so he recommended that she begin taking medication for both hypertension and diabetes. When the attending physician, however, went over Tweedy's treatment plan, he did not approve of his drug recommendations.

Although Tweedy prescribed Pearl standard medications, because Pearl was being seen at this pop-up clinic, they had to make some considerations about her financial and social status. For instance, they did not know whether Pearl had health insurance, and her visit to a free clinic was a big indication that she did not. They also had to consider that the clinic would not be back in the area for at least another month, meaning that Pearl would go at least a month before seeing a doctor again. When developing treatment options for Pearl, Tweedy did not even think about whether she could afford to purchase the medication.

The physician also found signs of nerve damage in Pearl's feet and was concerned about nerve damage in her eyes, both complications of diabetes. It was then that Pearl informed them that she did not have health insurance and could not afford the out-of-pocket costs treating her nerve damage would require. So, the best that the doctors could do was perform some basic lab tests. They gave her a prescription for the cheapest diabetic pill available and a sample pack of medication for hypertension, and test strips to check her blood glucose levels (using her brother's machine). They also gave her the name of a clinic a half an hour's drive away where she could obtain a free or low-cost eye exam. And with that and a recommendation to lower the weight on her 5 feet 4 inch, 210-pound body, they sent Pearl on her way.

At the same clinic, Tweedy also saw a patient named Tina. Tina was nearly 40, and she was a slender Black woman. She came to the clinic with complaints of excessive vaginal bleeding. Although Tina took steps to maintain her health like not drinking alcohol, nor using illicit drugs or smoking cigarettes, Tina had high blood pressure. The resident took charge of Tina's visit while Tweedy mostly observed. After an examination, Tina was diagnosed with uterine fibroids. The resident recommended that Tina see a specialist at Duke for care.

While Tweedy observed, the resident spoke with Tina about how to treat her high blood pressure. Tina informed them that she did not have health insurance. She once had temporary Medicaid when she was pregnant with her last child but she was removed from the program after delivery. Even though this was the only social history that Tina provided, Tweedy filled in the rest on his own. He assumed that she was unmarried and a single mother. He also assumed that she was uninsured because she did not have a job. But Tweedy was wrong. Tina was married to her husband for ten years, and he worked at his own business. Tina worked at a convenience store, but neither her job nor her husband's job provided health insurance. With their income of around $25,000, she was removed from Medicaid because, she was told, she and her husband made too much money to qualify for the healthcare program. Although Tina and her husband inquired about private health insurance, they could not afford the premiums. They felt secure that at least their two children had state-sponsored health coverage, even though they did not. With this information, the resident gave her a prescription for a low-cost diuretic pill (the clinic was out of free sample pills), told her someone would contact her with her lab results, and gave them a recommendation that Tina should return to the clinic when they are back operating next month.

From his first time at the clinic in rural North Carolina, Tweedy comments that three issues stood out to him: (1) all the patients were Black; (2) there was a stark difference in the care dispensed at the clinic and the care that he saw given to patients at Duke; and (3) all of the patients had chronic medical issues caused or worsened by their lifestyle. These observations seemed to create some conflict for Tweedy. Although he wanted to blame these patients for their health issues (e.g., the choice of eating McDonald's and watching TV rather than eating healthy and taking a walk), he saw this as a detached way of thinking about his patients that came from a place of limited perspective.

Pearl and Tina challenged Tweedy's way of thinking about Black people with poor health as well as people without health insurance. Despite coming from a working-class background, Tweedy's parents and brother had jobs that offered them health insurance, so his family life did not expose him to the trials of being uninsured. Because he was unaware how uninsured people lived, Tweedy believed that uninsured people were so because they did not work and that they must get healthcare from government-sponsored programs. So, when he met Tina and Pearl and many other patients like them at the clinic, he was forced to confront these biases.

Tweedy seemed to use his own experiences with hypertension to confront his biases about Black people being fully responsible for their poor health. For instance, Black people consistently have higher rates of hypertension than White people.[9] But what Tweedy discovered during his time in the clinic is that when he compared his own experience with hypertension to that of someone like Tina and Pearl, it was clear that socioeconomic status and education play a role in Black people's disproportionate experience of hypertension. Specifically, his higher socioeconomic status and education level gave him advantages that contributed to his better health outcomes. For instance, Tweedy had medical knowledge and worked within close proximity of physicians every day, who could impart knowledge when asked. Tina, on the other hand, had a high school diploma, and Pearl had only a tenth-grade education—and neither woman worked with physicians. Tweedy, although a poor medical student at the time, also had the benefit of his social standing. Tweedy had access to Duke's gymnasiums for exercise and nearby grocery stores and restaurants that offered healthy food options. Tina and Pearl, however, had limited exercise and healthy eating options. Similarly, Tweedy also had health insurance in which his doctor visits and medications were covered. He also had one physician responsible for his treatment with whom he could establish a relationship. Tina and Pearl only received care at the clinic, and with each visit they may see a completely new physician. They also may need more expensive medication in the future to control their chronic disorders and had to worry about how to pay for them. Thus, although both Pearl and Tina had hypertension, just like Tweedy, and all three individuals are Black, their access to key social determinants of health put them worlds apart.

Critique

At this point in the text, however, I wish Tweedy would have given more attention to the social determinants of health. It's not that Black people are never to blame for our poor health. If we have the financial means, education, transportation, and other social factors necessary to eat a healthy meal, but instead we choose fast food, it may be right to consider our role in our poor health. However, for some people, eating healthily or exercising is just plain difficult if not impossible. And I wish Tweedy showed more curiosity in how a lack of access to social determinants of health affected Pearl and Tina's health. For instance, Pearl and

Tina both made efforts to care for themselves. With no nearby doctor in their rural town, they made an effort to seek care from the clinic. Tina even took health measures like avoiding alcohol and cigarettes. This indicates that they care about their health. So, I think they deserved the benefit of the doubt that if they had better and knew better, then maybe they would do better. I would have liked to know whether Pearl and Tina knew what foods are healthy and conducive to warding off hypertension and diabetes. Are there grocery stores in their neighborhood that sell healthy foods? And if so, did they have transportation to these stores? Do they have the income to purchase healthy food, which is oftentimes more expensive than high fat, sugary foods? Did they have access to safe recreation areas? From the little information we have about Pearl and Tina, we can conclude that some important social determinants of health are inadequate in their lives.

To be fair, Tweedy and his colleagues saw a lot of patients at the pop-up clinic. Many of the town's residents took advantage of the small healthcare team because it was their only access to healthcare providers, so they likely did not have the time to educate patients on healthy practices or ask them about their social health. The failure is not Tweedy's alone; it is the healthcare system, employment system, and food production system that failed Pearl and Tina and others like them. Where we live and the nature of our neighborhoods and communities is also a product of a social system, which has a great influence on our health, yet failed and continues to fail people like Pearl and Tina.

Rural communities are notoriously plagued by disparities in health outcomes and healthcare largely because of a lack of access to a number of particular social determinants of health. For instance, people in rural areas are more likely to die from suicide, heart disease, cancer, stroke, and opioid overdoses. Some reasons for these disparities are that people in rural communities have less access to healthcare, including specialty and emergency care facilities. People in rural communities also have higher exposure to environmental hazards, and limited access to healthy foods and recreation areas. In part, because of this, people in rural areas are also more likely to suffer from hypertension and obesity, have lower rates of exercise, higher rates of poverty, and are less likely to have health insurance. Rural residents also tend to be older, have lower incomes, and have less education when compared to people in more urban areas.[10]

When race and rurality intersect, the outcomes are worse for Black and indigenous people who live in rural communities. Black and indigenous residents of rural communities have higher mortality rates than Black urban residents.[11] This is another instance of how the intersection of race and social determinants of health could have played a bigger role in Tweedy's stories about his encounters with Black patients. Doing so would help readers understand the invisible yet prominent forces that are driving his patients' poor health.

Lessons for Black scholars, students, and healthcare providers

Tweedy uses his patients' stories to show that often the result of the intersection of race and inequities in social determinants of health is poor health for Black individuals. But another running theme in his text is Tweedy's contemplations on what it means to be a Black doctor. From being one of the few Black students in his medical school to White and Black patients doubting his abilities and requesting White physicians, the fact that he is a Black man was a constant fixture in his career. As a result, Tweedy was always aware that he was not just a physician, but a Black physician. And what did this mean for him, his colleagues, and his patients? What did this mean for the advancement of his career? Did he have a special obligation to his Black patients? This contemplation of what role race played in his own story is one of the most salient features of the text that can benefit Black medical students, interns, physicians, and other current and future healthcare providers.

Although I am not a clinician, I connected to Tweedy's thoughts on what it means to be a Black physician. I frequently think about my obligation to Black people and their pursuit of better healthcare and better health outcomes. My specialty in bioethics is Black health. I study the ways inequities in social determinants of health contribute to poor health for Black people, but this wasn't always my specialty. In fact, early on in my career I made it a point to *not* study any topic related to race. But I changed career path and became a researcher of Black health because I felt a strong obligation to help this group of people, who were vulnerable to unequal power structures and unjust social institutions. Simply, I wanted to help. And I think many Black healthcare providers who want to help Black patients have better health outcomes also feel this pull, or what some may say is a calling. But this doesn't mean that Black physicians and scholars don't have other interests. To balance my calling to research Black health and my other scholarly interests, I make sure to devote time to expanding my research efforts to areas outside of Black health. This was my takeaway message from Tweedy's own story but there are many other messages that would help any Black professional.

Another lesson that Black students and physicians could learn from Tweedy's story is the value of vulnerability. It took courage for Tweedy to open up about the biases he held against Black and White people and biases he held against gay people. Him sharing this information gives permission for other Black professionals to share and confront their own biases so that they don't affect their patients. Tweedy's willingness to be vulnerable made him a better caregiver and I suspect it allowed him to come to terms with his own story in medicine. All healthcare providers have a story; the story of how they came to medicine and the story of how they think about their role in medicine. Being vulnerable can help individuals come to terms with their story, even the not-so-great parts. But it can also help healthcare providers connect to their patients who they see during the most vulnerable time in their lives. This connection could be one way to acknowledge race, class, gender, and sexual orientation differences that may exist between provider and patient while still connecting on a human-to-human level.

Another lesson in Tweedy's text comes from his successes as a story-teller as well as from his failures. For example, Tweedy saw a patient named Sean. Sean, an 18-year-old Black male, came to the emergency room for wounds related to gun violence he suffered while playing basketball in a neighborhood park. Although

Tweedy uses Sean and other patients' stories to take a critical look at the ways healthcare disadvantages Black people via medical racism, he does not apply this same critical lens to other social institutions that contribute to poor health, such as our governments that enact laws that affect people's lives. For instance, even a brief discussion of unsafe neighborhoods or laws that govern access to firearms would have enriched readers' understanding of Sean's story.

Rather than examining how people ended up in his care, however, Tweedy frequently placed the blame on Black people for their experiences of consequences conferred upon them by unjust social institutions. This way of thinking makes it seem as if Black people choose to be poor and choose to live under conditions that contribute to poor health, and all they have to do is work harder to fix their situations. This way of thinking also ignores the deliberate and structural steps institutions that govern people took to intentionally disadvantage Black people in an effort to maintain White supremacy, also known as structural racism.[12] Tweedy places an undeserved amount of moral responsibility on patients like Sean and, therefore, contributes to a lack of understanding of structural racism in medicine. This means that when discussing patients like Sean, where he and his family lived, how they came to live in that poor and disadvantaged neighborhood, and what institutional policies and laws kept their family in that neighborhood is just as important to his story as the gunshot wound itself. When discussing Black individuals' health, we cannot start with an examination of healthcare; we must start with an examination of all the unjust social institutions that contribute to their poor health. We also must consider the compounding effects of unjust institutions and the difficulties they pose to social mobility and good health.

In the stories of Pearl and Tina, we see some sympathy for this way of thinking about Black health when Tweedy gives some attention to the sociocultural roots of their life decisions. But at the end of the text he seems to fall back on the habit of moralizing Black people's decisions and telling Black people to do better. Tweedy is correct that Black people have to take some responsibility for their own health despite institutions that work against their achievement of good health. But the obstacles created by those institutions that govern so much of our lives must be a part of the story of how Black people came to have health outcomes that are inferior to White people. Given that Black people, even when they are wealthy, generally have poorer health outcomes than White people with lesser incomes and lower education levels,[13] an examination of Black health must be all-encompassing and not narrowed to just the effects of unjust healthcare but also include the institutions that maintain White supremacy and act as a barrier to proper health for Black people.

Conclusion

In the stories that Tweedy tells in *Black Man in a White Coat*, we frequently see Tweedy's frustrations with medicine and its limited ability to help patients experience well-rounded health. Tweedy's frustrations are oftentimes a result of him grappling with his own limitations as a steward of medicine and his thoughts about whether he has a special duty to his Black patients as a Black physician. In doing so Tweedy shows us how being Black adds another layer to the patient experience for Black people but it also adds another layer to the experience of being a physician. Although race played a role in both the lives of Tweedy and his Black patients, because of their class differences, his patients had an extra barrier to proper health.

The social determinants of health are an extra character in Tweedy's stories. They wield their power over people like Tina, Pearl, Gary, and Sean, making their homes unsafe, their food unhealthy, and their access to healthcare limited. In Tweedy's text we only get a snapshot of the ways his story as a Black doctor intersected with some of his Black patients. But in these snapshots, we see two different perspectives summed up into one question: do we ignore race and treat all patients and physicians alike, or do we treat patients and physicians differently, acknowledging their race and using it for decision-making? We see these dueling perspectives when Tweedy contemplates race-matching, i.e., Black doctors with Black patients. How we answer this question can create a rich discussion about the role race ought to play in healthcare, and Tweedy's text contributes to this discussion. Although Tweedy does not directly answer this question (and I'm glad he does not), he does give us a glimpse at what he finds important and that is the belief that everyone, regardless of race, wants to be seen, heard, and treated with respect, especially when sick and seeking care from medicine's gatekeepers.

Notes

1 Damon Tweedy, *Black Man in a White Coat: A Doctor's Reflections on Race and Medicine* (New York: Picador, 2015).
2 "Social Determinants of Health," Office of Disease Prevention and Health Promotion, accessed August 20, 2021: https://www.healthypeople.gov/2020/topics-objectives/topic/social-determinants-of-health.
3 Michael C. Stein, Chim C. Lang, Hong-Guang Xie, and Alastair J. J. Wood, "Hypertension in Black People: Study of Specific Genotypes and Phenotypes Will Provide a Greater Understanding of Interindividual and Interethnic Variability in Blood Pressure Regulation than Studies Based on Race," *Pharmacogenetics* 11, no. 2 (2001): 95–100.
4 Mark S. Eberhardt and Elsie R. Pamuk, "The Importance of Place of Residence: Examining Health in Rural and Nonrural Areas," *American Journal of Public Health* 94, no. 10 (2004): 1682–1686; Thomas C. Ricketts, *Rural Health in the United States* (New York: Oxford University Press, 1999).
5 Tweedy, *Black Man*, 12–13.
6 Ibid., 219.
7 Ibid., 129.
8 Ibid., 56.
9 Flacio D. Fuchs, "Why Do Black Americans Have Higher Prevalence of Hypertension?" *Hypertension* 2011, no. 57 (2011): 379–380; Vincent B. A. Chen, Hongyan Ning, and Norrina Allen, "Lifetime Risks for Hypertension by Contemporary Guidelines in African American and White Men and Women," *Journal of American Medical Association Cardiology* 4, no. 5 (2019): 455–459.
10 "About Rural Health," Centers for Disease Control and Prevention, accessed August 20, 2021: https://www.cdc.gov/ruralhealth/about.html; "Rural Health," Centers for

Disease Control and Prevention, accessed August 20, 2021: https://www.cdc.gov/chronicdisease/resources/publications/factsheets/rural-health.htm.

11 Carrie E. Henning-Smith, Ashley M. Hernandez, and Rachel R. Hardeman, "Rural Countries with Majority Black or Indigenous Populations Suffer the Highest Rates of Premature Death in the US," *Health Affairs* 38, no. 2 (2019): https://www.healthaffairs.org/doi/abs/10.1377/hlthaff.2019.00847.

12 Richard Rothstein, *The Color of Law* (Chicago, IL: University of Chicago Press, 2017).

13 Chandra L. Jackson, Susan Redline, and Ichiro Kawachi, "Racial Disparities in Short Sleep Duration by Occupation and Industry," *American Journal of Epidemiology* 178, no. 9 (2013): 1442–1451.

10 Fady Joudah

An exploration of borders and boundaries

Andrew Childress

Introduction

Borders are more than lines on a map. They can allow strangers to cross into unfamiliar lands, but they also can exclude both strangers and friends alike. Boundaries serve to define the limits, not just of nation-states, time zones, and biological structures but also of relationships and cultural norms. Fady Joudah's poetry asks numerous important questions about the purpose of borders and boundaries. Who mans these border crossings? What does life look like on the other side? How do we move beyond stereotypes to a more nuanced understanding of different cultures? Taken as a whole or individually, his poems serve as "internal maps or orienting devices" that can help physicians and patients navigate through the borderlands of medicine.[1]

Born in Austin, Texas, to Palestinian parents, Joudah's family would give him coins for memorizing Palestinian poetry as a child. His father left Palestine at the tender age of 14 (during the Palestinian exodus, also known as the *Nakba* or "catastrophe"), while his mother was born in a refugee camp in Gaza. His Palestinian heritage, which he describes as a "lineage" of exile, contributes to the nomadic feel of his poetry as it abruptly shifts from place to place.[2] When he was almost a teenager, his family relocated to Libya and then Saudi Arabia. He grew up speaking Arabic but became fluent in English before moving to Georgia for pre-med and medical school. He completed his medical residency training at The University of Texas Health Science Center Houston before practicing emergency medicine at Michael E. DeBakey VA Medical Center. He is currently an internist at Baylor St. Luke's Medical Center. Despite a series of demanding day jobs, Joudah has published four volumes of poetry dealing with a wide range of subjects from Middle Eastern geopolitics to deeply personal reflections on his nervousness as a father to a newborn.

There are some schools of literary criticism that discourage readers from making connections between a writer's background and their work. Proponents of this view argue that what is being said in the text matters independently of its relationship to an actual person's life.[3] However, Joudah's identity as a Palestinian-American and as a physician shapes his poetry to such a large extent that ignoring the tension between his personal and professional identity would almost certainly

DOI: 10.4324/9781003079712-10

lead to an impoverished understanding of his work. As this chapter will show, the social location of the poet and the speaker plays a significant role in crafting the borders and boundaries between the subject and the reader. As readers, we want to believe that these boundaries are both necessary and permeable. But we also need a reliable and self-aware guide to navigate them with us. For these reasons, the question of identity for Joudah plays a key role in his writing and what he thinks about his writing. It should also inform the reader's interpretation of his poems.

In interviews, Joudah gives conflicting opinions on how he views himself. Most of the time, it's his Arabic or Palestinian heritage that is important, more than his occupation or his American citizenship. For example, when asked for his five-word biography during an interview, he placed "Palestinian-American" first and "doctor" last.[4] On other occasions, he bemoans the contradiction inherent in the "amazing American obsession: actually reducing one's humanity to one's difference under the guise of celebrating one's difference."[5] Making sense of how assumptions about cultural barriers obstruct the recognition of our common humanity is the goal of many cultural engagement practices.[6] Reading poetry that emerges from writers like Joudah who incorporate multiple cultural identities into their sense of self can help inform explanatory models of illness that can then be used to navigate cultural barriers. The tension between speaking up for displaced or marginalized people and trying to avoid usurping their voice is apparent in Joudah's poetry.

In addition to asking questions about his cultural background, nearly every interviewer comments on Joudah's dual occupation of poet and physician. They seem to assume that the two are diametrically opposed in some way or that the relationship is particularly complex. When he's asked about what influence medicine has on his poetry, his answers are often a bit cagey or cryptic. For him, the "question of the doctor-poet has an algorithmic answer to it: a conversation about healing, science, eros, thanatos, William Carlos Williams or Gottfried Benn, etc."[7] To answer the question in an unscripted fashion, Joudah feels compelled to implicate himself in the power structures inherent in medicine, while speaking out against being a "physician in empire and of it."[8] In this response, there is a strong sense of guilt for being a victim of imperialism and the asymmetries of power that permitted imperialism to thrive. Joudah also reflects on the asymmetries of power within medicine, in which he considers himself complicit while simultaneously being a survivor and a critic of these larger forces.

As part of his education on the effects of imperialism and capitalism on the practice of medicine, Joudah served in refugee camps in Zambia and Darfur as part of Doctors Without Borders. He writes about some of these experiences in *The Earth in the Attic*, for which he won the Yale Series of Younger Poets competition in 2007, and *Alight*, his second poetry collection. He has won multiple awards and prizes, including the Banipal Prize for Arabic Literary Translation for translating works by Mahmoud Darwish, PEN Center USA Literary Award, and a Guggenheim Fellowship.

Why read poetry?

Despite the instrumental and intrinsic value of poetry and the fact that most of the high-impact medical journals have sections dedicated to poetry, some students and healthcare practitioners simply refuse to engage with a poem. They see poetry as disconnected from their experience—not clinically relevant, or too abstract to be worth investigating. At first glance, someone reading Joudah's work may agree with these critiques. But a second, or even a third, reading can reveal insights and develop capacities that are easily translatable into improving the practice of medicine. Poetry "encourages readers to entertain several possible interpretations without necessarily finding a 'correct answer.'"[9] It promotes tolerance of ambiguity, which is a key skill given the problem of prognostic uncertainty in decision-making.[10] Tolerance of ambiguity also opens up space for "getting into ignorance, surrendering oneself to the mercy of someone else's voice."[11] Spending time absorbing the unique language and rhythm of poetry can help physicians and students become more skilled communicators. They learn to dissolve boundaries that exist between strangers by listening for each other's "inner voice."[12] As Raphael Campo, a poet-physician, notes, physicians "who lack a passion for language or who fail to see beauty will be at a loss to translate those wonders in the most meaningful terms for their lay patients."[13] Finally, poetry provides a needed complement to the scientific manner of thinking that students cultivate as part of their medical training.

Medical education is intended to produce physicians who can draw on scientific knowledge, clinical experience, and excellent communication skills to diagnose and treat disease. Part of this education involves learning a new language: medical science. To the novice speaker, the vocabulary and syntax of this language may seem strange, oddly formal, elegant, and obscure. It has been developed over millennia, based on scientific reasoning and classification systems, to create a common language for diagnosing and treating disease. Everyone in the clinical setting knows what "myocardial infarction," "He's coding!" or "Defibrillator, stat!" means. They've all learned the same vocabulary and agreed that these terms represent scientifically proven facts about the world that require immediate action. Without clear and precise language in this setting, healthcare workers could become confused, make serious mistakes, and accidentally harm patients. For students, medical jargon provides shelter from the messier aspects of medical care. It gives them a sense of objectivity, cultural authority, and confidence. They may also feel that it shields them from worries about making an error. This language is not just spoken but also pervades the medical literature such that it almost entirely consists of "pieces of writing that are models of rationality and logic, and that require stripped-down, clinical language and do away with anecdote and allusiveness."[14] Only recently has poetry invaded this space as well.

Outside of the clinical setting, students and healthcare workers revert back to their usual ways of speaking and thinking. They tell stories instead of presenting cases. Words are allowed to have multiple meanings and convey emotions.

In their native tongues, medical students and others use metaphors, symbols, imagery, and other creative ways of speaking to tell stories and develop personal connections with one another. Outside of the clinic and the classroom, they are much more comfortable admitting that they are feeling uncertain or ambivalent. What some students fail to realize is that these feelings are actually part of the clinical experience as well, yet they remain hidden underneath the cloak of objectivity and detachment. Joudah and other physician-writers demonstrate that it is possible to live in both words simultaneously.

They can do this because they have developed what John Keats described as "negative capability," meaning that they are "capable of being in uncertainties, mysteries, doubts, without any irritable reaching after fact and reason."[15] Physicians who have developed this capacity can admit uncertainty and speak openly of their own vulnerability and fallibility without losing their patients' trust in their competence. They see their patients as people, not as instances of a case of influenza or heart disease. Reading poetry opens up spaces for multiple perspectives and interpretations of the same patient's story. Negatively capable physicians are quite comfortable with questioning their own assumptions about the meaning of illness or the right thing to do for a patient without reaching for the latest statistical evidence to support their viewpoints.

All that being said, I'll be the first to admit that my personal relationship with poetry has been a bit rocky. Though I believe that to be seduced by poetry is to be drawn in by an art form that distills the essences of what makes life meaningful in a way that no other art form can, I haven't always felt this way. As a young man, reading and writing poetry helped make sense of my angst and feelings of dislocation. I was smitten by love poems and even thought I could write my own. At my wedding, I read my bride-to-be an original poem instead of a list of vague promises. Yet, as I spent more time reading Aristotle than Auden, my poetry palate weakened substantially. I had fallen out of love with poetry, but I didn't realize how rocky our relationship was until a colleague accused me of being a "philistine" for turning my nose up at a William Carlos Williams poem (for the record, it was "This is Just to Say").

One morning, I was scouring the internet for poems that I could use in my medical humanities class when I stumbled upon Max Ritvo's "Afternoon." I remember casually glancing at the first stanza and suddenly feeling what the British call "gobsmacked." It reads: "When I was about to die/my body lit up/like when I leave my house/without my wallet."[16] The image was perfect. I sat in my office for a solid half hour reading and rereading the poem. Somehow, this 20-something-year-old cancer patient had captured the essence of our fear of dying. But his perspective was limited. Ritvo was speaking from the cold metal end of the stethoscope. I wondered what the poets with the earpieces and the white coats might have to say. So, I continued my search.

I had previously used Martha Sierpas's "The Diener" and Brendan Galvin's "Fear of Grey's Anatomy" in a section of the course called "Visualizing the Body in Health and Illness." As the title suggests, the goal of that class was to explore anatomical, artistic, literary, and philosophical representations of the body. One of my previous students had mentioned that they were spending their mornings in the anatomy lab before heading to my noontime class. No doubt they would be eager to discuss their experiences, if given the right nudge. Fortunately, serendipity struck again, this time in the form of "Progress Notes" by Fady Joudah.[17]

Unlike the works by Sierpas and Galvin, Joudah's poem speaks from the perspective of a physician reflecting back on his first anatomy lesson. This poem is not only about the final entry in a series of progress notes but also the speaker's encounter with beauty, death, and what lies beyond. The first two lines describe the modern obsession with beauty and documenting one's physical appearance as intoxicating experiences that can lead to narcissism and overindulgence. The speaker explains that beauty is defined by the endless pursuit of perfect proportions, then examines his self-portrait for potential flaws. His teeth? So perfectly arranged, they resemble sacred images of devotion. But his eyes are different sizes and a corner of his mouth hangs asymmetrically. He thinks it might be Bell's palsy. These questions of aesthetic value prepare the reader to judge the beauty of two cadavers: an elderly woman who died of natural causes and a soldier who committed suicide. To the nascent medical student, the soldier's bullet wound is beautiful.

Joudah's speaker vacillates among empathy, awe, and self-pity. Shared among the living and dead is the sense of isolation. The student desperately studying to keep up with his classmates and the soldier who took his own life felt the same way at one point. The despair and exhaustion extend so deeply that the speaker wants to join his subjects on the laboratory table. Death, beauty, macabre acts of rebellion—Joudah's poem leaves no lab tank unopened. His poem asks important ethical questions as well, particularly around the kinds of physicians we in the medical education business seek to send out into the world. What do we owe the dead? Does anatomy lab teach students to objectify others? How can students retain their humanity in the face of so many personal and professional challenges? I knew after reading "Progress Notes" that Joudah was the poet I was seeking.

Contributions to the literature

Before discussing a few of his poems in detail, I will give a brief overview of his poetic contributions to the literature. Most of his four collections of poetry cover common topics like love, death, sex, friendship, war, and parenthood. Though the themes may be universal, Joudah's lines are infused with a wide range of intriguing imagery, biological and religious metaphors, and clever uses of scientific language. He is given to flights of fancy, making abrupt turns that leap out of one context and into another, and weaving back and forth between interiority and exteriority. These are not clear-cut stories and easy to follow fables. They are moral tales, impressions, half-digested moments, and fading memories. They are evocative and mesmerizing daydreams.

In his time spent as a physician with Doctors Without Borders, Joudah bears witness to the suffering of the people he was called to help, but not without bitterness about his own inability to foster lasting change. For example, the speaker in "Pulse 14" describes the "humanitarian man" who adopts a stray dog but can't take him back home because of bureaucratic red tape. Regret for the ultimate futility of sporadic humanitarian aid appears in the line: "He came and loved, then he went."[18] Palestine is also never far from his mind. A dying carpenter in a hospital bed in "An Idea of Return" tells the speaker "I know your people. /They're good people, they/Have suffered enough/And the city is theirs."[19] Although the specific city is not specified—he could be referring to any number of (metaphorical or literal) cities—it's most likely Jerusalem. Joudah continues to draw on some of these themes in his second collection.

Alight features poems that are even more personal without devolving into cloying sentimentality or navel-gazing. Poems drawn from patient encounters are scant but more intimate and conversational. Readers get the sense that they are privy to the kinds of closed-door confessions and vulnerable moments that only transpire between strangers in healing environments. Soldiers share secrets normally reserved for their brothers in arms, while Joudah encourages them to find some form of hope instead of dwelling on the trauma they've endured. His gaze returns again to Palestine and his dual identity. Memories of olives, lemons, apricots, and events from his childhood fill the pages with bittersweet reminiscence as well as an embittered view of his displacement.

Textu, a portmanteau of "text" and "haiku," is a volume perfectly designed to fit in a coat pocket, whether that coat is white or purple. Most poems are exactly 160 characters, though some poems have multiple stanzas with the same meter. One imagines a white (or perhaps purple)-coated Joudah ducking into a dictation room after having just delivered bad news or examined another fuzzy CT image, his thumbs tapping rapidly in the Notes section of his iPhone. Placing limits on the character count (as opposed to the number of syllables) forces precision, but also allows the writing process itself to become more transparent. The result is a series of concentrated bursts of insight, breathlessness, and awe. Compared to his earlier work, there is less freedom here, but more depth of observation.

Footnotes in the Order of Disappearance is filled with allusions that are often elusive, leading ultimately to dead ends and furrowed brows. At some points, reading Joudah's verse requires an encyclopedia and a thesaurus to keep up. As with his other collections, he freely mixes words and images from a variety of sources: botany, ornithology, Islam, Arabic poetry, and medicine. He continues a conversation across civilizations that began in the Dark Ages, when Arab physicians and natural philosophers preserved and added to Greek and Roman science. Terms normally reserved for discussing diagnoses fill in as adjectives to describe both the banal and fantastic. The only reasonable thing to do is to give chase, follow him through the backstreets of Gaza, and hope that the footnotes lead somewhere wonderful. Spoiler alert: they do.

Aside from its aesthetic value, Joudah's poetry touches on a number of social concerns and experiences that hold great importance for the practice of medicine. His work is vital to the project of understanding and critiquing the borders and boundaries that separate and connect patients to care providers. Thematically, his poetry offers multiple opportunities to explore the liminal spaces in medicine, asymmetrical power dynamics, and the burdens of caregiving. From his perspective as someone who has inherited a sense of displacement and exile, Joudah questions the value of borders and boundaries, especially those that create barriers that disrupt human relationships. As a physician, he explores the power of medical language to obscure but also reveal truths about the human body. As a poet, one of Joudah's aims is to raise critical awareness through poetry of the imperial forces of scientific power and control over the body, and dangers of dehumanizing the Other. In the following sections, I will discuss how individual poems relate to these themes.

Liminal space between health and illness

In "Translation," Joudah explores the effect that living with uncertainty has on patients and physicians.[20] Like the characters in the poem, we are all perched between what Susan Sontag calls the "kingdom of the sick and the kingdom of the well."[21] We are dual citizens, shuttling back and forth across the border. While awaiting a diagnosis, we become stuck in a liminal space between the two kingdoms. Healthcare workers are customs agents. They review (and revoke) our passports, interrogating us and our bodies. If we are admitted to the kingdom of the sick, our belongings from the other kingdom are confiscated at the border. The speaker compares this boundary separating kingdoms to the borderlands between dreams and waking life.

> You live in a dream
> biopsy is set within hours racemes
>
> will bloom inside your flesh
> in LaserJet graphic
>
> or disseminate smudge
> into transfigurines

The title refers to the "LaserJet graphic," which translates the living body into text and imagery that can be dissected. Like a gardener trimming a bonsai tree, the physician plans to probe and extract delicate tissue from the body in order to find the root of disease. Biopsies are commonly used for identifying and staging diseases, normally some form of cancer, which is often referred to as "blooming" within the body. The fleshy growth will not end with a single flower, but, like racemes, will continue to bloom uncontrollably. Racemes develop in acropetal succession, meaning that new flowers are at the top and old flowers are at the bottom. The physician likely will witness a new lexical ordering where cancer or some other disease casts a shadow over the bloom of youth.

The fact that a biopsy is scheduled suggests that the abnormality has almost been identified. After all, malignant cells can also be described as "disseminating" throughout the body. That the smudge could be disseminated might suggest a laboratory error or false positive instead of an infiltration of malignant cells.

Unbeknownst to the patient, the speaker thinks he will discover something insidious that will soon be brought to light. Meanwhile, the patient lives within the dream of wellness. She may believe being asymptomatic means she is free from disease. Or that the symptoms she is experiencing are transitory, perhaps even hallucinatory in origin. Alas, soon the dream of infinite health may be shattered by the reality of disease. Hope blooms and withers in the space between the biopsy and the news.

Recasting medical ethics

My mentor in graduate school loved to ask the question: what do we owe each other as human beings? Joudah answers this by describing what can occur when we ignore our obligations to each other because of political, cultural, or other perceived differences. "Mimesis" is a simple, uncluttered, and direct poem that opens up questions about immigration and human rights.[22]

My daughter
                 wouldn't hurt a spider
That had nested
Between her bicycle handles
For two weeks
She waited
Until it left of its own accord

If you tear down the web I said
It will simply know
This isn't a place to call home
And you'd get to go biking

She said that's how others
Become refugees isn't it?

Joudah's transposition of the roles of victim, savior, and oppressor invites exploration of how each character in the poem adopts or considers adopting one or more of these roles. The central conflict is over how to respond to a stranger's intrusion into the daily routine. Who has the right to occupy the bicycle? This question of rights is important as it frames this community's obligations to treat each other fairly. To the humans in the poem, the spider is an Other. It is an insect, which is traditionally a trope used to describe inferior beings. But if we set the derogatory connotations aside, we can also see why the daughter thinks of the spider as a potential refugee. It is a nomad who has managed to find a home in an unfamiliar and inconvenient—for her—place.

The daughter clearly sympathizes with the nomadic spider. She recognizes the value of a life lived according to one's own choices and chooses to recognize the value of the Other. Seeing the spider as a refugee places a moral responsibility on her to prevent further displacement, even at the cost of her own happiness. She is both victim and savior in this microcosmic drama.

Enter the father figure as the oppressor who suggests a violent solution to the problem. If Joudah has cast himself in this role, it is surely with a sense of irony. Rather than simply allowing the spider time to resettle, he favors destroying its home. Even if the spider has no "right" to occupy the space, the consequences for the spider and his daughter's moral growth are high. He seeks not only to expel the refugee but also to teach him a lesson so that he will "simply know" that the oppressor can and will intervene whether his authority is recognized or not.

Recast in a medical context, the poem opens up questions about the right to healthcare. One might imagine a hospital administrator playing the father's role, upset that an uninsured patient is taking up resources that won't be reimbursed. The caring physician (in the role of the daughter) wants the patient to stay and be treated and is unwilling to write the discharge order. Some would argue that the spider's right to spin his web wherever he chooses is no different than an uninsured person's right to healthcare. Others would agree with the father: if the spider can't afford the rent, he shouldn't be allowed to stay. Many ethical dilemmas in the hospital setting center around competing sets of rights and duties: the right to access care, determine when care is medically inappropriate, and make autonomous decisions about a treatment plan. Poetic parables such as this one can move our thinking forward regarding medical ethics.

Suffering on both sides of the exam table

Joudah's poetry confronts the issue of whose suffering is recognized or ignored. Though his aim in writing about refugees (as he does in "Mimesis," "An Idea of Return," "Immigrant Song," and elsewhere) is not to prioritize their suffering over others', he raises a larger question about what those in power owe those who are suffering. Two poems in particular highlight the suffering of patients and physicians.

"Also" is a harrowing poem. It pulls nightmarish wartime imagery of scorched and disintegrated bodies into view immediately, followed by a dispassionate, almost surgical description of a soldier's self-cutting behavior in response to trauma. His cuts are precise, not deep enough to sever any vital structures, "but enough/for conversation and suture of two."[23] The expected phrase here would be "a suture *or* two" as a way to describe medical necessity and the soldier's desire for sustained attention. Instead, Joudah inserts the preposition "of" to indicate that the shared story connects the speaker and the veteran in a bond of recognition. Conversation, not surgery or pills, binds them together and may be the only way to repair the soldier's injuries. Likely drawn from his experience treating veterans, Joudah's verse foregrounds the soldier's isolation from his family as he attempts to reenter civilian life. His sons "want to be closer to him more/Than he can let them."[24] The soldier's choice to transform the mental scars into physical wounds arouses compassion in the physician, but he is powerless to sew together the veteran's broken life. And yet, the veteran isn't the only one who has experienced loss.

Joudah's verse demonstrates how the burden of caregiving can cause suffering, especially as personal and professional losses (time, patience, and patients) accumulate. Losses are often unexpected, always unwanted. They arrive as erasures from life, perhaps, but not from memory. The speaker in the titular poem "Footnotes in the Order of Disappearance" tries to brace himself for the next round yet recognizes that he is not immune to others' grief or his own.[25] His white coat is not thick enough to protect him. Physicians often try to hide their grief from patients and their families. After all, the death of a patient belongs to the family, not the physician. Yet, the speaker holds these losses close because they are related to him, if not by blood, then by virtue of being invested in the dying process. Too often, physicians suffer these losses in silence.

Power dynamics and social determinants of health

Few of Joudah's poems focus as steadily on the patient-physician relationship as "Luke Cool Hand I'm Your Father." Joudah intersperses pop culture references throughout the six stanzas, which keeps the reader invested as the speaker grapples with paternalism, social determinants of health, and power dynamics. Two of these references emerge from the title: the movies *Cool Hand Luke* and *Star Wars: The Empire Strikes Back*. Both are about rebellion against oppressive institutions: the prison system in the former and an evil space empire in the latter. *Cool Hand Luke* is probably best known among baby boomer fans of Paul Newman and Gen X fans of Guns N Roses, who sample the famous phrase "What we've got here, is failure to communicate" in the song "Civil War." The reference to *Star Wars*, specifically everyone's favorite dad, Darth Vader, reads as an allusion to paternalism in the patient-physician relationship.

The identity of the speaker of this poem is unclear, at least initially. His observations about how "pills & fear/& salt & sugar & grease" turn people into "junkies" could come from the nightly news just as easily as a medical chart.[26] Social determinants of health (poor diet, drug abuse, and mental health issues) are distilled into discrete emotional and physical elements, which are "softly killing them softly."[27] Yet, the speaker's position on whether people are entirely responsible for choices that affect their health is unclear. According to the speaker, "[t]hey did have a choice."[28] A literal reading would suggest that humans will always indulge in pills and junk food when presented with other options because we derive comfort from consumer goods. This libertarian version of personal responsibility (or lack of it) that is unaffected by socioeconomic and geopolitical boundaries is not uncommon among physicians, who feel that they are sometimes burdened by other people's bad decisions. Alternatively, the speaker may be acknowledging these boundaries and their effect on decision-making.

As the poem progresses, the speaker is identified as a physician who has become cynical and jaded about what his profession has become. He questions the assumption that the infirm should be referred to as *his* patients "as if I own them/as long as they're nothing/but patients."[29] Paternalism is built into this assumption that patients belong to their doctors or that doctors should be responsible for what happens to them once they leave the clinic. This tension is captured in the line "In tyranny there's also love/As gesture & as such/compassion is easy."[30] Compassion may be easy, but are the accompanying gestures justifiable? The tyranny he speaks of is the assumption that doctors know what is best for patients and that they make decisions and recommendations from a place of love. But this isn't so clear to Joudah, especially if the patient is nothing more than that to the doctor.

Ultimately, he rejects this idea of ownership. To him, they shouldn't be called patients, but "lives." Put another way, patients are the "authors" of their own life story. What doctors are really trying to do when they save lives is preserve patients' authorship of those lives. Authors of lives give each other "newsboy cap[s]" and "gift card[s] for fancy steak."[31] Patients do none of these things if they are simply seen as their doctors' property.

Joudah's speaker also bristles at the idea of omniscience within the patient-physician relationship. He remarks, sarcastically, "we-anoint-you-demigod." This is not false humility, but guilt about the asymmetrical power dynamic and resistance to the idea that the physician is omniscient and omnipotent. Those entering into the field should pay close attention to these lines. In anointing physicians with cultural authority by bestowing the white coat, society creates a tightly circumscribed social role for the physician. It is the contract that gives them privileges and wealth in exchange for their time and to a large extent, their lives outside of medicine. As the speaker in Joudah's poem indicates, some physicians may feel they are getting the worse end of that deal.

Discussion and criticism

Joudah's lyrical style can be very abstract, idiosyncratic, and elliptical. Some poems are particularly hard to follow as they bounce from image to seemingly unrelated image. Contrary to Galway Kinnel, who thought that poetry is someone saying "with as little concealment as possible, what it is for him or her to be on earth at this moment," much is concealed in Joudah's work.[32] Some reviewers have found themselves caught in a "dense lyricism that forces the reader to become a 'footnoter.'"[33] The title of that particular volume can be somewhat misleading as these footnotes convolute, rather than unpack or explain. Others have found his refusal to name places "registers as a kind of frustrating decorum."[34] Likewise, Curdy is frustrated by his "use of a medical lexicon that is natural to him as a doctor, but that doesn't always feel fully naturalized to the poems."[35] Pre-medical and medical students will likely not have the same objections. In fact, they may enjoy seeing some familiar terms used in unique ways.

Reading poetry as dense and complex as Joudah's may bring out some limitations in the reader. They may be tempted to try to dissect and overanalyze his poetry, to assume there is a deeper meaning that others grasp that they aren't qualified to find. Billy Collins writes in "Introduction to Poetry," "I ask them to take a poem/and hold it up to the light/like a color slide/or press an ear against its hive" "But all they want to do/is tie the poem to a chair with rope/and torture a confession out of it/ They begin beating it with a hose/to find out what it really means."[36] Some medical students may try these enhanced interrogation techniques because they are sure that a poem means only one thing, just as there is only answer to the question: how many carbon atoms in CO_2? With assistance from patient and knowledgeable humanities and clinical faculty, these problems may be less likely to occur.

As much as he tries to avoid the "deeper sin of appropriation" of the patient's suffering, one could argue that he fails to do so.[37] Pieces like "Also" and "Listening" paint veterans as deeply disturbed individuals who relish the disproportionate use of deadly force. Readers may assume that every veteran who returns from war has PTSD and may make hasty judgments about the credibility of their stories based on that assumption. Given that this is the only Western patient population that is clearly represented in these volumes, one may also wonder why this somewhat marginalized group was selected, rather than others whom Joudah could have chosen. Writing about patients will always be fraught with these kinds of questions of appropriation. As long as writers are transparent about their intentions and treat their subjects with respect, as Joudah does, the goal of giving voice to voiceless patients will remain worth pursuing.

Permission statements

Notes

1 Raphael Campo and Mark Doty, "Teaching Physicians Not to Be Afraid of Poetry," *JAMA* 320, no. 15 (2018): 1520.
2 Fritz Lanham, "Palestinian-American Doctor Turns Suffering into Song," *Houston Chronicle*, April 13, 2008.
3 W. K. Wimsatt and M. C. Beardsley, "The Intentional Fallacy," *The Sewanee Review* 54, no. 3 (1946): 46.
4 Paulette Beete, "Meet the 2013 Poetry Out Loud National Finals Judges," last modified April 29, 2013, https://www.arts.gov/art-works/2013/meet-2013-poetry-out-loud-national-finals-judges

5 Fady Joudah, "The Big Idea: Fady Joudah," Interview by Suzanne Koven, *The Rumpus*, November 18, 2013, https://therumpus.net/2013/11/the-big-idea-7-fady-joudah/.

6 Michele A. Carter and C. M. Klugman, "Cultural Engagement in Clinical Ethics: A Model for Ethics Consultation," *Cambridge Quarterly of Healthcare Ethics* 10, no. 1 (2001): 16–33.

7 Fady Joudah, "It's All Personal for Me," Interview by Kaveh Akbar, *Dive Dapper*, February 2, 2015, https://www.divedapper.com/interview/fady-joudah/.

8 Joudah, Interview.

9 Felicia Aull, "Poetry in the Borderlands of Medicine," *Family Medicine* 37, no. 10 (2005): 698.

10 Lois Leveen, "Finding Purpose: Honing the Practice of Making Meaning in Medicine," *The Permanente Journal* 21 (2017): 17.

11 Angela Andrews, "Lean Forward and Listen: Poetry as a Mode of Understanding in Medicine," *Perspectives in Biology and Medicine* 58, no. 1 (2015): 21.

12 Raphael Campo and Mark Doty, "Expanding the Time We Have with Patients through Poetry," JAMA 320, no. 17 (2018): 1734.

13 Raphael Campo, "Why Should Medical Students Be Writing Poems?" *Journal of Medical Humanities* 27, no. 4 (2006): 254.

14 Alstair Gee, "Ode on a Stethoscope," *The New Yorker*, January 14, 2015.

15 John Keats, "On Negative Capability: Letter to George and Tom Keats," 21/27 December 1817, https://www.poetryfoundation.org/articles/69384/selections-from-k eatss-lettersKeats 1817.

16 Max Ritvo, "Afternoon," *Four Reincarnations: Poems* (Minneapolis, MN: Milkweed Editions, 2016), 50.

17 Fady Joudah, "Progress Notes," *Footnotes in the Order of Disappearance: Poems* (Minneapolis, MN: Milkweed Editions, 2018), 6.

18 Fady Joudah, "Pulse 14," *The Earth in the Attic* (New Haven, CT: Yale University Press, 2008), 18.

19 Fady Joudah, "An Idea of Return," *The Earth in the Attic* (New Haven, CT: Yale University Press, 2008), 35.

20 Fady Joudah, "Translation," *Textu* (Port Townsend, WA: Copper Canyon Press, 2014), 35.

21 Susan Sontag, *Illness as Metaphor and Aids and Its Metaphors* (New York: Picador, 1978), 3.

22 Fady Joudah, "Mimesis," *Alight* (Port Townsend, WA: Copper Canyon Press, 2013), 14.

23 Fady Joudah, "Also," *Alight* (Port Townsend, WA: Copper Canyon Press, 2013), 17.

24 Joudah, "Also."

25 Fady Joudah, "Footnotes in the Order of Disappearance," *Footnotes in the Order of Disappearance: Poems* (Minneapolis, MN: Milkweed Editions, 2018), 79.

26 Fady Joudah, "Luke Cool Hand I'm Your Father," *Textu* (Port Townsend, WA: Copper Canyon Press, 2014), 39.

27 Joudah, "Luke Cool Hand I'm Your Father."

28 Ibid.

29 Ibid., 40.

30 Ibid., 41.

31 Ibid., 40.

32 Daniel Lewis, "Galway Kinnell, Plain-Spoken Poet, Is Dead at 87," *New York Times*, October 29, 2014.

33 Grant Schatzman, "Footnotes in the Order of Disappearance by Fady Joudah," Review of *Footnotes in the Order of Disappearance* by Fady Joudah, *World Literature Today*, 92 no. 3 May/June 2018.

34 Averil Curdy, "Do I Dare Disturb the Universe?" *Poetry* 193, no. 5 (February 2009): 473.

35 Curdy, "Do I Dare Disturb the Universe?" 474.
36 Billy Collins, "Introduction to Poetry," *The Apple that Astonished Paris* (Fayetteville, AR: University of Arkansas Press, 1996), 58.
37 Joudah, Interview, 2015.

11 Louise Aronson

Using facts and stories to improve medical care for older adults

Craig M. Klugman

Introduction

For Louise Aronson, her dual identities as a physician and as a writer are intimately intertwined. Aronson chose to specialize in geriatrics because,

> I just love stories. Thinking in terms of story led me to geriatrics because you really need to have to know who the person is and what they value and who is in their environment and what have they done in the past to provide good geriatric care. I had license to ask about the larger context of lives.[1]

Aronson's personal story is closely related to the people and place she loves, San Francisco. She was born in November 1963 at the University of California San Francisco, a place where she later trained in her residency and practices medicine. Her father, Samuel Aronson, completed his residency at UCSF as well (died 2013). He was a physician-scientist in ophthalmology and shared his love of medicine and science with his daughter. Her mother is Mary Ann Goldman Aronson, an avid reader who gifted her daughter with a passion for words and stories. Mary Ann graduated from Stanford University and worked in the nonprofit world, including founding her own business to assist organizations to determine where to give their money. Her sister Margot is two years younger. For 20 years now, Aronson has been married to Jane Langridge, a native of Britain who trained as a radiation physicist and works in nonprofit health technology.

A conversation

I had been a fan of Aronson's work since I first heard her interviewed on NPR in 2013 on the occasion of Oliver Sacks's 80th birthday.[2] Her writing quickly became a mainstay in my Health Humanities classes, speaking directly to my students' experiences of choosing a career, starting a family, and discovering what kind of person they want to be. For this writing project, I knew as a medical anthropologist that to understand the published author, I had to meet the author-as-real-person. On January 10, 2020, I dialed Aronson's 415 phone for a conversation, to which she had graciously agreed. In preparation, I reread both

DOI: 10.4324/9781003079712-11

of her books: A *History of the Present Illness* (AHPI), which is a collection of fictional short stories, and her most recent volume, *Elderhood: Redefining Aging, Transforming Medicine, and Reimagining Life*. Stories in AHPI are based on tales told by her patients, by the residents she teaches, and by her own friends during their medical school days. *Elderhood* is a nonfiction act of activism seeking to establish an "anti-ageist" medicine.[3] Aronson wants nothing less than to change how we view getting older and how we treat our elders. In *Elderhood*, Aronson weaves her life's story alongside facts about elders and caring for them. She wants her book to do for aging what Atul Gawande's *Being Mortal* has tried to do for the dying—to recenter the conversation onto a marginalized population. While a noble goal, *Elderhood* has not made traction in the same way as Gawande's book. Perhaps, this is because he was a [male] household name before his publication, so people paid attention not because of the topic but because of the author. Aronson's best work in recentering conversations on aging comes from her short nonfiction that appears in popular outlets. In such public forums as *The Atlantic*, *Vox*, *The New York Times*, and *The Washington Post*, she advocates for anti-ageist medicine, inclusiveness in research, and more recently on how the COVID-19 pandemic has starkly shown us the disparities against our elders.[4]

Making the world better

"I grew up in a family where science was a big deal," Aronson told me during our interview.[5] Her father regularly shared his passion for medical research and treating patients. When it came time for college, however, Aronson chose Brown University, where she double majored in history and independent study (that was similar to medical anthropology).[6] Medicine was the furthest career from her mind as she was more interested in pursuing her childhood dream of being a writer. In her junior year of college, Aronson volunteered to work with Southeast Asian refugees in Providence, RI, an experience that appears often in her short stories. Watching the healthcare staff interact in the clinic, she was taken with how nurses and social workers engaged with patients holistically, but physicians concentrated solely on biological functions. She also saw how everyone deferred to the physician, even if they were wrong. Aronson felt that physicians could have a different kind of role: "So I went to medical school because I wanted skills that would help people, and also enough power that I didn't have to be subservient to someone just because of our genders or roles in the health system."[7] After she submitted her medical school applications, Aronson became director of special education in a refugee camp on the Thai-Cambodian border (Khao-I-Dang). "Doctors were consulted about everything: not just medical issues but psychological, social, and existential problems as well. That reinforced my view of doctoring as a human enterprise in the broadest sense."[8] Aronson attended medical school at Harvard (graduated 1992) and continued her training at UCSF. These experiences, though, left her feeling that "the humanities part of myself had atrophied, becoming barely a twitch."[9]

Being a writer, however, was scary. Many writers work hard and still fail. Aronson wanted the security of a career in medicine and the knowledge that every day she was helping to make the world better, before taking on the high risk of failure of being a writer. She writes:

> I didn't have the confidence to suck at something long enough to be good at it. Once I got back into writing, I could comfort myself with being bad, but I could be bad at it because I knew that I got up most days and I made a difference in the world. I had income, health insurance, and was helping people as a doctor. I wanted to be a person who made the world better, some writers do that and some don't.[10]

Immediately after completing her fellowship training, she enrolled at UC Extension to take classes in mystery writing and graphic design. She pursued an MFA at the Warren Wilson Program for Writers (2001-2006), where she crafted many of the stories that are in A *History of the Present Illness*.

Aronson's experience and approach to finding stories follows a similar path to physician-anthropologist Arthur Kleinman, who learned to listen for patients' stories while living in China. He discovered that the contextualization offered by the story invited the physician into the patient's illness narrative.[11] The stories allowed the physician to access the patient's cultural reality. For Kleinman, the story helped him to diagnose and treat. For Aronson, the story helps her to know the person and how to care for them.

A History of the Present Illness

Aronson's collection of short stories was published in 2013 with Bloomsbury press. At 259 pages, A *History of the Present Illness* contains 16 short stories and an acknowledgment from the author. The volume was a finalist for both the Chautauqua Prize and the PEN America Bingham Award for debut fiction. Aronson started writing this book in the late 1990s and it took her over a decade—and her MFA program—to complete it. The title comes from "the critical first portion of the medical note that describes the onset, duration, character, context, and severity of the illness. Basically, it's the story."[12] Kathryn Montgomery agrees that the case note is a particular kind of story, and that medicine is a narrative practice. The physician's task is to take a subjective tale and to translate it into medical language, which is assumed to be more objective and pathophysiological.[13] But it is a highly proscripted form of narrative, having to adhere to a specific and minimal narrative structure, often stripping out the richer context and details that a story needs. A good story needs to incorporate "imagery, analogy, and metaphor ... and settings"[14] to be relatable in a way that the medical anecdote is not.

Aronson criticizes the way most doctors share stories—as cases, war tales, and teaching examples—as not being proper stories. "What most doctors call stories aren't really stories at all. They're anecdotes, which my Webster's dictionary tells me are 'usu. short narrative(s) of an interesting, amusing or biographical incident.'"[15] Her view differs remarkably from her medical humanities colleague at UCSF, Marilyn Mcentyre, who believes that poems best reflect the clinical encounter because they capture the "discontinuity, surprise, and the uneasy relationship between words and the life of the body."[16] Mcentyre holds that familiar narrative structures in stories prevent one from hearing patients, whereas in poetry, the dislocation of words allows one to hear new ambiguities and possibilities.[17] In a sense, both are correct. When a person is in the moment of a crisis or an illness, they usually cannot make sense of what is happening; they are living what sociologist Arthur Frank calls the chaos narrative: "Stories are chaotic in their absence of narrative order. Events are told as the storyteller experiences life: without sequence or discernible causality."[18] But after the events have passed, a person can look back and put them in some sort of order, add in symbols and meaning. This act of ordering the chaos constructs the narrative experience. In other words, a person's experience is created after the events have transpired. Aronson's work creates meaning afterward, while Mcentyre uses poetry to capture the chaos during.

As a writer, Aronson tries to craft atypical doctor's narratives. In most fiction, a physician is often a hero who comes in and saves the day by saving a life, or is an anti-hero in that they are flawed and "behaving badly according to certain widely accepted though rarely articulated codes of physician conduct."[19] She does not write to elicit sentimentality, humor, or outrage. For those of us used to more ordered writings with clear beginning, middles, and ends, Aronson's writing may frustrate. Her writing is experimental, trying out different narrator perspectives and storytelling styles. She moves from a discussion of empirical data to telling stories of her patients to examining her own biography in a few short pages. This means that a topic is often revisited several times over a volume. We see this in both her nonfiction and her fiction from her earliest work. For example, in "Fires and Flatlines," the reader sees the internal experience of multiple characters from the same events (a Rashomon tale):

> All the characters are having a traumatic experience, each in a different way, and what tends to happen with trauma is that some things stand out vividly and indelibly and others are lost. Life takes on a staccato character, and I wanted the experience of reading the story to mimic that and also for the reader to be able to see all the different perspectives, the narrator-doctor's, the boy's, his father's, his aunt's, the narrator's wife's, even the critically ill Vivian's.[20]

In AHPI, some chapters are straightforward narratives, others are lists, letters, and even a diagnostic entry. For example, "Blurred Boundary Disorder" is a letter describing a new diagnostic condition common to physicians whose professional work takes over their entire lives. While the text is mainly a DSM diagnostic entry, the story of what happened (an attending engaging in an inappropriate sexual relationship with a trainee) plays out in the footnotes. "Twenty-five

Things I Know About My Husband's Mother" is a list of facts a physician-and-wife writes about her mother-in-law.

Aronson tells us that her models for writing medical stories actually come from war books where there are "stories of good deeds and bad, but no heroes or villains. ... In other words, they were honest."[21] She points out that these are stories where people can do the right things and still have bad outcomes. She cites a sense of honesty in stories that put people through a "boot camp" (literal and figurative) where they are forced to do impossible, horrific things to human bodies in both war and medicine. She wants to capture this grey area of flawed people doing their imperfect best to the limits of human endurance (sleep deprivation, overworked, too many demands).

Like a soldier, Aronson describes physician's lives as ones where personal life is sacrificed for professional duty and career promotion. In "Heart Failure," Marta Perez feels that she is failing as a mother, spouse, and daughter-in-law because her work as a doctor demands so much of her. Her eldest daughter (15 years old) has anger issues and often takes them out on her mother. Abuelo is 76 years old with heart failure and Abuela, who has mobility issues, needs support in deciding whether to withdraw her husband's life support. Marta feels many of the problems are a result of her being absent from the family so often. "Psychiatrist's Wife" is told from the perspective of a surgeon who develops generalized anxiety disorder and quits her job when she realizes she no longer wants to operate. Her husband is a famous psychiatrist and seems more interested in his success than his family. Similarly, "Blurred Boundary Disorder" features a physician finding that her personal worth depends on a professional reputation earned while giving up a personal life. In "Lucky You," Perla Weldon is a resident who quits medicine in the second year of her residency after treating a gangbanger. The reader is told that she is smart and capable, but a chaotic personal life may have demanded too much attention for her to sacrifice all that is necessary to be a doctor. A life in medicine is all-demanding, all-consuming, and draining. In the real world, depression affects 27.2% of medical students and 11.1% have had suicidal ideation.[22] In terms of medical residents, 43.2% report depression. Male physicians' suicide rates are 40% higher than the general population, and for female physicians', the rate is 130% higher.[23]

These stories show the damage to individual lives caused by physician burnout, the physiological response to long-term stress "marked by emotional exhaustion, depersonalization, and a lack of sense of personal accomplishment."[24] Medicine today demands a great deal of one's time, is chaotic, and is controlled by others (including electronic records). Forty-two percent of physicians report signs of burnout.[25]

Literature is always personal

Being a doctor, a daughter, and a San Franciscan largely influences the stories that Aronson tells. Her patients and their families, her classmates, her students, and her family are the basis for her characters. In the short story, "Days of Awe," a husband and wife have moved to a large Jewish retirement home for the wife's health needs. Harold is an active 80-year-old who is happy with the move and has become a "big macher" (in Yiddish, an influential person). His wife, Ruth is severely depressed and rarely leaves her bed. Harold arranges to get his own room in a different part of the home; he is leaving his wife. The story shows that even an older couple can grow apart and want different things. In a twist, Ruth becomes more social after being treated with antidepressants and then suffers a fall and a broken hip. Harold then feels that he cannot leave her and becomes an attentive spouse. The basis for this story likely comes from Aronson's own parents who moved to an assisted living community when her father needed more care than her mother could provide at home. Samuel developed dementia and had multiple medical problems, mostly related to his heart failure and related surgical complications. By changing the genders of the characters, Aronson may be trying to protect the privacy of her family, but seeing the two stories (fiction and nonfiction) side by side, the inspiration becomes evident.

Mining her own biography can also be seen in the story "Giving Good Death." Robert is a physician arrested for allegedly helping a patient die. Much of his tale includes sharing with his therapist a list of books he has read while in prison. "On Becoming a Doctor" offers snapshots of life during four years of medical school and each scene is titled with a published story or book important in feminist politics and thought. Aronson and her mother used to exchange lists of books. This real practice made its way into these stories.

Boundaries

In medicine, a physician is supposed to keep clear boundaries between patient and physician; right and wrong; personal gain and helping patients. Most boundary crossings are rarely black and white but instead occupy a blurred line that one only sees once it has been crossed. For instance, in "A Medical Story," Aronson blurs the boundary between a fictional narrator and the real-life author. The narrator grew up in the Midwest and found palliative care after being a locum tens physician. The narrator and the author both found themselves taking a writing class. Even the narrator's penchant for writing down patients' stories paralleled what Aronson described to me that she used to do before the electronic medical record made that more difficult. The narrator, and perhaps Aronson, discuss the challenges of being a physician-writer from the difficulty of fictionalizing real events to the autobiographical turn:

> It seemed that in the process of becoming a doctor, I'd also become quite literal, unable to bend fact for the sake of drama or significance. ... To my surprise, most of my earlier stories contained a protagonist who could invariably be described as a young female doctor who was always having to adjust to new hospitals and patients and couldn't quite figure out what she wanted to do with her life.[26]

In our conversation, Aronson admitted that this story was the closest to her real life.[27]

Another way that Aronson blurs boundaries is through her style. In "A Medical Story," Aronson writes that doctors are discouraged from using the first person to give a sense of objectivity and accuracy in their case reports.[28] In a play on this cardinal rule, Aronson's stories frequently flout this prohibition. While many stories are told by a limited third-person narrator, several stories are told by an unnamed first-person narrator ("Third Wave," "Twenty-five Things I Know About My Husband's Mother," "Lucky You," "The Promise," "Blurred Boundary Disorder," and "A Medical Story"). Aronson told me that this playfulness in perspective comes about from different voice assignments she was given in her MFA program.[29]

Taking care

A second theme in this collection is taking care of seniors at the end of life with their complex medical conditions and need to make end-of-life decisions. In "Snapshots from an Institution," we are introduced to Jiao, who has dementia, and her doting husband Quingshan. When the doctor suggests a DNR order for Jiao, their son Charles refuses it even though everyone else desires it. Ricardo Perez is at the end of his life following a heart attack in "Heart Failure," where the family makes the decision to withdraw life support. In "Vital Signs," 101-year-old Edith Picarelli ends up dying alone in a hospital room with a DNR order signed by a resident who does not remember seeing her previously. In "The Promise" and "Giving Good Death," two physicians struggle with terminally ill patients asking for help in ending their lives. In one case, the physician does help and is arrested. In the other story, the request comes from Hattie Robinson, a 90-year-old patient that the physician believes has a poor quality of life after she is given aggressive stroke care because the resident did not see an advance directive and did not want to make assumptions simply based on the patient's age.

Diversity and inclusiveness

Aronson brings into her stories her experiences from working with refugees in Providence and in the camp on the Thai-Cambodian border. Consider the Asian couple in "Snapshots"; the Khmer family in "An American Problem"; the El Salvadoran patient in "The Promise"; the Hispanic family in "Heart Failure"; the medical students who are Asian, Black, and gay in "Becoming a Doctor" and "Lucky You"; the Indian physician in "Twenty-Five Things I know About My Husband's Mother"; and the Jewish couple in "Days of Awe." Aronson is not only being inclusive in delivering a picture of the diversity of people in medicine and in San Francisco, but also pushing us to question our assumptions. This attempt is clearest in a joke a patient tells a med student in "Soup or Sex." The joke is about a daughter yelling upstairs to her elderly father from whom she does not hear a response. She finally goes upstairs and asks him the question, to which he responds that he has already answered four times. As the patient explains, the problem was not in the elderly father's hearing, but that the younger daughter was deaf.[30] The joke requires us to acknowledge our cultural assumptions that equates "elderly" and "decrepit." Other stories force the reader to abandon the idea that death only happens to those who are very old. In "Soup or Sex," newly graduated medical doctor Chira Agarwal has to talk with her 22-year-old cystic fibrosis patient about completing a "Preferred Intensity of Treatment Form" (a DNR), which he ultimately rejects. These vignettes force us to check our assumptions about what it means to be old—while there is usually slowing, it is not a period of decline and disability for everyone—and dying—a 22-year old is assumed the be healthy with most of their life waiting in front of them.

Linking

Within the volume, many of the stories link to one another. For example, a resident rounds in the VA in "Becoming a Doctor" and the very next story, "After," is from a VA patient's point of view. "The Psychiatrist's Wife" occurs at a Caribbean psychiatry conference, and "Blurred Boundary Disorder" mentions that all of the psychiatrists in town are at a Caribbean conference. Althea is a fellow medical student, friend, and roommate of the narrator in "Becoming a Doctor," who is also mentioned as a classmate in "Lucky You," a story about residency told by a different narrator. Lenore is a clinical social worker at the Tenderloin Family Clinic in "An American Problem" and is referred to as the wife's therapist in "Giving Good Death." The faculty advisor in "Lucky You" is Dr. Ernest Westphall, who is the narrator in the next story, "The Promise." On first look, a reader might assume that these are snapshots of the author's life or an intention to tell an epic from the perspective of a number of patients (what would be called an ensemble drama in television). The connections, however, feel forced and inconsistent. For instance, Althea has one personality in "Becoming a Doctor" and seems like a different character, even though just mentioned in passing, in "Lucky You." Aronson told me during our interview that she deliberately added these links on the advice of her agent, who said that linked stories were all the rage when she was trying to publish.[31]

Elderhood

Transitioning from a fiction writer to a nonfiction writer is something that Aronson credits to her own aging and the electronic medical record. With paper records, she would write a few lines in the appropriate places and then craft a "narrative note" that told the patient's story. With the transition to electronic medical records, she could no longer write in the same way. She began using these patient stories and photos in her talks to make them entertaining, a process that increased her interest in moving toward nonfiction. Aronson discovered that she could use these stories to move people toward action. "I could use my fiction skills to write and do advocacy. I realized I could combine those parts [medicine and fiction] of myself. I think of my writing now as a public health tool; how I change the world."[32] Certainly, other scholars view her writing as a form of advocacy. Thomas Cole calls Aronson's book *Elderhood* "the richest and most comprehensive source for understanding healthcare for, as well as broad social and historical aspects of, aging and old age."[33]

Being an elder in the United States

My father was the only child of an entire generation of his family. This meant that much of my childhood was spent taking care of our elderly family members who aged in very different ways. There was my aunt Lil and uncle Sam, who were artists and political activists working into their 90s. Uncle Sam was one of the last remaining concertina players, and he would give concerts in nursing homes (to people 20 years his junior) while convincing them of the benefits of socialism. My grandfather died from a heart attack in his 60s brought on by diabetes, when I was only 8 years old. For the next 8 years, we were the primary caregivers for my grandmother, visiting her in a posh nursing house every Sunday. An earlier experiment in her living with us did not end well—a busy household did not make her happy. In the beginning, all four of us (my parents and younger sister) would pile into the car and drive the 40 minutes to the home. There we would load grandma Klugman in the car (which in later years involved adding a walker and then a wheelchair) to take her for lunch, shopping, or to a park. Several times a year, we brought her to our house for a holiday dinner. We would spend a few hours and then bring her back. My father visited her daily since the home was near his office. In the later years, she was unable to go on these outings and visits meant sitting with her in a common room, or standing around her bed once she was no longer mobile. As my sister and I grew up and visits became about seeing elderly people who were decrepit or had been dressed up and left in a wheelchair in one of the fancy common rooms to stare at each other (or at nothing), the experience left less and less to be desired. We would have preferred to spend Sundays with our friends, watching TV, or doing homework, and often did.

These experiences taught me that our senior years are a time for withdrawing from the world. It was a space to become something smaller where you became a burden on your family, began to wear funny clothes (and shoes, always the orthopedic shoes), and developed a funky odor. These elders regressed to a child-like state where other people had to make their decisions and take care of their needs because they no longer could do that for themselves (not considering, as a child, that perhaps these choices were removed from them). Old age is viewed as something "'less than' compared with youth, and aging came to be associated with decline and obsolescence—conditions people distance themselves from even today."[34] This notion of othering elders is a modern, Western idea that differs from the exalted station the aged held for most of human history:

> Aging was removed from the ancient provinces of religion and mystery and transferred to the modern terrain of science and mastery. Old age was

removed from its place as a way station along life's spiritual journey and rede-fined as a problem to be solved by science and medicine.[35]

Rethinking being an elder

Aronson wants us to return to thinking of elderhood as a time of spiritual and psy-chological growth, a journey she lays out in her OpEd writing and in *Elderhood*. Her work as an author, a medical educator, and a geriatrician is to show that "elderhood" is a vibrant stage of life ripe with possibilities of spiritual growth, enjoying our bodies, and having meaningful relationships. Isaac Chotiner says this book "examines Americans' fraught relationship to the aging process, from our enthusiasm for supposed anti-aging cures to our troubled health-care system and the persistence of ageism among employers."[36] Aronson wants to reclaim the senior years because for too long we have tried to put aging out of sight and out of mind, similar to how I viewed my grandmother's nursing home. "People look at geriatrics and old age as the thing that happens before you die," she adds.

> No. It lasts decades and has all these stages and substages and most of them are quite wonderful for most people. A big message of the book is that so much of what's horrible about old age isn't about aging nearly as much as it is about our dysfunctional approach to it.[37]

In fact, Aronson notes that the senior years are often among the happiest of a person's life.[38] The problem is that her vision is a white, upper socioeconomic idealization of aging. In communities of color, elders often take on child and home care because parents are working or unavailable. The vision that Aronson provides comes from her Jewish, urban, upper SES upbringing, but may not be familiar to or even desired by many.

The 15-chapter book is divided into 3 major and 2 minor sections that are titled with different stages of life (childhood, adulthood, elderhood, death, and coda), though the titles have nothing to do with the content except to organize Aronson's autobiographical tales. Naming chapters after life stages makes the book more confusing: these titles reflect her experiences with those stages of life and then tries to fit in facts, studies, and other examples into that framework. The attempt is less than successful from an organizational standpoint. *Elderhood* explores four interrelated themes: (1) stories of patients she has treated in her geriatrics practice; (2) vignettes of her caregiving for her own father as he ages from his 70s to 80s and struggles with heart disease, orthopedic challenges, surgi-cal complications, and death; (3) a critical study of ageism[39] and how the ways society is setup and medicine is practiced fails the elderly; and (4) an autobiogra-phy of her own career from being a child and noticing age (in her grandmother's body) to being a medical trainee to her medical practice and personal challenges as a person who is aging.

Growing older herself introduced her to the lived reality of aging from being treated differently due to her greying hair (a conscious choice not to dye it) to seeing her friends and family being diagnosed with illness and dying: "I could not have written elderhood if I had not been in my 50s."[40] As someone who has cared for patients and her father, she learned that the United States needs to change how we take care of older people. Historically, medicine has struggled to take care of seniors, leading to frequent problems of misdiagnosis, undertreating, overtreating, and ignoring their needs. Elders often have multiple health issues, a complication that confuses doctors who were trained to only look at one disease at a time and frustrates insurers that limit how much time people can have with their physician. However, the number of physicians choosing to specialize in geriatrics is trending down at the moment when we have need of more of them.[41] Federal estimates show that the United States will be short 26,000 geriatric physicians by 2025.[42]

Aronson shows us that ageism is overt as well as subconscious. For example, she points out that putting "aging" or "geriatric" in a program title will make students, patients, funders, and administrators flee.[43] Such bias against aging decreases their quality of care. After all, drugs and procedures are rarely tested on "older bodies," and diagnostic norms rarely consider the age of patients who may metabolize differently and take multiple medications. Similar to criticisms espoused by disability scholars, Aronson says the problem is not growing old, but a society that is built without aging in mind. Consider the built environment that may not be friendly to people with slower walking gaits, who need a grip bar in the shower, or who no longer lift their leg as high to take a step. Consider the culture that celebrates youth and views being over age 50 as no longer useful. Consider workflows and patient quotas that do not permit the time to hear a patient's story or to consider all of their concerns. Consider language where the connotation of elderly is "outdated" and means "People who are stupid and fun to kick." In contrast, "young" is described as a modifier that makes its noun "10× better."[44] Even the recent phrase "OKboomer" is supposed to be an insult, dismissing criticism from an older generation that is viewed as misunderstanding, irrelevant, and judgmental.[45] The solution is to see aging as a natural part of life and rewire society to embrace our elderhood as a positive time of life. Aging in place should be a concept behind design and architecture (something I was very aware of during my recent apartment hunt, seeing many fourth-floor walkup units). Most of us all will grow old, our bodies will change, and our interests will mature, so why not make this a source of celebration, of honoring, and of respecting?

Discussion

One of the ethical challenges in writing about patient stories is whether one should get permission from the patient before writing and publishing. In *Elderhood*, Aronson writes:

> When I lacked a patient's or family's permission to tell their story, I have changed select telling details. Those measures were taken not only in keeping

with core tenets of medicine and the stipulations of federal health privacy laws but also out of profound gratitude for the many people who entrusted me with their well-being and in so doing taught me about what old age is, what it should be, and what it could be.[46]

Aronson told me that her characters tend to be amalgams of people she has known—patients, friends, patients of friends, and her students. She rewrites stories and changes details multiple times, which means that her characters bear passing resemblance to the real people on which they may be based. Other physician-writers, such as Rita Charon, approach this issue as if they are a coauthor with their patient. Charon shares copies of her stories with her patients.[47] Without gaining permission, a former patient or friend who knows a story well could recognize the written tale and experience distress and loss of privacy. Arthur Kleinman holds that he should preserve the story and use the patients' words as much as possible in the retelling: "*The Illness Narratives* told stories of sickness much as they had been told to me. I felt a deep compulsion to retell these accounts."[48]

During our conversation, Aronson and I found that we have a lot in common. She grew up in the Bay Area and moved to the Northeast for college. I grew up in the Northeast and moved to the Bay Area for college. She was a humanities major who moved to medicine, only to rediscover literature and the medical humanities. During our talk, Aronson said she sometimes wonders what if she had chosen to work in publishing in New York or been an anthropologist instead of being a doctor. I responded to her that my college major was human biology and in my sophomore year I walked away from the idea of medical school. My first career was as a journalist in magazine publishing in New York City, and later I earned a degree in medical anthropology. In a sense, we lived each other's youthful dreams. Despite these different roads, we both ended up in the medical humanities, working with health students and trainees. For me, I use stories and writing in medicine and health to "inoculate" pre-med students against the loss of empathy, the burnout, and the blurred boundaries that they will face in their future training. Aronson told me that writing and the medical humanities,

> have enabled me to more fully inhabit the patients' experience. I would say I am this empathetic doctor, which I try to be, and in putting their life into a character [in her writing], I know inhabiting someone's reality takes more practice and effort. Being a writer helps me to see alternative perspectives as a doctor.[49]

Notes

1 Louise Aronson, "Personal Interview," interview by Craig Klugman, January 10, 2020.
2 Tom Ashbrook, "Oliver Sacks on Growing Older," *On Point* 46, July 18, 2013: https://www.wbur.org/onpoint/2013/07/18/oliver-sacks-on-growing-older.

3 Louise Aronson, "Koppaka Family Foundation Lecture in Health Humanities," Webinar, University of Virginia's Medical Center Hour: Medicine & Society Conversation, March 3, 2020.

4 Louise Aronson, "Coronavirus Reveals Just How Little Compassion We Have for Older People," *Vox*, March 27, 2020: https://www.vox.com/the-highlight/2020/3/27 /21195762/coronavirus-older-people-quarantine-loneliness-health; Louise Aronson, "We Can Help Men Live Longer," *The New York Times*, November, 7 2019: https://ww w.nytimes.com/2019/11/07/opinion/men-health-crisis-.html; Louise Aronson, "I'm a Geriatrician. There's No Clear Age that Is 'Too Old' to Be President," *The Washington Post*, June, 12 2019: https://www.washingtonpost.com/outlook/2019/06/12/im-ge riatrician-im-fine-with-an-year-old-running-president; Louise Aronson, "Ageism Is Making the Pandemic Worse," *The Atlantic*, March 28, 2020: https://www.theatlantic .com/culture/archive/2020/03/americas-ageism-crisis-is-helping-the-coronavirus/608 905/.

5 Aronson, Interview.

6 Louise Aronson, *Elderhood: Redefining Aging, Transforming Medicine, and Reimagining Life* (New York: Bloomsbury, 2019); Monique Williams, "Louise Aronson," *Fourteen Hills, SFSU Creative Writing Program*, December 30, 2012: https://www.14hills.net/i nterview-louise-aronson.

7 Williams, "Loiuse Aronson."

8 Aronson, *Elderhood*, 43.

9 Aronson, Interview.

10 Ibid.

11 Arthur Kleinman, *The Illness Narratives: Suffering, Healing, and The Human Condition* (New York: Basic Books, 1988).

12 Aronson, AHPI, 257.

13 Kathryn Montgomery Hunter, *Doctors' Stories: The Narrative Structure of Medical Knowledge* (Princeton, NJ: Princeton University Press, 1991).

14 Aronson, AHPI, 252.

15 Ibid., 241.

16 Marilyn Chandler Mcentyre, *Patient Poets: Illness from Inside Out* (San Francisco, CA: University of California Medical Humanities Press, 2012), 1.

17 Ibid.

18 Arthur Frank, *The Wounded Storyteller*, second ed. (Chicago, IL: University of Chicago Press, 2013), 97.

19 Aronson, AHPI, 245.

20 Williams, "Loiuse Aronson."

21 Aronson, AHPI, 249.

22 Lisa S. Rotenstein, et al., "Prevalence of Depression, Depressive Symptoms, and Suicidal Ideation among Medical Students: A Systematic Review and Meta-Analysis," *Journal of the American Medical Association* 316, no. 21 (2016). doi: 10.1001/ jama.2016.17324.

23 Molly C. Kalmoe, et al., "Physician Suicide: A Call to Action," *Missouri Medicine* 116, no. 3 (2019): 211–216.

24 "Physician Burnout," Agency for Healthcare Research and Quality, 2017, accessed August 20, 2021: https://www.ahrq.gov/prevention/clinician/ahrq-works/burnout/inde x.html.

25 Leslie Kane, "Medscape National Physician Burnout & Suicide Report 2020: The Generational Divide," *Medscape*, January 15, 2020: https://www.medscape.com/slide show/2020-lifestyle-burnout-6012460#1.

26 Aronson, AHPI, 243–244.

27 Aronson, Interview.

28 Aronson, AHPI, 249.

29 Aronson, Interview.

30 Aronson, AHPI, 110.
31 Aronson, Interview.
32 Ibid.
33 Thomas R. Cole, "A Job I Never Expected," *OUPblog, Oxford University Press,* January 6, 2020, https://blog.oup.com/2020/01/a-job-i-never-expected.
34 Aronson, *Elderhood,* 68.
35 Thomas R. Cole, *Old Man Country: My Search for Meaning among the Elders* (New York: Oxford University Press, 2020).
36 Isaac Chotiner, "How Old Is Too Old to Work," *The New Yorker,* March 8, 2020: https://www.newyorker.com/news/q-and-a/how-old-is-too-old-to-work.
37 Christina Ianzito, "How to Embrace the Stages of Aging," AARP, American Association of Retired Persons, 2019, accessed August 20, 2021: https://www.aarp.org/entertainment/books/info-2019/elderhood-embraces-stages-of-aging.html.
38 A. S. Karlamangla, et al., "Biological Correlates of Adult Cognition: Midlife in the United States (MIDUS)," *Neurobiol Aging* 35, no. 2 (2014): 387–394.
39 "Ageism" is a term coined by Robert Butler, which means, "prejudice by one age group toward other age groups … a deep-seated uneasiness on the part of the young and middle-aged—a personal revulsion to and distaste for growing old, disease, disability; and fear of powerlessness, 'uselessness,' and death." Robert N. Butler, "Age-ism: Another Form of Bigotry," *The Gerontologist* 9, no. 4 (1969): 243.
40 Aronson, Interview.
41 Paula Span, "Older People Need Geriatricians. Where Will They Come From?," *The New York Times,* January 3, 2020: https://www.nytimes.com/2020/01/03/health/geriatricians-shortage.html; A. H. Petriceks, J. C. Olivas, and S. Srivastava, "Trends in Geriatrics Graduate Medical Education Programs and Positions, 2001 to 2018," *Gerontology and Geriatric Medicine* 4 (Jan-Dec 2018): doi: 10.1177/2333721418777659, https://www.ncbi.nlm.nih.gov/pubmed/29796406.
42 Health Resources and Services Administration, U.S. Department of Health and Human Services, National Center for Health Workforce Analysis, "National and Regional Projections of Supply and Demand for Geriatricians: 2013–2025," Rockville, MD, 2017.
43 Aronson, *Elderhood,* 73.
44 Urban Dictionary, *Urban Dictionary* (San Francisco, CA: Aaron Peckham, 2020): https://www.urbandictionary.com.
45 Aja Romano, "OK boomer" Isn't Just about the Past. It's about Our Apocalyptic Future," *Vox,* November 19, 2019: https://www.vox.com/2019/11/19/20963757/what-is-ok-boomer-meme-about-meaning-gen-z-millennials.
46 Aronson, *Elderhood,* xii.
47 Rita Charon, *Narrative Medicine: Honoring the Stories of Illness* (New York: Oxford University Press, 2006).
48 Arthur Kleinman, *Writing at the Margin: Discourse between Anthropology and Medicine* (Berkeley, CA: University of California Press, 1995), 14.
49 Aronson, Interview.

12 Marc Agronin

Into the heart of growing old

Jill Yamasaki

Introduction

You can't list the problems of aging without also tallying the hopes and promises.[1] If I had to capture the heart of Marc Agronin's work in one sentence, that would be it. As a communication scholar invested in matters of health and aging, I examine how language shapes personal and social meanings and experiences of old age. Like Agronin, I acknowledge the inherent challenges of age but usually gravitate toward the good. Unfortunately, in a culture that equates value with youth, that's not always the typical—or natural—perspective of others. People, including students, colleagues, and friends, often ask why I'm drawn toward time-intensive qualitative research (i.e., narrative interviews, participant-observation, guided reminiscence, photovoice) with participants over the age of 75. I always shrug and simply say, "I enjoy spending time with older adults."

By his own admission, Agronin also enjoys "talking with very old people."[2] A geriatric psychiatrist, he serves as the Vice President for Behavioral Health and Clinical Research at Miami Jewish Health (MJH), one of the largest nursing homes in the United States—and one often dismissed as "God's waiting room."[3] On average, his patients are 90 years old and psychotic, depressed, infirm, or demented; each year, he loses to death almost as many as he gains. Throughout his career, though, Agronin is regularly "reminded that when we see only the silent darkness of old age, we miss the sparks of life still present."[4] These patients come to him with rich histories comprised of people, places, experiences, and—despite frail bodies and diminished minds—the potential to persist, live with meaning, and even thrive at the end of life. "I could confess to occasionally feeling depressed," writes Agronin, "but in truth with each patient I have a different state of mind—delight, disappointment, curiosity, consternation, *wonder*."[5]

It's this wonder that inspires his writing and animates his clinical work. Like others, including myself, who seek to understand aging from the inside,[6] Agronin explores the experience of old age through his patients and offers a more balanced perspective on aging in his publications. Two of his books in particular—*How We Age: A Doctor's Journey into the Heart of Old Age* and *The End of Old Age: Living a Longer, More Purposeful Life*—champion a multifaceted understanding of old age that challenges dominant narratives of aging as decline or death.

DOI: 10.4324/9781003079712-12

More than that, they articulate Agronin's alternate view of old age as a time of emerging strengths—most notably, wisdom, purpose, and creativity—for mitigating loss and moving forward regardless of impairment or disease. From this perspective, Agronin joins other pioneers in gerontology who assert that people have unimaginable potential as they grow old not in *spite* of age but *because* of it. To those who question this potential or fear a miserable late life, he insists: "I work in a nursing home day in and day out, and I see how life goes on and even flourishes. Under the right circumstances, the imagined grim reaper of old age can seem more like an angel."[79] Agronin's devotion to these circumstances is his life's work and passion, reflected in the stories of his patients at the heart of growing old.

Old age reimagined

The first old person in Agronin's life was his great-grandmother, whom he remembers equally as "a very bright and beloved woman with a good sense of humor" and "an exotic and perfumed lady with long painted fingernails, a mysterious accent, and a thick purple coat and scarf surrounding her wrinkled and wizened face."[8] He was especially close to his grandfather, a doctor who "taught me with both an earnestness and a severity about caring for patients."[9] During Agronin's childhood, more than half of the residents in his grandfather's small town were either current or former patients, including Agronin himself, and he was renowned for his legendary perseverance and dedication to them all. Agronin counts both his grandfather and great-grandmother among the elders who populated his childhood, noting they "were all active, colorful, and beloved figures who conferred a delightful mystique on aging" and crediting them with "why I was always comfortable working with the elderly."[10]

I, too, enjoyed close relationships with my grandparents as a child and now have an affinity for working with older adults. For more than two decades, I've been fortunate to engage as a volunteer, employee, and/or scholar with diverse populations in a variety of excellent assisted living and continuing care communities. I have dear friends who are three and four decades older than I, and I purposefully seek out blogs, books, and media that highlight the voices of older adults. Indeed, I envision the old age of which Agronin writes.

Many people lack such vital figures in their lives, however. Agronin concedes their resulting vision of old age—which may be taken from decrepit grandparents in wheelchairs or agitated relatives with dementia—is often colored with dread or disgust. This constricted notion of old age is internalized throughout the life span and prevalent in society's stereotypes, stories, and experiences.[11] Indeed, chronological age may indicate the number of years we've lived, but social constructions largely shape how individuals or collective groups anticipate, experience, and represent age: from this perspective, age-centric perceptions of the "nuisances and miseries" of old age, as well as the tendencies to equate aging with dementia and to perpetuate an ageist culture in which the young are idealized, the old are stigmatized, and those who care for them are denigrated.[12]

These ageist thoughts and behaviors are also engrained in the teaching and practice of medicine. "*For nearly every doctor*, the very first encounter in medical school with an old person is with a corpse,"[13] writes Agronin, noting that the lesson is that *aging equals death*. "From a young doctor's vantage point, the aging process brought only decay, decline, and disease until the inevitable demise of the body," he explains. "This depressing view of aging, reinforced during my years of internship and residency in medicine, neurology, and psychiatry, was then coupled with a new equation: *Aging equals dementia*."[14]

The antidotes to these fears, Agronin claims, are equally harmful. While doctors are less sanguine about reversing the effects of aging as promised by the current multi-billion-dollar industry of products and clinics, they nonetheless view age as a disease that warrants treatment, seeking to preserve intellect and strength as long as possible before inevitable decline. For patients already in the throes of old age, frailty, or dementia, doctors may subconsciously dehumanize them, reducing them to labels, objects, or bodies that can be examined without much emotion. Remarkably, even providers attending to elderly residents in nursing homes experience ageism from their peers. Doctors like Agronin, working with patients who are both old and demented or psychotic, are typically "dismissed as either incompetent or overly sentimental individuals who couldn't hack more illustrious or challenging medical specialities."[15]

In the midst of these cynical and fatalistic attitudes toward aging and the old, Agronin advocates for a new paradigm: *aging brings strength*. Rather than focusing solely on the common and expected struggles of old age, he argues, people should recognize the immense potential in aging. Agronin proposes three emerging strengths that underlie this more balanced and inclusive paradigm. Wisdom, purpose, and creativity can both mitigate losses and guide people forward in a later life that is purpose-driven, personalized, and meaningful. "We must learn how to age in a creative manner that is both the antidote to feeling old and the elixir of aging well,"[16] he writes, joining renowned visionary Gene Cohen—the late American psychiatrist who pioneered the field of geriatric mental health—and Cohen's life partner Wendy Miller in understanding and promoting creative aging.[17] Cohen, and now Miller and Agronin, viewed aging as a source of strength for thriving and creativity as an essential resource for growth, development, and possibility in later life.

Importantly, Agronin insists that this paradigm applies even to individuals with severe physical and cognitive losses, like his patients, who are typically left out of models of aging that don't focus solely on decline. Popular paradigms of successful or positive aging explain how people can survive and change during a process defined by decline and loss; however, they don't cast aging itself as a source of strength. Agronin, like Cohen, has "seen the best and the worst of old age"[18,22] as a geriatric psychiatrist but still sees "a higher value, purpose, or accomplishment in aging regardless of its current state."[19] This viewpoint is inherent in the stories of memorable patients that populate his writing. *How We Age*, in particular, illustrates the inevitable psychological, physical, and social changes that make aging a challenge while also showing the many promises that transform late life into a time of positive change, adaptation, and even rejuvenation.

Creativity and the vital forces of old age

It is here where I as a social scientist and narrative scholar especially appreciate Agronin's sensibilities. As a medical doctor, Agronin draws masterfully from the humanities, using classic quotes, characters, poems, and parables to contextualize cultural meanings and possibilities of age. Literary luminaries like T. S. Eliot, John Updike, Herman Melville, Jonathan Swift, and Henry Wadsworth Longfellow figure prominently in his works. Agronin couples this extraordinary command of literature with tales from personal conversations with doctors and gerontologists who share similar sensibilities. In one of those conversations, renowned cardiologist and Nobel Peace Prize winner Bernard Lown detailed the paradox of aging that, at age 88, he had experienced and noted while growing older. Lown lamented declines in the cognitive skills deemed so essential to his role as a doctor and in the short-term memory needed to remember details of patient histories, the names of drugs, or the latest advances in his field. At the same time, though, Lown described acquiring

> the ability to commune and perceive an emotional dimension that is pre- or post- or extra-verbal. It's not words—it's gestalt. It's an ability to perceive, but more than that, a sensibility to nuance that is so trivial that it is overlooked.

Indeed, he told Agronin, "I was better in judgment, far better and far keener, and the patients sensed that. They would say to me, 'You're a far better doctor than you were twenty, thirty years ago.'"[20]

This paradox—that aging gives even as it takes away—is the central premise of Agronin's written work and a hopeful context for his clinical practice, where he seeks to recognize and leverage the inherently positive elements within his patients regardless of any disease or dysfunction. Here, Agronin joins Cohen and other eminent gerontologists, including Louise Aronson, Robert Butler, Thomas Cole, and George Vaillant, in championing the inherent capacity for creativity in old age and the importance of hope as a viable response to old age. "Compared to younger peers," writes Agronin, "centenarians cope better with stress, tend to be more confident and independent, are generally less anxious and depressed, and have increased levels of life satisfaction, even when functional limitations are greater."[21] For these gerontologists and other like-minded scholars, "human freedom and vitality lie in choosing to live well within the limits of aging even as we struggle against them."[22] They claim that resilience in later life is the capacity to not only handle adversities but also to learn, grow, and be positively transformed by them.[23] Ultimately, claims Agronin, lessons learned from the old "promise not the end of aging, but a new beginning even as we age."[24]

To illustrate, Agronin devotes most of The End of Old Age to explicating a better aging process in which "one can actively live a creative age as opposed to falling headlong into an uncontrollable old."[25] Using scientific understandings and patient experiences, he contends that aging changes people in fundamental ways. Specifically, individuals develop five core strengths: (1) a life of accumulated *knowledge*, experience, and skills; (2) lessons from trial and error that enhance *judgment*; (3) failure, which leads to humility, gratitude, and *empathy*; (4) ambition and motivation to build, compose, and *create*; and (5) the approach of death, which brings increased *insight* and a transcendent perspective on life. Put together, these elements "compose the greatest gift of aging: *wisdom*."[26] A multifaceted ability, wisdom enables people to grow and develop new abilities even in the face of age-related decline. These abilities are expressed through roles or identities that strengthen with age and bring greater resilience, purpose, and creativity. According to Agronin, it is up to each of us to identify, develop, and optimize these age-given strengths for living late life with more purpose and meaning. Fortunately, he delivers a specific course of action to do so.

Wisdom in late life

"Once upon an island I was happy. I was free," lamented Cuban American artist Margarita Cano. In 1962, she fled from Cuba, which she depicts in her painting *¡Libertad!* According to Agronin, it took 30 years of aging and then retirement for Margarita to find a way to express her nostalgia and ongoing sadness through painting. Now, her paintings are recognized for the vivid colors and symbolism of a lost world, and she continues to create into her 80s, declaring, "I will continue my quest in pursuit of a happy closure to this never-ending saga."[27]

Agronin shares Margarita's story to exemplify how creativity as a powerful and enduring lifelong attribute has great potential to bloom with increasing age. More than just artistic ability, the true strength of creators in later life "lies in thinking and acting differently from before, liberated from their past and willing to take risks for the sake of self-improvement, the good of their family or community, or sheer adventure."[28] Agronin characterizes this strength of age as one of five points on a crown that all people wear into later life:

> We can imagine this expansive notion of wisdom as a five-pointed crown … studded with precious jewels that are continually added each year. The crown and its jewels represent our *reserve*, and consist of all the mental abilities we accumulate over time. The ways in which we wear and use the power of this crown represents our *wisdom*. Each point of the crown is a subtype of reserve and wisdom based on the five cited strengths and can be labeled as *savant, sage, curator, creator,* and *seer*.[29]

Savants embody the most common and recognizable form of wisdom, characterized by a lifetime reserve of accumulated knowledge, skills, and expertise and the ability to show, share, and teach it (e.g., a family storyteller, expert seamstress, or master cook). Sages have this same wisdom but also insights, values, and virtues that they can apply to judgments and problem-solving (e.g., giving advice).

Curators possess a wisdom more distinct from the savant and the sage because its essence lies in the empathy, care, and concern for others at personal and community-wide levels (e.g., a caregiver, counselor, steward for a cause, or committed volunteer). The fifth point of the crown belongs to the seer, whose introspective, inquisitive, and spiritual mindset helps individuals cope with change and find meaning in life. "Each form of wisdom has corresponding verbs that represent their mutual interactions with others, especially younger generations," explains Agronin. "The savant *learns, shows,* and *teaches;* the sage *weighs* and *decides;* the curator *cares* and *connects;* the creator *imagines* and *makes;* and the seer *accepts* and *communes.*"[30]

Over the years, Agronin has guided patients, caregivers, and various audiences through an action plan that helps them age better by improving how they value the aging process, navigate stress, and find ways to creatively address change. To begin, Agronin encourages everyone to individually chart their current reserve of wisdom based on the five core strengths and their corresponding roles. Doing so means tallying a lifetime of experience, interests, and knowledge into a chart of wisdom, which is then followed by four additional steps:

(1) Review one or more major age points (i.e., a period of adversity that exposes a gap between the challenges or demands of a life event and an individual's existing strengths, values, skills, and connections) to identify personal modes of resilient coping.

(2) Consider pathways for renewal and reinvention by committing to age imperatives (i.e., actions based on the thinking and doing action verbs from the five types of wisdom) that demonstrate current activities, new activities, or contingency plans for anticipated limitations, including creative and meaningful activities, relationships, and pursuits. Agronin specifically notes that this step is similar to Gene Cohen's social portfolio of age, which consists of a personalized list of activities that one can do under two basic conditions: low or high mobility and individual or group pursuits. Agronin and Cohen both propose that age imperatives or social portfolios "be developed with the input of close family and friends, be as diversified as possible, and include activities as 'insurance' that can be pursued even in the face of more severe physical or cognitive limitations."[31]

(3) Consider, appreciate, and disseminate messages about your identity and legacy (i.e., the lives you've lived and the impact you've had), with an understanding that "the fruits of our aging—the crown of wisdom and the whole gown and scepter of our existence—extends far beyond our own lifetime."[32,37]

(4) Plan a ritual to celebrate aging itself as a positive and dynamic force, given that "aging individuals are left facing multiple later life transitions without the benefit of 'ritual, ceremony, or symbol.'"[33]

At each step, Agronin offers descriptive charts and illustrative examples from cultural figures (e.g., David Bowie, Matisse, Leonard Cohen), prior participants or patients, and his own social circle of family and friends.

Of course, it's tempting to dismiss this call to action as only applicable to so-called SuperAgers,[34] whose minds and bodies are extraordinarily bright and active well into their 80s and beyond; however, Agronin contends that the strengths comprising wisdom in late life apply to every aging person regardless of life circumstances—including those like his patients with limited abilities and choices. A sage, for example, might remain engaged in a mutually beneficial relationship or activity out of an inherent sense of its relevance or importance (e.g., a frail mother whose adult children suspend disagreements in her presence), while a curator could serve as a living display or cultural icon with specific knowledge, experience, or memories (e.g., World War II veterans in their late 90s). Savants could be meaningful community icons notable for their long-term memories, residual abilities, and even their very presence (e.g., a respected longtime pastor's wife with progressive dementia), and seers might be considered living relics with a powerful, residual presence that continues to inspire others (e.g., Pope John Paul II with Parkinson's disease in his later years).

Even people with dementia, Agronin insists, can be creators like Cuban artist Margarita Cano, but they may need help to do so. Consider, for example, Hilda Gorenstein, whose painting I solicited to grace the cover of my health communication text *Storied Health and Illness*.[35] Hilgos, as she was known professionally, completed hundreds of paintings in the last three years of her life while in the later stages of Alzheimer's disease. After worsening dementia seemingly ended her accomplished 75-year artistic career, Hilgos was able to resume painting with the help of students from her alma mater, the School of the Art Institute of Chicago, claiming, "I remember better when I paint." Her abstract watercolors allude to the nautical themes she specialized in throughout her career, and they represent opportunities for Hilgos—in the depths of a progressively isolating disease—to connect with others and be embraced and appreciated for her artistic spirit and innate creative impulse.

To that end, her daughter, Berna Huebner, created the Hilgos Foundation[36] to support and encourage art therapy for people with memory problems, dementia, and/or Alzheimer's disease. These experiences inspired Huebner to write a book that was later turned into an award-winning documentary in further celebration of Hilgos' expressive paintings and the therapeutic benefits of art therapy programs. It was Huebner who gave me her blessing to use Hilgos' painting, recognizing that we share similar sensibilities in our lives and work.

Agronin touts his action plan as encapsulating an alternate view of aging that is both experienced and celebrated by a rapidly growing segment of the population. For him,

> this message is a call to action for each one of us to begin shaping and reshaping aging in our own unique ways, guided and inspired by the lives of the most beloved, influential, and profound individuals who have gone before us.[37]

His evidence-based alternative provides both agency and autonomy to older adults—basic human dignities not always afforded to people when aging is viewed through the limited prism of decline.

Care and connection in old age

"I write about what people have taught me," explains Agronin. "These are not things I have made up on my own. I would never claim at age 52 to know what it is like to be 82 or 92."[38] As one of America's leading geriatric psychiatrists, his vita is impressive. A graduate of Harvard University and the Yale School of Medicine, Agronin completed his residency on adult psychiatry at Harvard University's McLean Hospital and then a geriatric psychiatry fellowship at the Minneapolis VA Medical Center. He is a recognized national expert in Alzheimer's disease and geriatric mental health issues as well as a prolific scholar, having published numerous scholarly articles and books that integrate his clinical expertise in psychiatry, medicine, and neurology. Currently, he is the driving force in MJH's EmpathiCare philosophy (i.e., an innovative approach to patient-centered care with a focus on empathy and connection) and the future EmpathiCare Village—a first of its kind in the United States—for adults living with cognitive changes and memory disorders.[39]

Having spent most of his career in what he deems "the epicenter of aging that is South Florida,"[40] Agronin has

> a deep and enduring fascination and affection for these aged souls. Their care is my life's work and my passion. But many of the countless older patients whom I have treated have tested me as a doctor, and I have sometimes failed. And they have forced me to admit that old age is not always what I want it to be.[41]

Throughout both How We Age and The End of Old Age, Agronin balances the promises of aging with the understanding that the experience of aging is circumscribed by physical health, personal resources, cultural norms, and historical events. He notes this reality for many of the patients he sees at MPH:

> It is tempting to dismiss the late-life course of many older individuals labeled with chronic mental illnesses. In this scheme we focus instead on the "personality disorder" or the "schizophrenic" or the "demented" as if they were no more than a stereotyped disease. ... Being old and being mentally ill are a double whammy, bringing derision and discrimination from two different directions.[42]

Nonetheless, Agronin writes that he has seen "how sparks of humanity persist until the final moments, and I must state, 'Perhaps we are missing something.' Even without mental rationality, there are perception, emotion, and imagination."[43] Agronin practices medicine in the same way he saw his grandfather tend to patients in a small Midwestern town for more than 50 years—with empathic attention, personal connection, and total dedication.

Consider the story he tells of Aron, an 84-year-old Auschwitz survivor with a recent diagnosis of Alzheimer's disease. He arrived at Agronin's office at the urgent pleading of his adult children. There, he shuffled into the office, had a baffled expression on his face, and only spoke a few phrases in a mix of English, Yiddish, and Hebrew. The family was deeply concerned at his rapid deterioration, given that Aron had been functioning independently and driving a car only four months earlier, and furious with his primary care physician who would not authorize a brain scan, reasoning it would not change the diagnosis or management of Alzheimer's disease. Instead, he sent Aron to a psychiatrist, who diagnosed depression and prescribed medication.

Agronin, however, realized that the clinical picture looked nothing like Alzheimer's disease but instead suggested a rapidly progressing neurological disorder that warranted immediate attention. Indeed, after fighting the insurance company on Aron's behalf, Agronin got a report from the radiologist that the new brain scan indicated a large mass on Aron's brain. More struggles with bureaucracy ensued until Aron was finally admitted to the hospital for surgery and completely cured. Three weeks after surgery, he drove himself to Agronin's office, strode into the office with a steady, normal gait, threw his arms around him, and thanked Agronin in perfect, fluent English. "In every doctor's life there should be at least one such moment of satisfaction, one shining opportunity to witness the miraculous glory of healing the seemingly incurable,"[44] Agronin mused a year later at Aron's 85th birthday party.

Agronin shares this story not out of arrogance or boastful pride but rather to demonstrate how easy it can be for doctors to dismiss the concerns of older adults and their families when they present with the trappings or afflictions of old age, and also how important a doctor's presence—when imbued with a sense of commitment and caring—can be for older adults and their families. Agronin writes often about the importance of cultivating empathy by listening closely, responding with physical attentiveness, resonating emotionally, and sometimes just being attentively present with his patients. Even as he shares his vision and practice of humanizing care, Agronin takes great pain to ensure that he writes about his patients "in a manner as humane and respectful as possible."[45] He does so by seeking permission, focusing on the human being rather than simply portraying him or her as a disease, and changing identifying names and biographical details in order to retain the basic condition without allowing identification by even clinicians or caregivers who know these individuals personally.

Unfortunately, Agronin notes that "we simply ignore, avoid, or neglect our most debilitated elderly,"[46] exacerbating the relentless loss of persona inflicted on sufferers of dementia with human-made problems of abandonment and loneliness:

> I have found over the years as I speak, lecture and write about aging that I always hear the common refrain: "That's well and good but once you have dementia or go into a nursing home it's terrible." I want to push back on it. It conflates old age and aging with absolute misery, and it is simply not true. If that is how we think about aging, it will have a profound negative effect on our lives.[47]

Agronin's work with very old, very sick, and/or very frail patients has convinced him that while some conditions "evade our most intensive and compassionate efforts to help," the loss of hope engendered by those conditions is always more devastating.[48] "We cannot reverse death," writes Agronin, "but dementia, depression, delirium, and destitution are challenges we *can* do something about."[49]

To that end, Agronin's patients have taught him two important lessons: (1) it is easy to miss sparks of the person hidden under the burden of disease; and (2) we can step in to discover and even help rejuvenate the person behind the lost memories. He espouses personal connection as an antidote to the first and as an opportunity for the second. Connecting with patients in the throes of dementia requires imagination and creativity. Studies—and Agronin in his clinical work—demonstrate the humanizing potential of meaningful interventions like guided reminiscence, artmaking, and memory boxes that both personalize patients and help caregivers honor, celebrate, and connect with them beyond the debilitating effects of dementia.[50]

I endorse and practice this inherently dialogic perspective in similar settings. A biographical approach to long-term care acknowledges the power of stories for making sense of lived disruptions, including corporeal and social threats in long-term care. Most of all, it embraces the storied nature of aging. Valuing older adults, in general, and long-term care residents, in particular, as biographical selves with complex histories, meaningful presents, and futures alive with possibility can ultimately shape thicker versions of late life and inspire new normals in long-term care.[51] For Agronin, such humanizing practices mean "the difference between settling for the achievement of some physical comfort and striving to enable life *and* positive growth, comfort *and* meaning. It's about not giving up."[52]

Limitations

Ever the steadfast optimist, even Agronin admits that "I could easily be accused of painting an overly rosy picture of what I want growing old to be."[53] As described at the beginning of this chapter, I share his hopeful enthusiasm. And, for Agronin, that's exactly the point: our experience of aging will be influenced by how we imagine it to be.[54] "We imagine the pains of late-life ailments but not the joys of new pursuits," he writes. "We recoil at the losses and loneliness and fail to embrace the wisdom and meaning that only age can bring."[55] While I agree with this premise, I can see how those who dread their own aging might dismiss Agronin's work as largely untenable or unrealistic, especially given the patient population from which he draws examples. Miami Jewish Health—due in significant part to Agronin's leadership and vision—employs an innovative care model centered on empathy, strives to be the leading source of healthy aging through a continuum of care, and offers renowned memory care services. It's easy to forget as you read Agronin's work that many people do not have the material, financial, social, or emotional resources available to them for this type of care in later life. His books offer an important treatise of meaningful old age for providers and caregivers, which is an important step in challenging and disrupting negative societal views of aging; however, even with the action plan he delineates in *The End of Old Age*, I suspect lay audiences may appreciate his inspired view of aging without adopting it as their own.

Conclusion

Regardless, Agronin ultimately claims that "it is the failure of our own creativity and willingness to conceive that life up until its last minutes has its own ways and meanings."[56] The patients he presents as examples often seem both the exception and exceptional, but he notes that he's seeing more like them every day. Although older and with more daunting medical and psychiatric issues than those he saw at the beginning of his career, Agronin's average patients are now "less concerned about living a long life and more focused on living a life full of purpose and meaning."[57] Even those with significant cognitive and/or physical impairment are thriving with the help of empathic others who imagine alternative ways to work around barriers and identify best approaches.[58] From these lived experiences, Agronin asserts that "we can all hope for a vital and meaningful old age—for our elders, ourselves, and our children. In the end, we may actually get what we wish for."[59]

Agronin is not alone in championing a new perspective of aging (see the chapters in this volume about Louise Aronson or Atul Gawande, for example). He is a leading, often poetic voice, however, in transforming how Americans view old age and experience late life as a time of strength and creativity. "I have encountered hundreds of wonderful sayings and aphorisms," writes Agronin.

> There is one that stands above them all in my mind because it speaks to the essence of my beliefs. It comes from Psalm 92: *Even in old age they will still produce fruit; they will remain vital and green.*

He notes with amazement that this insight comes from a time when old age was rare and, when it did occur, quite difficult. His admiration of the psalmist who wrote the passage likely mirrors what I think of him as an imaginative doctor-writer at the heart of growing old:

> I offer my gratitude to this ancient, wise, and charitable soul who decided to inspire us toward what we could be as we aged, rather than to denigrate us for what we might become when illness, injury, and loss are at hand.[60]

Notes

1 Marc E. Agronin, "For Anyone Interested in Aging," accessed August 20, 2021, https://www.marcagronin.com/book/how-we-age/.
2 Marc E. Agronin, *How We Age* (Cambridge, MA: Da Capo Press, 2011), 279.
3 Ibid., 12.
4 Ibid., 277.

5   Ibid., 20.
6   Jan-Eric Ruth and Gary M. Kenyon, "Introduction: Special Issue on Ageing, Biography, and Practice," *Ageing and Society* 16 (1996): 653–657; Gary Kenyon, Ernst Bohlmeijer, and William L. Randall, eds., *Storying Later Life: Issues, Investigations, and Interventions in Narrative Gerontology* (New York: Oxford University Press, 2011); and Jill Yamasaki, "Aging by Surprise: Navigating the Unexpected or Unimagined in Late Life," *Communication Monographs* (in press).
7   Agronin, *How We Age*, 43.
8   Ibid., 23.
9   Ibid., 21.
10 Ibid., 27.
11 Agronin, *The End of Old Age* (Cambridge, MA: Da Capo Press, 2018), vii; Margaret Cruikshank, *Learning to Be Old: Gender, Culture, and Aging*, 3rd ed. (Lanham, MD: Rowman & Littlefield, 2013); and Jill Yamasaki, "Age Accomplished, Performed, and Failed: Liz Young as Old on *The Biggest Loser*," *Text and Performance Quarterly* 34 (2014): 354–371.
12 Agronin, *How We Age*, 8–9.
13 Ibid., 1.
14 Ibid., 7.
15 Ibid., 8.
16 Agronin, *The End of Old Age*, vii.
17 Wendy L. Miller and Gene D. Cohen, *Sky above Clouds: Finding Our Way through Creativity* (New York: Oxford University Press, 2016).
18 Agronin, *The End of Old Age*, 4.
19 Ibid., 133.
20 Agronin, *How We Age*, 198.
21 Ibid., 41.
22 Thomas R. Cole, *The Journey of Life: A Cultural History of Aging in America* (Cambridge: Cambridge University Press, 1992).
23 Jennifer E. Ohs and Jill Yamasaki, "Communication and Successful Aging: Challenging the Dominant Cultural Narrative of Decline," *Communication Research Trends* 36 (2017): 4–42; and Miller and Cohen, *Sky above Clouds*.
24 Agronin, *How We Age*, 13.
25 Agronin, *The End of Old Age*, 12.
26 Ibid., 48.
27 Ibid., 62–63.
28 Ibid., 64.
29 Ibid., 49.
30 Ibid., 68–69.
31 Ibid., 182.
32 Ibid., 184.
33 Ibid., 187.
34 The idea of SuperAgers is scientifically recognized by scholars, neurologists, and psychiatrists, including Agronin, and celebrated by anti- and healthy aging experts in the popular press.
35 Jill Yamasaki, Patricia Geist-Martin, and Barbara F. Sharf, eds., *Storied Health and Illness: Personal, Cultural, and Political Complexities* (Long Grove, IL: Waveland Press, 2017).
36 For more information, visit http://hilgos.org.
37 Agronin, *The End of Old Age*, 195.
38 Sally Abrahms, "Let's Get Rid of Those Tired Notions of Aging: In 'The End of Old Age,' Dr. Marc Agronin Challenges Americans," *NextAvenue*, January 19, 2018, https://www.nextavenue.org/get-rid-tired-notions-aging/.

39 For more information, visit https://www.miamijewishhealth.org/giving/empathicare-donations/.
40 Agronin, *The End of Old Age*, 3.
41 Agronin, *How We Age*, 236.
42 Ibid., 136–137.
43 Ibid., 236.
44 Ibid., 247.
45 Ibid., ix.
46 Ibid., 144.
47 Abrahms, "Let's Get Rid of Those Tired Notions of Aging."
48 Agronin, *How We Age*, 44.
49 Ibid., 236.
50 Jill Yamasaki, "The Poetic Possibilities of Long-Term Care," in *Imagining New Normals: A Narrative Framework for Health Communication*, edited by Lynn M. Harter (Dubuque, IA: Kendall/Hunt, 2013), 107–124; Anne D. Basting, *Forget Memory: Creating Better Lives for People with Dementia* (Baltimore, MD: The Johns Hopkins University Press, 2009); and Miller and Cohen, *Sky above Clouds*.
51 Yamasaki, "The Poetic Possibilities of Long-Term Care."
52 Agronin, *How We Age*, 118.
53 Marc E. Agronin, "Shedding a Protective Cocoon, Woven by Delusions," *The New York Times*, February 14, 2011, https://www.nytimes.com/2011/02/15/health/views/15cases.html.
54 Agronin, *How We Age*, 43.
55 Ibid., 19.
56 Ibid., 11. Agronin expands on this sentiment in Abrahms, "Let's Get Rid of Those Tired Notions of Aging": "I'm not ignoring the challenges [nor do I] have a Pollyanna view. I think it's a more accurate view. If you believe that aging is a disease and a process of decline and decay, it may lead you *not* to take steps that will enhance your own life or that of others. That's only half the picture. Aging is a precious part of life and we need to do everything possible to engage with it, embrace it and use it as a positive force."
57 Agronin, *How We Age*, 4.
58 Yamasaki, "The Poetic Possibilities of Long-Term Care."
59 Agronin, "Shedding a Protection Cocoon, Woven by Delusions."
60 Agronin, *The End of Old Age*, 197.

Part IV
Alternative models

13 David Watts and Frank Huyler

A tale of two patients

David Elkin

What do patients want from their doctors? And what do their healthcare providers expect in return? In this chapter, we will analyze, compare, and contrast two physicians' accounts of interactions with two very different patients. We will consider the definitions of the medical humanities, and the tools that this interdisciplinary field provides to potentially improve our ability to understand what is being transacted in clinical interactions. We will consider how the medical humanities and narrative approaches can augment our ability to understand and connect with patients and better understand the providers who care for them.

The author's path to narrative medicine

Before I begin to consider these issues, I would like to discuss my own path to both medicine and the medical humanities. I offer a summary of my experiences for several reasons. First, I believe that they are instructive about the call to the medical field and simultaneously illustrative of the changes that medicine has undergone in the past half century. I also think that it is important for readers to understand the potential biases of anyone sharing their views on a subject—including mine. And lastly, the medical humanities, which will be highlighted in this chapter as a skill set for understanding patients, is an essential tool for shedding light on the inner lives of clinicians. One of the key methods of narrative medical approaches is to stress the importance of story, so I'll begin with my own.

As a child, I was fascinated by science, but I also loved reading, the arts, and history. As a college student, I majored in biochemistry, intent on being admitted to medical school and pursuing a career in medicine and infectious diseases. Exploration of the humanities appeared extraneous and distracting. Medical school proved challenging, and I struggled to keep up with the enormous amount of information that we had to learn. My experiences in clinical rotations revealed a central conflict of a yearning to connect with patients and their families, and to understand the social and cultural contexts of their lives and illnesses—a desire that was antithetical to the emphasis on efficiency and biomedical factors. My stressful first year of residency in internal medicine highlighted the gap between my ideals and the crushing reality of internship.

DOI: 10.4324/9781003079712-13

Eventually, with the help of unexpected peer mentors, and some surprising clinical encounters, I realized that I needed to change course. I made the fortuitous discovery of a field that would give me time and training to work with patients in the same clinical setting: consultation-liaison psychiatry. Immediately after graduating from my psychiatry residency, I started as a faculty member at San Francisco General Hospital, working part of the time with patients with HIV at the height of the AIDS epidemic. This proved to be the perfect place to combine my clinical interests in public health and teaching, and I loved the challenges of the work, and the support of like-minded colleagues.

My love of reading, film, history, and philosophy remained separate from my clinical work, until some fortuitous exposure to the medical humanities in a multi-day national workshop in 1998. I came to learn that the humanities are essential in understanding and connecting with patients, for enlivening teaching sessions, and reclaiming parts of ourselves that are otherwise extruded or barred from our professional lives as physicians. In my case, that has meant a fuller, more rewarding experience being a physician and teacher. And my growth has not stopped. A few years ago, I participated in a workshop on improv comedy that transformed the way that I interact with patients. I would like to share with readers a sense of the richness of human experience that lurks around many corners of clinical interactions that the humanities can help to illuminate.

The medical humanities

The medical humanities draw on the expertise offered by history, philosophy, sociology, and anthropology. Literature, the visual arts, poetry—all of the disciplines that examine what characterizes human behavior, thought, and creativity. The skills of close readings of works, careful reasoning reflection, and critical thinking are tools from these fields that can be deployed when examining patient-clinician interactions.[1] Rita Charon, an internist and literature professor at Columbia University, is a seminal figure in the field. She has championed the centrality of the story in understanding our patients' lives and experiences, as well as our own. In her article,[2] and her powerful TEDx talk,[3] Charon describes the nomenclature, rationale, and power of narrative competence and the practice of narrative medicine. She compellingly argues for applying the same skills utilized in literature to closely attend to the patient's account of their life and their experience of illness to strengthen meaningful connections and understanding between patients and their treating clinicians.

I don't remember when we first paired the two essays that I would like to explore in depth here. I do know that they were two of my favorite essays in books that I read in the beginning years of the twenty-first century, works that I admired for their candor and clarity in portraying clinical encounters. It was a pleasant surprise to discover that they were short enough to be read aloud by a small group with plenty of time left in the hour to discuss their portrayals of doctors and patients in conflict, the conclusions that they drew, and the mysteries that they left unresolved. The two are in some ways mirror images of each other, complementary in their depictions of physicians and patients. The first essay portrays a patient who is seemingly so anxious about having an illness that he almost certainly does not have that he will repeatedly request and tolerate invasive and potentially dangerous procedures by his experienced and increasingly frustrated physician. The other renders a glancing contact between a young emergency room resident with a patient who is so remarkably nonchalant about his very serious medical problems that he is well-known to staff for refusing further medical care and leaving against medical advice after each brief encounter. Together, they offer remarkable insights into clinical encounters, the cultural construct of illness, and the inner lives of patients and physicians alike.

A synopsis of the essays

"White Rabbits"

David Watts is a gastroenterologist, National Public Radio correspondent, and poet. An adjunct professor of medicine at UCSF, he leads classes on poetry and the "Healer's Art" for medical students. He has published numerous essays about his interactions with patients. In "White Rabbits," from his collection *Bedside Manners*,[4] Watts recounts an encounter with a challenging patient, Frank, who believes that he has colon cancer and requests multiple colonoscopies despite constant reassurances from Watts that he does not have cancer. Watts shares his mounting frustration with his patient, who goes so far as to record his bowel sounds to play back to his incredulous doctor. Watts is candid in his desire to distance himself from Frank:

> Without thinking, my body has stood up and is leaving the room. I babble something polite like I have to see someone down the hall and am gone before I can laugh or burst out with something I'd be sorry for. I am tempted to relate this story to those in the hallway, but who would believe that there's a guy in my office playing a recording of his own bowel sounds?[5]

He chides Frank for being concerned about an imaginary illness, when he has a verified and more serious problem. Frank, who apparently has a cardiac disease, is scheduled for bilateral carotid endarterectomies to clear atherosclerotic plaques that block the main arteries to his brain. At the end of their encounter, Watts is insistent on shutting down his patient's concerns, stating definitively and emphatically: "'You don't have cancer.' Since he cannot shut that door, I shut it for him."[6] Frank is shocked and disappointed and ends the interaction with a plaintive request: "Can we talk about this again?"[7] Watts is certain that Frank will return in the near-future, undeterred by any prior negative tests or explanations, with continued concerns about his gastrointestinal tract.

The Invitation

An emergency room is the setting for Frank Huyler's sparse and enigmatic tale of Mr. Santana, a patient who presents while Huyler is working a shift as a relatively inexperienced resident in New Mexico. Huyler, who also trained as a poet, has published two novels and two nonfiction accounts of medicine and medical training, the first based on notes that he kept during medical school, residency, and as an emergency room physician. In "The Invitation," from Huyler's book of collected essays *The Blood of Strangers*,[8] Mr. Santana "cheerfully" presents with chest pain: "And, it's ten out of ten," he offers, before he can be asked. He flirts with a nurse, who alerts Hulyer that his new patient is well-known for his presentations to the medical emergency room, as well as a repeated history of signing out against medical advice. Mr. Santana recounts a history of coronary heart disease, multiple stents, CABGs (cardiac bypass surgeries), heart attacks, and an episode of a nearly fatal arrhythmia, treated successfully in the same hospital. He went on to say that he died and that the hospital workers saved him. Huyler, disbelieving, reviews the multiple volumes of records and finds that Mr. Santana has indeed given a very accurate rendering of his medical history. Humbled by this information and the realization that his patient may be experiencing another life-threatening myocardial infarction, Huyler tells his patient that he will need to be admitted, but Mr. Santana refuses. "I'm always having a heart attack," he replies cheerfully. He asks for the AMA paperwork. Somewhat dumbfounded, Huyler complies, but then Mr. Santana takes the interaction into an unexpected direction. "Bury me in the Pecos,"[9] he abruptly instructs an increasingly mystified Huyler. He says that his family has a cabin in the Pecos wilderness, with "real adobe walls, four feet thick—a single candle can keep it warm in the winter. One candle, that's all you need."[10] He holds up a finger to illustrate this image. Huyler again gently pleads with his patient to stay, but Mr. Santana is dismissive: "I'm always having a heart attack."[11] And he concludes his mysterious emergency room visit with an apparently sincere invitation to come to the Pecos as his guest, and to "bring your girlfriend up there."[12] He hands Huyler his business card, which features only Mr. Santana's last name and telephone number, but no address. And with that, Mr. Santana departs the emergency room, leaving a befuddled Huyler—and the reader—in his wake to contemplate the interaction with his enigmatic patient.

Introductory notes and observations

How do we best approach a discussion of these two works? Rita Charon has advocated five factors in the use of the narrative medical approach. These include learning about the lives and stories of people who are ill; weighing the power of the physician in the relationship; assessing ethical concerns; exploring how writings conform to genre; and to using text or other works to "strengthen the human practice of doctoring."[13] She also suggests considering concerns about mortality, the narrative context of illness, the patient's causal explanation of their illness, and "shame, blame and fear."[14]

We can begin by thinking about what these two clinical tales have in common. At a superficial level, these two patients are repeatedly seen for health complaints whose likelihood of physiologic causes range from the highly unlikely to the very probable. Frank believes that he has colon cancer despite multiple negative workups, while Mr. Santana is experiencing chest pain with significantly abnormal electrocardiogram findings and a verified chart history that places him at high risk for death, either acutely or in the near future. Frank and Mr. Santana seem to have little in common, with one man desperately intent on wanting more time and procedures from his physician, while the other is content with a brief encounter before departing.

Physicians are trained to begin with the question, "What brings you to the clinic (or hospital)?" Neither physician appears highly comfortable or competent probing this. Watts constructs his own explanatory model of what drives Frank's obsession and requests for repeated colonoscopies. "Now we've come to it, I thought. This is the root of the multitudinous colonoscopies, the driving force for the unseen locomotive: failure to believe negative data. Failure to temper the fear that something is wrong somewhere."[15] After accusing Frank of solipsistic thinking, Watts's own thoughts appear to suffer from similarly circular reasoning. The patient's main problem, in Watts's view, is that he does not believe his doctor! Watts, an experienced physician, appears especially perturbed at not being fully in control of his interactions with Frank in his office.

Huyler, in contrast, is writing as a young physician who is quietly perplexed and decidedly outmatched by his much-older patient. Mr. Santana, upon learning that Huyler is 28 years old, comments, "You're young, I can tell. You have a lot to learn. I remember when I was your age. I held the world in the palm of my hands."[16] His patient's age and experience, including his knowledge of the medical system and ability to wield autonomy and power in the emergency room, clearly intimidate Huyler, who demonstrates considerable humility—and confusion—in the face of an unexpectedly challenging situation.

From a psychological perspective, these interactions are rich with both metaphor and meaning. Frank seems to be repeatedly seeking reassurance from his gastroenterologist, but also paradoxically wanting to have him find a physical finding to corroborate his fears. A psychodynamic framework would lead a clinician to hypothesize that Frank's constant worry about having colon cancer stems from unconscious psychological conflict. Frank is somatizing a psychological defense mechanism that leaves him stubbornly convinced that he is having physical problems, when in fact his symptoms likely have a psychological origin. A psychiatrist would consider diagnosing illness anxiety disorder, formerly known as hypochondriasis. Maladies such as hypochondriasis drive a high proportion of clinical encounters—a significant proportion of patients in primary care settings have been shown to experience psychologically based symptoms that manifest with physical symptoms such as chest pain, palpitations, back pain, and dizziness. Evaluation and tests fail to reveal a physiologic etiology in an astounding 90% of these cases, and the causes are believed to be psychologically based.

Mr. Santana's psychology, on the other hand, remains more mysterious. What motivates him to return repeatedly to the medical emergency room, only to sign out repeatedly against medical advice? On the one hand, he seems pleased with his care from the emergency room based on his past experiences: "'Yes … this hospital saved my life. I owe my life to you.' He looked pleased."[17] But why does he repeatedly return, only to leave again against medical advice? Is it to flirt with the nurses, or to enjoy the consternation of young emergency room residents? Because he is lonely, or because he wants to touch base, however briefly, like a talisman, with the institution that saved his life once before? Modern psychology would posit that there are both superficial and deeper meanings and intentions to any action, some of them conscious and some of them outside of any individual patient's awareness. This could be what is taking place for both Frank and Mr. Santana. Their physicians appear to struggle to comprehend that possibility, stubbornly engaging with only the more explicit or manifest levels of their patients' behavior and awareness. They consider the concrete meaning of their patients' words, but not the symbolic or metaphorical nature of communication, and the richness of unconscious meaning that their words suggest. The resulting communication gap between patient and clinician is what is most intriguing, yet remains largely unexplored in both clinical vignettes.

How might a humanities perspective help clinicians with their understanding and efficacy in these clinical encounters? First, a more holistic approach to medicine, better informed by philosophy, anthropology, and sociology, would consider the context of the doctor-patient encounter as the interaction has been defined historically and culturally. The narrative approach would focus on the stories of the patients and their physicians, examining the chain of events that brought each to the encounter. The narrative approach also includes attention to the symbolic meanings of symptoms, of the rich communication between physicians and patients, and the psychological needs of both parties. A reasonable place to begin is the possible psychology responsible for interpreting physical symptoms, as a starting point for what brings Frank and Mr. Santana to their clinical encounters.

Somatization as a psychological defense and a social construct

What is causing Frank to be so obsessed with the conviction that he has colon cancer or something else wrong in his gastrointestinal tract? Recall Watts's sense about what is driving Frank's obsession: "We've finally come to it, the roots of the multitudinous colonoscopies . . . failure to believe negative data."[18] Watts is attempting to model Frank's psychology but does so closely based on his own.

In fact, there are a wide range of conditions that can cause someone to fixate on bodily sensations. Depression, anxiety, anger, and alexithymia—a diminished awareness or ability to express one's emotions—are all associated with patients developing a somatic focus.[19] Certain brain lesions, including strokes, a condition for which Frank is at risk because of his carotid artery disease, can also cause somatic preoccupations. Or he could have a psychologically based preoccupation. But Watts shows no sign of considering this range of possibilities, or differential diagnosis for Frank's ruminations, and has apparently settled on a psychological explanation, a reasonable interpretation if the other possibilities were first excluded. This raises the question, how do we model someone else's psychology?

Over a century ago, the novelist Edith Wharton addressed what happens when we attempt to understand the inner lives of other people: "We live in our own souls as in an unmapped region, a few acres of which we have cleared for our habitation; while of the nature of those nearest us we know but the boundaries that march with ours."[20] In other words, we don't really know ourselves completely and, when we try to understand other people, we tend to overemphasize areas that appear similar to our own psychology. We fail to acknowledge or understand features of ourselves and others that exist outside of conscious awareness, the larger uncleared region of our minds to which Wharton alludes.

Around the same time that Wharton wrote these words, at the beginning of the twentieth century, Sigmund Freud, a young neurologist, was struggling to understand his patients' physical complaints. He gradually began to appreciate these physical symptoms as manifestations of their unconscious anxieties, conflicts, and traumatic experiences. Physicians had ventured hypotheses about somatic manifestations of distress for millennia. The term "hysteria" is based on the ancient Egyptian notion of a "wandering uterus," an almost 4,000-year-old gender-stereotyped effort to pinpoint the anatomical source of common maladies.[21] Freud made numerous errors and blunders in constructing his model of human psychology, but some of his theories were accepted and are now deeply ingrained in our culture and understanding. We speak with relative ease about "Freudian slips," the concept that dreams may reflect a hidden aspect of our psychology, and expect that each person has blind spots in their perceptions. Some parts of his theories prefigured studies of unconscious mental functioning.[22]

Psychoanalysis owes its roots to patients—mostly young women—who had unexplained medical symptoms. A key insight of psychoanalysis was to cite the use of defense mechanisms to deflect unconscious conflicts into other thoughts and behaviors.[23] In "White Rabbits," Frank appears to be displacing his concerns about his carotid artery disease onto an imagined problem in his colon. His insistence that something is wrong with his colon is an example of the defense mechanism of somatization. His focus on somatic complaints hypothetically serves to avoid presumptive unconscious conflicts. Thus, the person who uses somatization finds a physical problem on which to fixate and defends against conscious awareness of the more anxiety-producing cause.

The decrease in intrapsychic anxiety from blocking conscious awareness of a conflict is referred to as primary gain. Secondary gain is an interpersonal benefit that is realized by taking on the "sick role," a term first coined in the 1950s by the sociologist Talcott Parsons.[24] Cultural factors also play a significant role, as they have direct bearing on how people express distress, shape somatic complaints, and influence secondary gain.

In contrast to hypochondriacal patients, physicians are wary of patients who consciously simulate physical problems and who are aware of their goals, usually to obtain financial compensation for their problems, or opioid pain medication. This is malingering, and in extreme states is associated with antisocial personality disorder. Frank is presumably not aware of the origin or goal of his symptoms, and he does not appear motivated by a desire for financial gain or pain medication.

The root cause of his obsession with having colon cancer remains unknown, and his doctor does little to illuminate them. Most readers would probably agree that he is in some type of distress, but the exact nature of that distress is a mystery, presumably one with psychological causes. I am reminded of Napoleon's army discovering the Rosetta stone, a tablet that bore Egyptian cuneiform symbols as well as hieroglyphs and a Greek translation. For the first time in two millennia, it became possible to read ancient Egyptian hieroglyphics. What we are lacking for Frank, and others like him, is a way of decoding the symbolic nature of their physical symptoms, which despite their presentation in a medical setting, lack a physiologic explanation.

Many clinicians may have firsthand familiarity with somatization. "Medical student syndrome" has been observed in a significant portion of second year medical students, who develop the conviction that they have a disease just as they are learning about pathology, and the many ways in which the human body can malfunction. I have to acknowledge my own bout with this syndrome. During my second year of medical school I developed lower back pain, an episode which I became convinced was ankylosing spondylitis, an autoimmune disorder that causes a progressive and inexorable calcification of the spine that I happened to have learned about a few weeks before. It was only after a long week of dread in which I contemplated my likely death from that disorder that I sheepishly realized that the soreness in my lower back was actually the result of a new exercise routine: riding my bike over 10 miles a day to and from class, with a heavy textbook-laden backpack.

Anxiety among healthcare providers was understandably high during the COVID-19 pandemic.[25] Anecdotally, I had numerous colleagues tell me of minor episodes of panic, believing that a cough or other minor symptoms meant that they had contracted COVID-19. Somatization is a defense mechanism that can manifest in anyone, including healthcare workers, under stressful conditions.

While Frank may suffer from illness anxiety disorder, full psychiatric disorders are actually not that common in clinical practice. What is exceedingly common is the scenario where a patient presents to a clinical setting with a vague or mild symptom for which no physiologic cause is detected. These are referred to as "medically unexplained symptoms" by some researchers and are believed to be psychologically mediated and are believed to be extremely prevalent in healthcare settings.[26]

It is striking that neither Drs. Watts or Huyler consult with a psychiatrist or psychologist about their patients. The current medical model has been faulted by its tendency to focus on biological factors at the expense or exclusion of psychological, sociocultural, and spiritual considerations. George Engel's biopsychological model was expected to be widely adapted and deployed to restore the focus on nonphysiologic processes in medical presentations, but it appears to have drastically failed to find purchase in medical practice.[27] However, the concept of "embedded psychiatry" is finding utility, as psychiatrists and psychologists deploy to clinics and emergency rooms to help providers understand and treat their patients in real time.

The psychology of clinicians

Healthcare professionals have their own unique psychology, and clinicians have been the subject of increasing scrutiny, through studies as well as autobiographical writing and fiction. These works offer glimpses into the inner lives of physicians. What are they really thinking and feeling during clinical interactions? What is it that physicians struggle with? What are their needs, and their emotional responses to their patients?

Both studies and the writings of physician-authors offer windows into the inner lives of physicians. Like all human beings, physicians have basic needs, and they want to feel competent, autonomous, and connected. They are selected and trained to be emotionally stable, and to be able to modulate their emotions as needed, to attain emotional distance as needed when breaking bad news to patients or performing invasive procedures such as inserting tubes into veins or orifices, or performing surgery. They remain vulnerable to feelings of frustration, of loneliness, of powerlessness, and also of fear of illness themselves. Unmet or unexamined emotions may "affect both the quality of medical care and the physician's own sense of well-being, since unexamined emotions may also lead to physician distress, disengagement, burnout, and poor judgment."[28]

While the psychodynamic model focuses on the importance of unconscious mental processes in how our patients experience the world, we should also note that clinicians are human beings, and have the same psychological structures. The work of Daniel Kahneman and Amos Tversky (summarized in Kahneman's best-seller *Thinking Fast and Slow*[29]) considers the role of unconscious forces in economics and in other fields, including medicine. Medical training has moved to incorporate these findings in an attempt to better educate physicians about the role implicit bias plays in misunderstandings across cultural backgrounds. But there are broader implications for how physicians may be influenced in their assessments and reasoning based on many unconscious forms of influence. Thus, physicians have responses to their patients that encompass both conscious and unconscious thoughts, beliefs, biases, and feelings. In psychological terms, we refer to patients' responses to their doctors as transference, and physician's reactions to patients as countertransference. Modern definitions describe each of these as the sum of conscious and unconscious responses to the other party. Transference and countertransference are not just important factors in psychiatric encounters, but are universal features of all human interactions, and may powerfully affect healthcare workers in all clinical settings.

Thus, while it is incredibly helpful for Watts and Huyler to relate their emotional responses to their patients, there may be other thoughts and feelings occurring outside of their conscious awareness.[30] "White Rabbits" and "The Invitation" offer clues about this phenomenon. Both Watts and Huyler display moments in which they are not quite in control, and it is a credit to their candor that they both recount these incidents honestly to the reader. Watts writes of his mounting frustration with Frank, as he attempts to locate the section of audiotape with noises that he believes will convince his physician that he has colon cancer:

> I realize I am most amazed not by the weirdness it takes to record one's own bowel sounds, not by his solipsistic assumption that I will find this of such great and compelling interest as to arrest my whole practice while we await the multimedia presentation, but that I will tolerate his time-consuming fiddlings with this bowel-noise recording device of his while patients fully deserving my attention wait their turn. Were it not so humorous, it would be maddening. ... I am tempted to relate this story to those in the hallway, but who would believe that there's a guy in my office playing a recording of his own bowel sounds?[31]

These sentences may result in laughs from readers, but this response also raises the issue of the function and ethics of humor in medical practice.[32]

Thanks to Watts and Huyler's candor, we see examples of their conscious and unconscious emotional responses in their interactions with their respective patients. At one point, Watts, becoming increasingly frustrated with Frank, writes: "Without thinking, my body has stood up and is leaving the room. I babble something polite ... and am gone before I can laugh or burst out with something I'd be sorry for."[33] This is a fascinating statement, as Watts is enacting his own mind-body dichotomy, in an apparently less-than-conscious decision to leave the exam room. Similarly, in "The Invitation," Mr. Santana asks Huyler after reviewing his chart history, "You didn't believe me, did you?" Huyler replies: "'I believed you,' I lied, 'but I needed to make sure exactly what was done.'"[34]

Thus, we see complex interplay of thoughts, feelings, and needs on the part of physicians and patients alike. For better and worse, doctors and patients exist in a dyadic relationship. Ideally, patients want to be helped, are clear in their communication and boundaries, respectful of their physicians, and adherent to medical recommendations. Physicians in turn would be patient, knowledgeable, empathic, and available. In reality, of course, both parties have unrealistic expectations of the other; some needs may be met, while others are not, leading to disappointment. Empathy may be greatly strained. Again, Western medicine can be seen as being its own culture, with values, communication patterns, and established normative behavior. Both essays examine what happens when patients deviate from these expected norms.[35]

Ethical concerns

Ethical issues and moral reasonings are essential components of clinical work, involving critical decisions about care, weighing patient autonomy and provider beneficence, the proscription to "first, do no harm" and to treat patients fairly. Not surprisingly, ethical issues manifest in both "White Rabbits" and "The Invitation," but sometimes implicitly, and they are worth highlighting here.

In "White Rabbits," Frank wants multiple colonoscopies despite a lack of evidence that this will be beneficial, and there are clearly risks involved. Watts, an experienced gastroenterologist, is aware of these risks, and relates that Frank wrote a long letter releasing everyone this side of Kansas from any kind of liability connected with colonoscopy. This is a man who knows what he wants even if it doesn't make sense. We did it, but not before I secretly cleared it with the cardiologist. And we survived. All three of us.[36]

While it seems that Frank is making an informed decision about having another colonoscopy, one could object to whether this type of consent is truly informed. The use of the term *secretly* in a clinical interaction has significant implications. "Secretly clearing" any procedure with a specialist out of deference to potential risk and danger implies keeping vital information from the patient, and Watts may have a reason for this. But there is a notable lack of reflection about why Watts follows a clearly nonnormative path to "give that patient what he wants," after informing the reader that Frank wants more colonoscopies than are either safe or medically indicated.

In "The Invitation," Huyler does not seem to consider the possibility that Mr. Santana's ability to make an informed decision to leave the emergency room might reflect impaired judgment on his patient's part. Some patients in the process of experiencing an acute myocardial infarction psychologically defend against their anxiety by using denial.[37] In both cases, a better understanding of each patient's life experience and values would assist the reader—and presumably the clinician—in deciding if Frank or Mr. Santana has impaired judgment about their medical problems, and if so, how to approach the consequent ethical dilemmas.

Huyler, after reading Mr. Santana's chart, realizes that he has erred in his initial assessment that Mr. Santana's chest pain was not serious, and asks his patient to consider admission to the hospital for further workup. "You didn't believe me, did you?" Mr. Santana asks perceptively. "I did," Huyler responds, before acknowledging to himself—but not to his patient—that he is "lying" when he says this. Thus, Huyler catches himself in the act of committing a falsehood, a courageous admission for a physician-writer to share with their audience, and one that is worthy of more exploration and discussion with readers. How common is the practice of "white lies" in clinical work? Are we always ethically bound to be truthful, or are there ethically justifiable exceptions? Are we brave enough as clinicians to admit to when we have erred, or do we lie to protect our employers against liability, or our own egos from being bruised?

Another unaddressed concern is whether either Frank or Mr. Santana have advanced care directives and whether either has been asked about their wishes for invasive care, including intubation and cardiac resuscitation if needed. Both have cardiac conditions, and Frank is about to undergo a surgery to remove carotid artery blockage, during which he could experience a stroke. What are their advance directives? Have they been addressed by their healthcare providers? When Dr. Watts advises him to ask his surgeons, Frank replies, "They don't hold still as long as you do." Ideally, advance care decisions would be discussed out with patients in nonacute settings, with providers who know them and can take the time to fully discuss the implications of these decisions and ensure that patients' values are being reflected in their choices. The field of narrative ethics highlights the importance of knowing the patient's preferences based on their life stories and lived values.[38]

The principle of justice or fairness is relevant to both essays. Mr. Santana's emergency room visits are quite cost-intensive, as are Frank's repeated colonoscopies. Funding sources may have a significant bearing on either patient's access to these evaluations; patients in a public setting who lack insurance might not be eligible for these. Thus, there are inherent ethical choices and sources of moral quandaries implicit in structuring of healthcare in the United States. The medical system provides far greater financial incentives to perform invasive procedures than for patient education and communication. Given the tremendous financial burden of healthcare annually in the United States, it is reasonable to suggest that there are indeed resources to accomplish both. Thus, health policy, advocacy, and politics are highly relevant to discussions about ethics and care.

How the humanities can help

Because the medical humanities are firmly rooted in the goals and methods of literature, they place a preeminent role on the importance of story and narrative. But in both essays, there is a curious absence of information about each patient beyond their current presentations to their respective clinical settings. It is as if they exist solely in the clinic or emergency room for the physician to interact with, like a video game character. We know little about either Frank or Mr. Santana beyond the confines of the medical setting. Nor do we gain any information about their personal histories. What sorts of employment did Frank and Mr. Santana have? How was their childhood, their young adulthood, their lives through the present day? Do they have friends, romantic partners, or children? We have little sense of them as people living full lives, and the experiences that must have shaped them and their values. In Mr. Santana's case, this is partially due to his decision to abruptly sign out of the hospital, leaving an enigmatic human-sized hole in his absence as he walks out of the emergency room. But Huyler fails to mention any previous social or personal information that might have appeared in his many charts about his background. Instead, the focus is on purely biomedical data, while the more human details are omitted.

Frank is an irritating patient, but Watts is dropping us into one of many office visits. What preceded these is left unspoken. Does Watts know his patient's background? If so, he does not share any details with us. It is left unclear as to whether Frank has family, has a partner, if he works, or other salient details. This lack of information seems both curious and harmful, as Frank is reduced to a near-stereotype of a hypochondriacal patient, rather than a complete person with his own experiences and values—views that would be essential in his charting his upcoming medical challenges and life-threatening surgery. Referring to this phenomenon of reductionism in clinical settings, Foucault summarized one of the core problems with modern medicine's overemphasis of biological factors: "Disease is perceived fundamentally in a space of projection without depth, of coincidence without development. There is only one plane and one moment."[39]

Or to frame this question positively, how can we as clinicians help patients and their providers to find meaning in the face of illness when the stories that we tell are stripped of any context? One of the essential goals of the medical humanities and the narrative approach is to restore a sense of meaning through the integration of life stories that match clinical encounters with illness with lived, personal experience. The medical humanities may hold the answer, or at least an important component of a solution, by supplying a vital extra perspective on illness.[40]

A medical humanities perspective would also help to explore the meaning and use of metaphor and symbolism that occur in both clinical encounters.[41] For example, in "White Rabbits," Watts makes at least two allusions to a possible explanation for his patient's suffering. He tries to emphatically reassure Frank about his conviction that his symptoms constitute evidence of a serious gastro-intestinal problem. Finally, in exasperation with Frank's continued requests, he exclaims: "We've been there. Done that. Checked you out, first class. All is well in loop-de-loop land."[42] An astute physician, steeped in the humanities, might focus on the use of the phrase "teeth to toenails," which very obviously describes someone's entire body, with the significant omission of the brain! Watts is, whether or not he is aware of this, vaguely describing a psychological explanation for Frank's health concerns. In medical parlance, these are sometimes referred to as supratentorial disorders whose origins reside in the higher levels of the central nervous system, a black box approach that carries little psychological specificity and is sometimes used in a pejorative sense. Later, the sentence "all is well in loop-de-loop" land should make the reader consider the other organ where loops are prominent in the body, the brain. The brain in fact shares many neurotransmitter systems with the gut, which is sometimes referred to as the body's "second brain," and thus a link to the expression, "I have a gut feeling about this." Could Frank know something in his gut that he is not consciously aware of in his head?

Similarly, Huyler's essay features extremely powerful imagery. Mr. Santana requests that Huyler bury him in the Pecos wilderness on his family's property, mentioning the house made of "real adobe, very rare, four feet thick," that has been in his family for generations. "'One candle can keep it warm in winter. One candle'—he held up a finger—'that's all you need.'"[43] Anyone who appreciates the use of language and literature will see the symbolism of "a single candle." Each of us possesses a single life, a candle that must, inevitably, burn down. As physicians, our job is to tend to that candle, to keep it brightly lit for as long as possible. But we must inevitably face the finite nature of the candle's wick, and life's end. This is true for all of us, including for those of us who work in the healthcare field. And it leads us to a consideration of existential issues, and how they manifest in clinical encounters.

Existential issues in patient encounters

One of the limitations of psychodynamic theory is a lack of attention to deeper concerns about mortality and death. Freud has been criticized for ignoring the way that death and dying haunts some of the case histories that frame his earliest cases.[44] As Iris Murchoch noted: "It is always a significant question to ask about any philosopher: what is he afraid of?"[45] What would it mean to engage with patients in honest dialogue about deeply philosophical questions in a clinical setting? Watts and Huyler provide examples of deflection and avoidance, if not the outright denial of existential issues in their essays.

One of the most striking examples of this avoidance of discussing death comes shortly after Huyler catches himself lying to Mr. Santana, falsely claiming that he believed his patient's medical history before confirming the account in his medical records. But he seems to miss the second and substantially larger lie that he utters shortly after this. When his patient enigmatically instructs the doctor to bury him on his family's property in the Pecos wilderness, Huyler responds, "You're not going to die, Mr. Santana."[46] This statement is, of course, patently untrue. Mr. Santana, Dr. Huyler, you, the reader, myself—we are all mortal and one day we all will die. Mr. Santana is at high risk to die at any moment. He's actually done so once before! He was resuscitated then, but his overall condition is dire and he appears to communicate this via his admittedly odd request. We can easily grasp that he is grappling with his mortality, and the existential issues that attend this.

The core existential issues, as philosophers and writers have charted, focus on four key areas: the meaning of life; the nature of death; the possibility of connection with others versus isolation; and the balance between freedom and responsibility.[47] The goal of the medical humanities is to place humanity—our patients', as well as our own—back at the center of medical practice. What appears diminished in "White Rabbits" is the appreciation for the patient's suffering, as well as the causes of that suffering as a human concern. Frank's age is not given in the essay, but one could easily surmise that he is old enough to have carotid artery disease, and thus likely to be in his mid-60s or older. Watts writes candidly about his own frustration with his patient, but does not—at least in this encounter—comment on the possibility that his patient is frightened of dying. Nor does he pose this possibility to Frank. Frank expresses only minor concern about his upcoming carotid artery surgeries, and the attendant risks of stroke and death. The fear of having colon cancer looms much larger and is potentially displaced from another life-threatening condition. Neither Frank nor Mr. Santana—or their physicians—ever appear to address the elephant in the room, but anxiety about death appears to haunt both of these essays.

The medical humanities can serve as a unique searchlight, useful in illuminating areas of medicine that frequently are left untouched and unexplored. What would such a practice look like? Clinicians who are familiar with the humanities would approach these encounters in different ways, bringing their own unique experiences and sensibilities to each patient, sensitive to the symbolic representations that might help them to better understand their patients. They would likely find common ground in a more flexible, intuitive, and improvisational ability to follow the threads of each clinical encounter. In the case of Mr. Santana, an emergency room clinician might model, with humility, their lack of having all of the answers. They might tell Mr. Santana,

> Yes, I'm young, and have a great deal yet to experience. But you have a wealth of experience. Could you share this with me? Please tell me more about your life. What role does our emergency room play for you? Why do you come here, and are we giving you what you need here? You said that you died once, and that we brought you back? That's extraordinary! Can you tell me more about how that experience changed you? You clearly display considerable courage in living your life, day after day, poised as you are on the brink of another heart attack. How has that been for you? Who are your allies in this? Is there no one else who could bury you in the Pecos? What are your beliefs about death?

Similarly, reading "White Rabbits" one wishes for a more candid exploration of Frank's fears. Why is he so terrified of having colon cancer? Has he recently, or not so remotely, lost someone to colon cancer? Is he anxious about his upcoming carotid artery surgery? If unconscious forces are causing him to overly focus on the possibility of colon cancer, can we get a meaningful sense of what those pressures are? We long to hear more about Frank's story of his life, his thoughts about and the possibility of death, and what this might mean for him and his family.

Is it even appropriate for medical professionals to be asking these questions? Some clinicians might argue against the exploration of spiritual issues in a medical setting, considering this territory that should be left to chaplains, separate from the purview of medical practice. But concern about the nature of death and the meaning of one's life are existential issues, and spiritual beliefs are only one aspect of these, albeit an important one. Social scientists have written about the growing epidemic of loneliness in America, despite the seemingly superficial appearance of greater connectedness through social media.[48]

Moreover, the decline of religious belief and attendance in the West may leave people searching for sources of meaning in their lives; in times of distress, some patients look to their physicians as spiritual guides[49] or at least want to talk about spirituality as an important coping skill,[50] especially if they are facing life-threatening illness. It is likely that many clinicians feel poorly prepared to take on such a responsibility, and with an overwhelmingly biomedical focus, physicians have been shown to fail our patients and their families as they approach death. Clearly, there is a significant gap in the expectations of our patients and the services that clinical medicine provides. Subcontracting emotional or spiritual tasks to psychiatric consultants or to chaplaincy services may leave patients feeling unsatisfied with the lack of integration of their care.

Asking a patient about their spiritual beliefs may seem daring. "What do you think happens when people die?" is one of the more provocative questions that a clinician can ask. Not only daring for the patient to answer, challenging for the provider to hear and engage with. This question poses the ultimate playing field: none of us, even physicians who work with dying patients, know the answer. Beliefs about the nature of death begs exploration by both parties, which may be unsettling for clinicians as they reflect on their own mortality and existential concerns.[51] This type of dialogue can eradicate any previous power dynamic, and would place both parties on equal ground—one in which they can share an exploration of the unknown, with respect, openness, and a desire to learn.

Physicians face their own existential concerns, beyond issues related to death and dying. There is also the question of living, of finding purpose and meaning in life, as well as meaningful connection to others. It is easy to see the links between these issues and the problem of burnout in physicians, who also grapple with the common and crushing issue of responsibility, and the difficulties of establishing boundaries around their work life after professional training to squelch the yearning for freedom on a regular basis: to delay rest, sleep, time off in the service of our patients. These are some of the salient existential issues that clinicians bring to each encounter.

Even if these queries are not posed aloud, existential philosophy teaches us to listen, as clinicians and individuals, for the questions that inhabit the spaces in our conversations with patients. What important points are not being said? Having the framework for key existential questions allows clinicians to attend to some of the most meaningful human issues.[52]

Conclusions

Watts and Huyler have written candidly about their interactions with their patients, and their essays reveal a great deal about the values, character, and quality of Western medicine in the early twenty-first century: its triumphs and strengths, as well as the blind spots inherent in our medical system, and the manner in which it fails to meaningfully connect and provide for patients at a personal, psychological or spiritual level. An astute student of the medical humanities will recognize the wisdom and value of broader perspectives, including narrative approaches to patient care, informed by the arts, the humanities, and social sciences.[53] Narrative practices could guide us toward a more holistic practice of medicine, bringing a greater sense of meaning in clinical encounters to both patient and physician.[54] The medical humanities can affirm and illuminate the subjective experiences of patients as well as those of physicians. For trainees in particular, medical humanities exercises are often anchored in exploring the values, emotions, individuality, and authenticity of participants.

It would be overly optimistic to argue the practice of narrative medicine would be enough to reverse the systemic problems in modern medicine. The essays by Watts and Huyler clearly illustrate that time is the enemy of the complexity and richness that accompany each clinical interaction. There is a clear need for reform of the larger systems of healthcare, to give greater time and weight to clinical interactions, to supporting patients, their families and communities as well as providers. Then again, the medical humanities offer powerful insights to help construct deeper understanding and more meaningful interactions between patients and clinicians. Narrative medicine can promote reflection, growth, and empathy, and possibly prevent burnout in trainees and professionals.[55] This approach to clinical care, steeped in the humanities and attendant to the needs of patients and physicians alike, represents an important component of the effort to regain the soul of medicine, and to help make the practice of medicine a richer place of meaning, understanding, and care.

Notes

1 Kathryn Montgomery Hunter, "Narrative, Literature, and the Clinical Exercise of Practical Reason," *The Journal of Medicine and Philosophy* 21, no. 3 (1996): 303–320.
2 Rita Charon, "Narrative Medicine: A Model for Empathy, Reflection, Profession, and Trust," *JAMA* 286, no. 15 (2001): 1897–1902.
3 Rita Charon, "Honoring the Stories of Illness," *TEDxAtlanta*, accessed August 20, 2021: https://www.ted.com/tedx/events/3334.
4 David Watts, "White Rabbits," in *Bedside Manners: One Doctor's Reflections on the Oddly Intimate Encounters between Patient and Healer* (New York: Three Rivers Press, 2005), 3–10.
5 Ibid., 8.
6 Ibid., 6–7.
7 Ibid., 10.
8 Frank Huyler, "The Invitation," in *The Blood of Strangers* (Berkeley, CA: University of California Press, 1999), 37–40.
9 Ibid., 38.
10 Ibid., 39.
11 Ibid.
12 Ibid., 40.
13 Charon, "Narrative Medicine."
14 George Zaharias, "What Is Narrative-Based Medicine? Narrative-Based Medicine 1," *Canadian Family Physician* 64, no 3 (2018): 176–180.
15 Watts, "White Rabbits," 6.
16 Huyler, "The Invitation," 38.
17 Ibid.
18 Watts, "White Rabbits," 6.
19 Kyung Bong Koh, *Stress and Somatic Symptoms: Biopsychosociospiritual Perspectives* (New York: Springer, 2018).
20 Edith Wharton, *The Greater Inclination, 1899* (Los Angeles, CA: Hardpress Publishing, 2012).
21 Cecilia Tasca, Mariangela Rapetti, Mauro Giovanni Carta, and Bianca Fadda, "Women and Hysteria in the History of Mental Health," *Clinical Practice and Epidemiology in Mental Health: CP & EMH* 8 (2012): 110.
22 Matt Ffytche, *The Foundation of the Unconscious: Schelling, Freud and the Birth of the Modern Psyche* (New York: Cambridge University Press, 2011).
23 George Vaillant, "Involuntary Coping Mechanisms: A Psychodynamic Perspective," *Dialogues in Clinical Neuroscience* 13, no. 3 (2011): 366.
24 Matthias Varul and Talcott Parsons, "The Sick Role and Chronic Illness," *Body & Society* 16, no. 2 (2010): 72–94.
25 Tait Shanafelt, Jonathan Ripp, and Mickey Trockel, "Understanding and Addressing Sources of Anxiety among Health Care Professionals during the COVID-19 Pandemic," *JAMA* 323, no. 21 (2020): 2133–2134.

26 Marianne Rosendal, Tim C. Olde Hartman, Aase Aamland, Henriette Van der Horst, Peter Lucassen, Anna Budtz-Lilly, and Christopher Burton, "'Medically Unexplained' Symptoms and Symptom Disorders in Primary Care: Prognosis-Based Recognition and Classification," *BMC Family Practice* 18, no. 1 (2017): 1–9.

27 Albert Farre and Tim Rapley, "The New Old (and Old New) Medical Model: Four Decades Navigating the Biomedical and Psychosocial Understandings of Health and Illness," *Healthcare* (Basel, Switzerland) 5, no. 4 (2017): 88.

28 Diane Meier, Anthony L. Back, and R. Sean Morrison, "The Inner Life of Physicians and Care of the Seriously Ill," *JAMA* 286, no. 23 (2001): 3007–3014.

29 Daniel Kahneman, *Thinking, Fast and Slow* (New York: Farrar, Straus and Giroux, 2013).

30 Danielle Ofri, *What Doctors Feel: How Emotions Affect the Practice of Medicine* (Boston, MA: Beacon Press, 2013).

31 Watts, "White Rabbits," 8.

32 See Katie Watson, "Gallows Humor in Medicine," *Hastings Center Report* 41, no. 5 (2011): 37–45. Also see Lorelei Lingard, "Language Matters: Towards an Understanding of Silence and Humour in Medical Education," *Medical Education* 47, no. 1 (2013): 40–48.

33 Watts, "White Rabbits," 8.

34 Huyler, "The Invitation," 39.

35 Western medicine can be seen as having its own unique culture, with specialized language, communication patterns, divisions of power, and values that are often unexamined by physicians steeped in their training and patients who enter into these expectations. These cultural values are all clearly on display in these two vignettes. Medical training is not just a gateway into a world of specialized knowledge. The "hidden curriculum" of medical training is thought to include indoctrination into this value system.

36 David Watts, "White Rabbits," 4.

37 Jennifer Covino, Thomas W. Stern, and Theodore A. Stern, "Denial of Cardiac Illness: Consequences and Management," *The Primary Care Companion to CNS Disorders* 13, no. 5 (2011). doi: 10.4088/PCC.11f01166.

38 See the following sources: Lindsay Holmgren, et al., "Terminology and Praxis: Clarifying the Scope of Narrative in Medicine," *Literature and Medicine* 29, no. 2 (2011): 246–273; Anne Hudson Jones, "Narrative in Medical Ethics," *BMJ* 318, no. 7178 (1999): 253–256; and Rita Charon and Martha Montello, eds., *Stories Matter: The Role of Narrative in Medical Ethics* (London: Psychology Press, 2002).

39 Michel Foucault, *The Birth of the Clinic: An Archaeology of Medical Perception*, trans. by Alan Sheridan Smith (New York: Vintage Books, 1973).

40 Alice Malpass, James Dodd, Gene Feder, Jane Macnaughton, Arthur Rose, Oriana Walker, Tina Williams, and Havi Carel, "Disrupted Breath, Songlines of Breathlessness: An Interdisciplinary Response," *Medical Humanities* 45, no. 3 (2019): 294–303.

41 Rita Charon, "Narrative Medicine: Attention, Representation, Affiliation," *Narrative* 13, no. 3 (2005): 261–270.

42 Watts, "White Rabbits," 9.

43 Huyler, "The Invitation," 39.

44 Irvin Yalom, *Existential Psychotherapy* (New York: Simon and Shuster, 1980).

45 Iris Murdoch. *Metaphysics as a Guide to Morals* (London: Chatto and Windus, 1992).

46 Huyler, "The Invitation," 38.

47 Yalom, *Existential Psychotherapy*.

48 Stephen Marche, "Is Facebook Making Us Lonely?" *The Atlantic*, May 2012: https://www.theatlantic.com/magazine/archive/2012/05/is-facebook-making-us-lonely/308930/.

49 Charles MacLean, Beth Susi, Nancy Phifer, Linda Schultz, Deborah Bynum, Mark Franco, Andria Klioze, Michael Monroe, Joanne Garrett, and Sam Cykert, "Patient

Preference for Physician Discussion and Practice of Spirituality: Results from a Multicenter Patient Survey," *Journal of General Internal Medicine* 18, no. 1 (2003): 38–43.

50 Randy Heabert, Mollie W. Jenckes, Daniel E. Ford, Debra R. O'Connor, and Lisa A. Cooper, "Patient Perspectives on Spirituality and the Patient-Physician Relationship," *Journal of General Internal Medicine* 16, no. 10 (2001): 685–692.

51 See Jerome Groopman, "The Last Deal," *The New Yorker* 8 (1997): 53–64; and Cornelus Sanders, "The Road," *The Lancet* 366, no. 9503 (2005): 2135–2136.

52 Aaron Saguil and Karen Phelps, "The Spiritual Assessment," *American Family Physician* 86, no. 6 (2012): 546–550.

53 Paul Crawford, Brian Brown, Victoria Tischler, and Charlie Baker, "Health Humanities: The Future of Medical Humanities?" *Mental Health Review Journal* 15, no. 3 (2010): 4.

54 Bradley Lewis, "Narrative Medicine and Healthcare Reform," *Journal of Medical Humanities* 32, no. 1 (2011): 9–20.

55 Gita Anjali Narayan, Penny Stern, and Alice Fornari, "Effect of Reflective Writing on Burnout in Medical Trainees," *MedEdPublish* 7, no. 4 (2018). doi: 10.15694/mep.2018.0000237.1.

14 Tending and extending

The long and short of Siddhartha Mukherjee

Sandhya Shetty

The world is full of cancer researchers and physicians, but none, arguably, as well-known as Siddhartha Mukherjee, an expert on blood cancers. In large part, Mukherjee's Pulitzer Prize-winning book *The Emperor of All Maladies: A Biography of Cancer*, a riveting account of cancer's appearances and treatment in the recent and remote past, accounts for his fame beyond the precincts of academic medicine.[1] The publication of *The Gene: An Intimate History* cemented his reputation as one of the best "explainers of science" in the United States today.[2] This book picks up where *Emperor*'s account of cancer genetics ends; Mukherjee spells out the conceptual relationship between the two as follows: "If cancer … is the 'distorted version of our normal selves,' then what generates the undistorted variants of our normal selves?"[3] As the story of the search for what generates these variants, *Gene* narrates the long struggle against the destructive alterities within us.[4]

Emperor's interest in the changing conceptions of cancer's nature takes readers back to the beginnings of human history. Providing a brief account of paleopathology before moving forward to the Egyptian physician Imhotep's description of cases, the narrative leaps forward two millennia to Herodotus's record of a lump in the Persian queen, Atossa's breast. Coursing on through the early modern period, the book arrives at the seminal years of the nineteenth century, when radical surgery emerged as the first major intervention in cancer treatment. By this point, readers have been disabused of the notion that cancer is a paradigmatically twentieth-century affliction. Yet, to get to what constitutes *Emperor*'s "real" scientific and philosophical core, we must persist through two final parts set in post-World War I America. While the early chapters on cancer's antiquity fascinate, the intimations of hope glimpsed in these final sections on advances in genetics seize our imaginations. Mukherjee's explanation of how genetics has redefined the nature of cancer and reconfigured scientists' imagination of cure is a *tour de force* of science writing.

Emperor has had the distinction of being called a "great and beautiful book"[5]; "the notion of 'popular science,'" Alexander Linklater exclaims, "doesn't come close to describing this achievement. It is literature."[6] No one has called *The Gene* "literature" or "beautiful" (yet). Not only that, a scuffle between its author and prominent geneticists over an essay that appeared ahead of the book's publication cast a pall over even its scientific credentials.[7] Drawn from *Gene*'s manuscript,

DOI: 10.4324/9781003079712-14

this essay, "Same and Different," is a lively presentation of new research in the field of epigenetics, but Mukherjee's "popular" representation of gene regulation and the field was deemed woefully mistaken. There is more to *The Gene* than the row over epigenetics (which I'll come back to). The book traces the history of genetics from its 1864 starting point in Mendel's pea-flower garden to the draft publication of The Human Genome Project in the twenty-first century. Even as it takes a historical view of genetics research and underscores ethical questions raised by new methods of editing and changing the human genome, *The Gene* does all this in an extraordinary, sometimes even beautiful, way. Mixing genres and registers, genealogy and history, Mukherjee experiments with fresh ways of retelling science, eschewing default narrative modes and Eurocentric cultural-historical locations in his explanation of biological concepts like human normalcy, identity, variation, and heredity.

As the foregoing sketches suggest, Mukherjee is partial to *longue durée* or "big picture" writing projects. Were he a creative writer of fiction, one imagines he would be a novelist—after the manner of a Salman Rushdie, known for subcontinental-sized novels, or an Amitav Ghosh, fond of transcontinental historical sagas. However, the scale of Mukherjee's operations frequently shifts. Some of his best works in fact take on the essay form. Confining himself to treading small plots, Mukherjee's essays range far, exploring among other subjects the contemporary resonance of Anton Chekhov on Sakhalin Island, the significance of epigenetics (refracted through stories of his mother and her identical twin), the feel of a corpse, and what that can convey about the heft and immensity of death.[8] But in so far as his book-length productions are concerned, the characterization of his aptitude in terms of amplitude is certainly justifiable. This chapter attends to both his small- and large-scale work.

Not only does this work move between different scales, but it also crosses divergent disciplinary borders, inviting flexible and eclectic analytic frames. Apropos of the question of aptitude, Mukherjee's own list of different types of actors/thinkers is worth noting: one sort "highly defined in their goals and their ambitions" [9]; another "profoundly interdisciplinary"[10]; the "systems thinker" (his example is fellow doctor-writer, Atul Gawande)[11]; the synthesizer; and so on. Of these, I believe, "synthesizer" best suits Mukherjee, *Emperor* and *Gene* clearly suggesting his preference for the pan back, visualization, and collation of the various and disjunct.[12] Equally striking is the depth of his interdisciplinarity in both these long narratives and in the essays. In his best moments, literary, narrative, and scientific language become *cognate* and reversible not opposed modes of *knowing* and speaking. This deep reversibility of the scientific and the literary manifests most powerfully in the shorter essays, two of which—"Tenderness" and "Love in the Time of Numbness; or, Doctor Chekhov, Writer"—are discussed below.

In a different mode, *Emperor* and *The Gene*, too, cross more than one genre and academic-disciplinary border. Their subtitles openly index their aspirations as histories of medicine/science although not perhaps in the way academic historians conceive that genre. On one level, both seem like traditional histories of medicine (albeit without the hagiographical touch), for they center the lives and work of surgeons, physicians, and scientists—usually "great men." Mukherjee's historical writing, however, has been shelved by academic historians (for reasons other than its implicit gender biases or provinciality). The discussion below elaborates this academic (non)reception of Mukherjee's forays into historical writing.[13]

Placed within the doctors-who-write rubric, Mukherjee's *oeuvres* turn in directions that buck the dominant trend in physicians' writings, which has been to individualize patients or detail adventures and errors in caregiving. Indeed, readers thinking about the illness experience and interested in affecting stories about his patients will have to look elsewhere. Vignettes of patients do of course surface from time to time in *Emperor*, as do the doctor's personal reflections "memorializing" patients who died under his watch, but overall neither *Emperor* nor *The Gene* (which does have much to say about psychiatric illnesses) is conceived as an examination of what doctors or patients fear or think or feel in the course of illness or caregiving. Mukherjee himself frankly acknowledges it is the biology of the cancer cell that moves him.[14] Remarkably, we are haunted by that as well. Who would have thought prose describing the mechanistic function of the cancer cell could be so strangely poignant? Here lies a key virtue of this physician's writing: the ability to illuminate the human condition and affectively move readers through careful explanation of the impersonal biology of cancer at the level of cell and gene rather than through the typical fare of patient cameos that reveal the good doctor's struggles.

This impersonal yet affecting mode of explanation is discernible in both *Emperor* and *The Gene*, books written for a mixed audience. Although this accessibility of Mukherjee's writing has been stigmatized as "popular" by experts in the nonscientific disciplines he traverses, it is nevertheless built on scholarly seriousness and executed without any exaggerated sense of the laity's desire for fast-paced, user-friendly, pitying, or uplifting narration. Instead, Mukherjee's many-stranded narratives proceed on the assumption that non-specialist readers have stamina and intellectual curiosity about conversations beyond their immediate ken, needing only willingness to traverse challenging terrain with a sure-footed guide. His prose thus pulls us along through the ins and outs of, say, cancer genetics arcana without ever letting us off the hook of concentrated effort. To reiterate Linklater's observation differently, the notion of "popular science" does not adequately signal the fact that Mukherjee's scientific writing spills ever restless past its medical-scientific remit, nor does it illuminate the challenging texture of its satisfactions.

Be it on cells or genes or on writing itself, then, Mukherjee's *oeuvre* lying athwart clinic, laboratory, archive, and library calls for supple reading. But, however we frame the forms and aspirations of his inquiries, his style remains a constant that merits special notice: always lucid and unforced, even modest. One senses no straining after the philosophical argument or the political point well within reach. Mukherjee writes without solicitude or condescension toward readers. And we follow, sometimes rapt in the wonder of cellular life, at other times, flailing against the irreversible, immanent tragedy of human biology that his prose unsentimentally, conscientiously explains. Literary science writing of this sort performs exactly the antidotal function Mukherjee's essay on Chekhov envisions as the *sine qua non* for writers in these times of numbness. In long and short pieces that keep readers awake and alert or render us tender (at once soft and raw), this writer-physician cultivates scientific and literary sensibility, nudging "beauty" in the literary aesthetic sense closer to *aesthesia* in this term's older medical sense.[15]

The prequel: "The blood of your parents is not lost in you"

Born and raised in New Delhi, Mukherjee is Associate Professor of Medicine at Columbia University Medical Center. He received a B.S. in Biology from Stanford University, a D.Phil. from Magdalen College, Oxford, where he was a Rhodes scholar, and an M.D. from Harvard Medical School. In 2006, he completed an oncology fellowship at the Dana Farber Center. A desolate year, this *annus horibilis* was nonetheless gestational with respect to his then new *avatar* as writer. Mukherjee emerged from this bleak phase of "stunned incoherence" with an urge to transmute a journal kept during his fellowship into a "less rehearsed and robotic" response to his patients, that is, into some language other than the stock idiom of "sympathy" he had learned to affect in the clinic.[16] *Emperor* is that other response, in another idiom, a performance of sympathy that awakens us readers as well to the many modes, moods, and scales in which one might write bodily life.

While the big questions that shape all of Mukherjee's writings are of general universal import, it is important to register the deep personal freight some of them carry. One does not have to ferret out this private history. As an explainer of science, Mukherjee has been refreshingly open about personal history in several essays, and most remarkably in *The Gene*, wherein he interlaces conceptual breakthroughs in genetics research with (auto)biographical prose sections that accommodate vivid family portraiture. Weaving genetic science with memoir, the book's innovative combination of genres and styles bursts the bounds of "science writing," conventionally understood.[17] Indeed, viewed as life-writing, *The Gene* consists of stories within stories, a narrative mode one is tempted to identify as Rushdiesque. Like the literary narrator in *Midnight's Children*, the science writer yokes family genealogy to national history. This knitting of (auto) biography, national history, *and* transnational history of science creates a many-stranded narrative of unrelated events that all accrete around the base concept of heredity (also a concept of significance in Rushdie's 1980 novel). In other words, uniquely, Mukherjee's history of the refinement of the scientific concept of the gene comes to us entangled with intimate histories of multigenerational life within a joint family in 1970s Delhi. Along with Mendel and Monod, Berg and Boyer, Gurdon and Yamanaka, and Jennifer Doudna, *The Gene* presents a gallery of Mukherjee's Indian kinfolk: uncles, cousins, parents, grandparents, and his mother's identical twin sister, Bulu, who lived in Calcutta but remained an important presence in his life.

Bulu's story initially appeared in "Same but Different," the essay that provoked geneticists' ire in 2016 just before *The Gene*'s publication.[18] Beginning with story and family memories of the twin birth, different natures and talents of aunt and mother, Mukherjee narrates how marriage separated Bulu from her twin, taking her to Calcutta where the fortunes of her well-to-do husband's family declined.[19] Mukherjee's mother, who had married a man in Delhi without family wealth, connections, or ancestral mansion, turned out, however, to have made the (economically) better match. The Delhi branch of the family prospered along with the capital city, while Bulu's husband's fortunes mimicked the downward spiral of postcolonial Calcutta. These personal stories modulate into the essay's consideration of how twins become different despite identical genomes. Exploring the specific idea that "an organism's individuality … [is] suspended between genome and epigenome," the essay explains recent research on histone modification and DNA methylation. It was Mukherjee's treatment of these topics that sparked anger and the disdain of geneticists for whom transgenerational epigenetics, a relatively new area of research, remains a dubious enterprise and the very notion of gene regulation by acquired or nongenetic factors carries with it the intolerable whiff of Lamarckianism (the theory of the heritability of acquired traits). Although to some the spat "seem[ed] overblown," it is true that had Mukherjee acknowledged, even briefly, foundational work on "transcriptional activators, repressors, and regulators," he might have given lay readers a sounder sense of "the primary mediators of the biological response to the environment" and parried accusations of misrepresentation. A summary of mainstream consensus on these primary mediators or even a brief note stating all biologists do not consider epigenetics and the role of nurture in shaping heredity or nature a settled matter may have pre-empted the wrath of some. In the absence of explicit caveats, "Same but Different" generated an uneasy-making kerfuffle over epigenetics. Even after Mukherjee acknowledged his omission of mainstream scientific opinion, some leading geneticists remained unforgiving, insisting he not only overemphasized the newer work of those researching epigenetic processes thought to alter gene behavior but that he also fundamentally misunderstood and/or ignored scientific consensus on theories of gene regulation.

Unqualified to weigh in on either the scientific consensus or the newer paradigm of epigenetics, I approach the public conversation around Mukherjee's essay conducted in various science blogs as a cultural event.[20] Some few scientist-commentators who contributed to the conversation have noted the tonal excess of certain remarks in Jerry Coyne's blog. *Ad hominem* or just angry, these remarks allege *The New Yorker*'s "cultural elitism" or sarcastically damn Mukherjee's essay as "fine writing," or dub it as "woo" (one commentator even going so far as to conflate Mukherjee with Deepak Chopra). Perhaps it is too easy to put this blog commotion down to the old two cultures debate, but the dudgeon and mocking idiom against "fine writing" and "cultural elitism" seems like a vestige of that cold war. To grant this is not necessarily to dismiss scientists' dismay over alleged flaws and the sins of omission in Mukherjee's exploration of epigenetics.

More significant, the blog eruption indexes the ongoing difficulty of writing across the science and literary divide, difficulties on *both* reception and production sides. As Tabitha Powlege points out, Mukherjee has been unusually successful at navigating the pitfalls of explaining science to nonexperts, but even he fails to escape the complaints of old-school molecular biologists.[21] The controversy around a lively essayistic presentation of epigenetics is symptomatic of precisely the challenge literary science writing (as distinct from medical or science journalism) poses in some constituencies. The risks and difficulty of treading the fine line between necessary scientific rigor and coverage, on the one hand, and the constraints of the essay genre, on the other, could not be clearer. What remains unclear at the end is where the lines are to be drawn, or who can be that arbiter acceptable across "the two cultures" divide? Doctor/scientist-writers who seek to enter meaningful interdisciplinary space in between "the two cultures" undoubtedly have, as the scientist-bloggers insisted, an extra responsibility to maintain the highest standards even as they appeal to a general readership. At the same time, the overstatement of the implications of Mukherjee's essay and peevish mischaracterization of it as just "fine-writing," "woo," "cultural elitism," or left sentimentalism *contra* the high standards of hard genetic science make it that much harder for the general reader to distinguish principle from peeve, or rigor from disdain for newer paradigms and alternate conventions, contexts, and modalities of knowing and speaking within (and beyond) the science in question.

Let us return to *The Gene,* a more sustained science writing experiment that pushes limits. Like the briefer "Same but Different," which eventually debouched into it, *The Gene*'s juxtaposition of seemingly out-of-place bits of personal family narrative and history of science seems destined, one imagines, to irritate certain denizens of not just science but also academic history. As a history of the science of heredity, *The Gene* travels back in time to the nineteenth century, but it also travels in other ways that impact its content and form. The opening chapter titled "Prologue: Families" sets the shifting tone and scales on which the book explores normalcy and malignancy, identity and variation, history, and heredity. We begin with family stories, learning that the youngest of five brothers, Mukherjee's father, Sibeswar "Shibu" Mukherjee migrated with his mother from East Bengal even before the Partition of India in 1947 when East Bengal became Pakistan (and later in 1970, Bangladesh). Employed by Mitsubishi in New Delhi, Sibeswar Mukherjee prospered, marrying Chandana "Tulu" Banerjee in 1965.[22] Their children, Ranu and Siddhartha, grew up in a household dominated by Sibeswar's mother who, along with an adult son, Jagu, lived with Sibeswar and his family. Jagu had schizophrenia. One other uncle who had died young in Calcutta also suffered from an "unraveling of the mind."[23] The first-person narrative voice puts it succinctly: "Madness, it turns out, has been among the Mukherjees for at least two generations."[24]

Locating his uncles' and cousins' maladies in the interstices of his historical account of phases of genetics research, Mukherjee provides glimpses of a novelist's genius for vivid characterization and compelling narrative, and not a little of soft wit with which he tempers the tragic impact of colonial history, the Partition of India, ancestry, and shame on individual family members and on their joint life together. Speaking of yet another uncle's son, Moni, he writes,

> Like most Bengalis, my parents had elevated repression and denial to a high art form, but even so, questions about this particular history were unavoidable. ... Had Moni [the author's cousin] inherited a gene, or a set of genes, that had made him susceptible—the same genes that had affected our uncles?[25]

It is a question about the family history of illness then that launches Mukherjee's historical investigation into genetic science in this his third book which tells

> a very personal story—an intimate history. The weight of heredity is not an abstraction for me. Rajesh and Jagu are dead. Moni is confined to a mental institution in Calcutta. But their lives and deaths have had a greater impact on my thinking as a scientist, scholar, historian, physician, son, and father than I could possibly have envisioned. Scarcely a day passes in my adult life when I do not think about inheritance and family.[26]

Fittingly, *The Gene* is dedicated to the writer's paternal grandmother, Priyabala Mukherjee, a woman who responded bravely to the impacts of history and heredity on her sons, and their sons. This was a woman, he writes, who

> embraced and defended the most fragile of her children from the will of the strong. She weathered the buffets of [political] history with resilience – but she weathered the buffets of heredity with something more than resilience: a grace that we, as her descendants, can only hope to emulate.[27]

Embodying human grace before the impassable alterity within, Priyabala, thus, frames Mukherjee's trajectory *and* affiliations as doctor-scientist-writer. Neither heredity nor history, nor filiation or migrancy are abstractions; rather, they constitute the stuff out of which this history of a concept, this doctor's writing on biological inheritance, cultural belonging, and professional affiliation, is spun.

Emperor of all maladies: patient or disease

Emperor opens in Mukherjee's first professional home, MGH, Boston. It is May 2004. Mukherjee is an oncologist in training at the Dana Farber Center. Only ten months into his fellowship, he is summoned to the 14th floor of MGH to the bedside of Carla Reed, a patient diagnosed with acute lymphoblastic leukemia. We learn, subsequently, Carla does not die in his care; her cancer goes into remission and Mukherjee would declare her cured. But that day in May, neither he nor she knew that. Carla's story gives Mukherjee's epic review of the search for a cure a singular twenty-first-century human face. While Sidney Farber and Mary Lasker are also cited as "characters" who "stand at the epicenter of the modern quest" for a cure, it is Carla's story that bookends his telling of that history begun with the Persian Atossa.[28] Although she does not exactly pull the massive tome together, her personal experience of treatment and cure constitutes a singular, small-scale world in which from time to time the narrative dwells.

> Cancer begins and ends with people. Amid scientific abstraction, it is sometimes possible to forget this one basic fact. ... Doctors treat diseases, but they also treat people, and this precondition of their professional existence sometimes pulls them in two directions at once.[29]

So reads the June Goodfield epigraph to *Emperor*'s Prologue. That doctors do not merely treat diseases but people is a medical humanities truism. What is interesting here, however, is the "confessional" aspect of the epigraph, which articulates *Emperor*'s own oscillation between the individual patient and the intellectual problem the disease presents, between an impulse to be imperial in scale and locally grounded in a case. By the time Carla the patient returns at Prologue's end, readers have been given both the elements of an individual patient's story— Carla waging her war—and a preview as well of the ups and downs and ins and outs of a collective scientific effort to cure "the most relentless and insidious enemy among human diseases."[30] The account that follows attempts a rapprochement between these two competing poles: both Carla and leukemia matter. This is what the Prologue suggests.

Yet, as *Emperor* progresses, shifting the scale from local (Boston MGH) to national-historical (nineteenth-century America, Baltimore) to global-historical (Egypt, Imhotep etc.), the disease itself looms larger and larger. Cancer gets top billing. Strung on a fragile thread, patient stories only occasionally intercept the juggernaut of Mukherjee's multilayered pursuit of answers to questions about cancer's origins and longevity.[31] Not only are patient stories brief, but Mukherjee's wording is impoverished too, sometimes strained by his reaching after effect and significance (as in his admiring description of Dr. Thomas Lynch chatting easily with Kate Fitz, a woman recovering from surgery on a large mass in her lung).[32] Fair to say, the "biography of cancer" rather than Carla's calls most powerfully to Mukherjee *as writer*.

In the time of his dejection, we've been told, a *longue durée* study of cancer's conceptual and therapeutic history constituted a lifeline, giving Mukherjee answers to questions posed by the grim clinical ground of illness and treatment: "How old is cancer? What are the roots of our battle against this disease? Or, as patients often asked me: Where are we in the "war' on cancer?"[33] Camidge Ross strangely characterizes this investment in studying the disease rather than telling patient stories as evidence of "Stockholm Syndrome."[34] Among other things, this casting of Mukherjee's captivation by the intellectual problem of cancer biology overlooks the heterogeneous springs of writerly enthusiasm. It assumes writers who are doctors will always or must always be writing about patients, hospitals, bioethics, and illness experiences in certain expected ways, an assumption that sometimes threatens to verge on dogma.[35] Narration of the patient's story, which has become a touchstone of humanist writing in medicine, is not for everyone. There is no one way to be a doctor-writer.

As Mukherjee tells it, *Emperor*'s broad historical canvas and emphasis on research were roads deliberately chosen. Admitting his predilection for research, Mukherjee identifies himself as "a lab rat."[36] This *in media res* declaration functions as a portal into the two final, challenging parts of the book, which meticulously delineate what scientists know about the biochemical workings of normal and malignant cells. The language of genes and mutations emerges to illuminate the tantalizing possibility that the book's prolonged, intense amassing of detail around shifting conceptualizations of cancer has all the while been broaching: the singular origin of all cancers and the hope of therapeutics based on this unitary cause. If *Emperor* reads like a history of medicine (a point to which I return), then it is also a kind of intellectual genealogy of the state of oncology research and therapeutics in the narrative present.

Enormously interesting as are the historical parts of Mukherjee's *Emperor*, what "we *now* know" about the biology of cancer emerges as in fact the most urgent and moving. For, it is this that conveys the powerful and disappointing truth the book's prologue has warned us about: the mechanisms of cell growth make cancer the "more perfect versions of ourselves."[37] *Emperor* is not a feel-good book; it pushes back on the "hype ... leveraged against an illness that was just three decades ago [in the 1970s] widely touted as being 'curable' within a few years."[38] Although Carla's story ends well, "cure," "curable," and "cured" are words we look for but rarely find in *Emperor*'s long recital of the history of a disease "terrifying to experience, terrifying to observe, and terrifying to treat."[39] We read *Emperor* for the kind of illumination and affect Mukherjee is able to generate not so much when he details individual suffering as when he explains the impersonal physiological causes of suffering that lie seeded in the very genetic framework of human being. We read *Emperor* for what it can tell us about the tragic irony of biology. That is where Mukherjee excels, making the tragedy apparent without posturing, breast beating, literary allusions, false hope, or false negativity.

The tragic key: the fault is in our genes

As an account of encoded disease threats—whether cancers or schizophrenia—that flower into *le mal*, *The Gene* speaks to the essential predicament of human being that biology reveals: the fault is in our genes (although the element of luck remains in ironic play). We come with a manual of instructions inside us. In this sequel-prequel to *Emperor*, Mukherjee asks "What if we learned to change [rewrite the manual] our genetic code intentionally? ... How would the acquisition and control of this knowledge—and its inevitable invasion of our private and public lives—alter the way we imagine our societies, our children, ourselves?"[40] Knowing how to alter what is built-in—the promise of medical genetics today—threatens in turn to alter our understanding of what it means to be human.[41]

Similarly, Mukherjee's history of cancer excites us about (without guaranteeing) science's ability to seed panaceas that work against cell division gone rogue.

As *Emperor* draws to a close, we are surprised by news that Carla's nightmare with which the narrative opened is over. It seems like a perfect, hopeful way to close the book with the patient's cancer in remission, but Mukherjee doesn't take his own bait as he considers how to end.[42] Even though he was sure when he first began that Carla's story would end with her "relapse and death," and he now finds himself five years later staring at a miraculous case of cure, somehow, he resists ending with this amazing story of hope as a sentimentalist (justifiably) might. Instead, Mukherjee takes Carla's words ("cancer … is my new normal") as a point of departure that leads to an alternative conclusion.[43] He pushes the idea of normalcy with respect to cancer away from the domain of the individual patient's subjectivity back toward the larger, more startling point introduced in the Prologue. The question of normalcy is rendered "ominous" as the narrative moves toward its last words on "the cancer cell's capacity to consistently imitate, corrupt, and pervert normal physiology."[44] Cancer is not just the individual patient's normalcy but "*our* normalcy as well," Mukherjee observes, meaning that "we [collectively as a species] are inherently destined to slouch towards a malignant end. … The question then will not be *if* we will encounter this immortal illness in our lives, but *when*."[45] Unlike other maladies, cancer in this final reckoning is as normal as death, indeed a synonym for the unremitting normalcy of the latter itself; in the end, we will all catch it.

Part 5, *Emperor*'s core, addresses fully this central conundrum: the inexorability of the mechanisms of normal cell division and the equally inexorable susceptibility of these processes (the body *must* undergo) to fatal mutations:

> The secret to battling cancer, then, is to find means to prevent these mutations from occurring in susceptible cells, or to find means to eliminate the mutated cells without compromising normal growth. The conciseness of that statement belies the enormity of the task. Malignant growth and normal growth are so genetically intertwined that unbraiding the two might be one of the most significant scientific challenges faced by our species. Cancer is built into our genomes. … And cancer is imprinted in our society: as we extend our life span as a species, we inevitably unleash malignant growth. … If we seek immortality, then so, too, in a rather perverse sense, does the cancer cell.[46]

That malignancy is simply the other side of normal cell growth puts a new cancerous spin on the predicament of the *pharmakon*, annotated as drug and poison simultaneously. It calls for therapies so elegantly light-fingered as to be able to unbraid without unraveling.

The profoundly endogenous nature of this disease limits what we can prevent by way of action against known carcinogens. If victories have been gained against the Emperor of all Maladies, they are bittersweet. As Germaine's story illustrates at the very end of this history of endless research and hope, medicine's armamentarium exhausts itself before the cancer does. The vault full of resources and resilience aimed against cancer is emptied out without an ultimate victory.

At moments like this, we are reminded of Atul Gawande's *Being Mortal*, which comes (albeit from a different angle) at the same desolating conclusion about the limits of medicine and the finitude of life.[47] Gawande critiques the endless application of medical technology and therapeutics to prolonging life, advocating instead for strengthening palliative care and hospice; coming at the same problem of finitude but from the researcher's bench, Mukherjee keeps the lab rat's faith, continuing to probe new frontiers of science. The questions that interest him in the fields of cancer and genetics take *The Gene* in a different philosophical direction. With Mukherjee the scientist, we do not navigate away from the limits of therapeutic medicine toward acceptance of finitude.

A biography of cancer

"Normalcy," "history," and "biography" are big words in *The Emperor of All Maladies: A Biography of Cancer*. If "normalcy" invites contemplation on its reversibility, the other two terms give the book its unifying formal conceit. The subtitle's identification of the historical narrative as "biography" deserves discussion if only because academic medical historians have long been wary of the "biography of disease" genre of historical writing.[48] In Mukherjee's case, as it turns out, not just historians, but book reviewers and medical journalists as well have raised questions about the biography designation, dismissing it as glib and reductive.[49] The blowback has come from other quarters too on the grounds that the term "biography" anthropomorphizes cancer. The characterizing of disease as a person about whom a biography may be written, the critique goes, makes cancer out to be "an animate enemy rather than a biological phenomenon."[50]

To these critiques I would add that the "Author's Note" in *Emperor* makes a big point about the biography label without clinching the argument for it:

> This book is a "biography" in the truest sense of the word—an attempt to enter the mind of this immortal illness, to understand its personality, to demystify its behavior. But my aim is to raise a question beyond biography: Is cancer's end conceivable in the future? Is it possible to eradicate this disease from our bodies and societies forever?[51]

The quotation marks that crown the term "biography" already suggest that a certain catachrestic usage of the word is being passed off as somehow not really so. The big, substantive questions the book is raising are certainly outside the purview of the (literary and historical) biographical problematic altogether. These address the domain of a cure for cancer. The stakes are so high that we find the author is himself compelled to drop the biographical conceit. One can forgive oneself for wondering whether it has not been from the beginning an unnecessary even mystifying distraction—a "hook" the writing does not carry through the body of the work in any compelling or sustained fashion.

Mukherjee has defended his choice on various occasions, saying the word "biography" made sense to him on account of its resonance with Susan Sontag's idea of "illness as the night side of life" and with cancer itself, an illness so integral to self-definition or at least so able at revealing "an alternative self."[52] The biography of this intimate, night side of the ill human self is what *Emperor* purports to be. This rationale, based on loose association rather than some scholarly theory of the genre or professional historian's view of it, deflects rigorous critique, suggesting flexible reception of a formal conceit, useful to an oncologist aiming to present the big picture for the public, may be in order. In other words, Mukherjee appears to be lightly borrowing the name "biography" for entirely nonbiographical ends, namely, to tell the *longue durée* story of cancer and cancer research in an animated and formally coherent way. "Biography" works metaphorically in the title. That is one defense. However, one cannot help noticing that lineaments of biography are visible in the body of Mukherjee's narrative of cancer research's development as well. Applied to cancer *the disease* itself—its alleged "mind" and "personality"[53]—biography acts as a principle of narrative construction, attempting to give shape to the growing body of knowledge and treatment. As such, biography/life-writing gives *Emperor's* account of science evolving over time the character of an old-fashioned *bildungsroman*. The different developmental stages of research come to be conceptualized in terms of infancy, adolescence, and adulthood/maturity in the late twentieth century. However, this sporadic execution of biographical narration to give form to the evolution of cancer research feebly props up the case for a "biography- of-cancer" nomination.

Finally, like its topic, cancer, and perhaps for that reason, *Emperor* remains a mercurial and ramifying production. Despite the failed quest for a genre to belong to, manifest in the Author's Note's multiple pronouncements of formal and generic coherence, the narrative survives. Chronicle, military history, an oncologist's coming-of-age, biography, it needs not any of these defining marks. Its actual expansiveness, incredibly, works for both a general and specialized readership. *The Emperor* is best seen, I would say, as a gift to every patient and to family members who want to understand what cancer is, what goes on, and how it might be stopped. In a strange kind of way, simply reading—even the toughest articles in scientific journals in order to understand what *is* or *might* be happening deep within a suffering brother or mother—can become an expressive act for those called upon to witness and identify yet without the capacity to act or intervene in the course of disaster. The passing, almost throwaway, claims that knowledge growth has an adulthood-like telos or disease a "mind" or "personality" are superfluities this book does not need.

The problem of writing a global history of the sort executed by Mukherjee is not a new one. The "Author's Note" indexes the difficulty of stabilizing genre when narrative scales shift: how to narrate adequately the ins and outs and various highs and lows, in short, the dynamic nature of a dreadful disease—actually several dreadful diseases that are iterations of the same pathophysiology of overproduction? And how to do this over a period of 4,000 years in a way that does not reek of ahistorical simplification and essentialism? Was Atossa's experience of breast cancer really the same as, say, Fanny Burney's in early nineteenth-century Napoleonic France? Or is this a case of retrospective diagnosis of the sort medical historians, like Roger Cooter, justly question?[54] Has only the treatment regimen changed? Does a global history such as *Emperor* require the reader to swallow something like an imperial authorial edict that compels the suspension of disbelief and enforces the analogy between cancer/disease and the human individual whose story may be told in the historical narrative genre known as biography?

Mukherjee is not the first to employ such a conceit for the sake of "unity" or definition of an ill-defined gigantically scaled narrative that sets out to provide a retrospective survey of humankind's experience with cancer. Philip Teigen reminds us that trade and academic presses have not been past employing the "Biographies of Disease" rubric as "aid[s] for the historical study of disease."[55] We might also say that to talk of a biography of cancer when one is after a *history* of cancer research is to confuse scales unproductively, to attempt to pretend that *longue durée* history can be bottled in terms that are inescapably micro historical, individual, and small scale. Mukherjee might have spared himself the awkwardness since the main text of his global history located on a millennial scale neglects to parlay the notion of biography or the interplay of differing scales into any substantive insight. As a conceit, "biography" is neither capacious nor sturdy enough to support Mukherjee's vision of a protean, imperial illness such as cancer.[56]

A history of medicine: practicing without a license

Viewed from an academic-disciplinary perspective, *Emperor* perhaps comes closest to history of medicine. While the latter is written for historians, Mukherjee's history, however, addresses a wider audience. Interestingly, it is precisely this accessibility that accounts for the book's relegation to a marginal status within academia, as evidenced by its scholarly (non)reception. When cited at all by academic historians, it is downgraded to the category of the "popular" or examined for scholarly missteps. Arguably, the rampant mediatization of health today justifies the distancing of academic history of medicine from the efforts of "doctor-scientist-writers" who write for trade publishers; tensions between clinicians and academic historians over the history of medicine of course have a longer history.[57]

A random search for discussions or reviews of *Emperor* in, for example, *Bulletin of the History of Medicine* fails to turn up much by way of interdisciplinary solidarity. Michael Stolberg's article on early-modern metaphors and images of cancer cites *The Emperor*, but only to note Mukherjee's mistaken etymological identification of the term "metastasis" and his "mistransla[tion of] both of its parts" which, Stolberg observes, results in a "rather curious conclusion" that metastasis literally means "beyond stillness."[58] James Wright's essay on an associate of William Stewart Halsted contests "general public" memory of Halsted, who appears prominently in *Emperor* as the surgeon who perfected "the radical mastectomy."[59] I have already mentioned Cooter's reference to Mukherjee, which identifies him as a prize-winning *journalist*. Finally, in an essay review, Agnes Arnold-Foster argues:

[C]ancer's history is relatively unwritten. ... Compared to the other great 'plagues' ... cancer has few dedicated pages in the general surveys, and its specialists have largely failed to convince the broader community of medical historians—or indeed historians of anything at all—that histories of the disease can tell us fundamental things about the science and practice of medicine, both past and present. Moreover, cancer has a remarkably stable profile over time, at least in terms of its definition, language and terminology—a detail that only makes the disease's absence from historical literature more surprising.[60]

After acknowledging "cancer has generated a few *longue durée* accessible and popular studies" and citing *Emperor* as an example, Arnold-Foster simply moves on, having planted adjectival kisses of death—"accessible" and "popular"—on a volume that might, arguably, have a bit to offer on the questions she raises.

Fuller reflection on this icy relationship between medical practitioners and historians of medicine on the issue of historical knowledge and writing requires more space than I have; hence, a brief review of the tensions must suffice. Writing sharply about the stalemate/debate between history/historians of medicine and physicians in the always-interesting French context, Corinne Doria's discussion might well apply to other national contexts. Doria's comment that the term "debate" itself may not be an entirely appropriate characterization is well taken since historians and physicians mainly tend to avoid any real dialogue altogether. The question of who can "legitimately write the history of medicine?" therefore remains underexamined.[61] One key problem is the demotion of history of medicine in the education of doctors today. Discussing American medical historiography, Plinio Prioreschi (physician *and* historian of medicine) observed long ago that "in general, historians know only their field of specialization and physicians know only how to treat diseases."[62] He doesn't mince his words: "These are the times of focused competence and general ignorance. ... Historians write for other historians who, limited by their ignorance of medicine, cultivate mainly its sociological and political aspects" while "physicians are not much better; they have no use for the past of their own profession, relegating everything that does not bear on cure as immediately irrelevant."[63] If any one of them should presume to "dabble" in history of medicine (*pace* Cooter, Stolberg, Foster-Jones, Wright), she will surely be considered an amateur appropriate for "the general public" but not for methodologically rigorous historians of science possessed of "knowledge and capacity for the task."[64]

Given this old disciplinary cold war, it seems fitting, as we appraise *The Emperor* and *The Gene* as works of a physician practicing history without a license, that we note these books do for cancer and mental health what has been done for other "plagues" such as cholera and tuberculosis. Ironically, these books are built on its doctor-writer's humanist tastes, which echo Oslerian assumptions that knowledge of past medical ideas and practices *should* matter to doctors and scientists in the present.[65] Although they do not profess to be academic-professional history and are, as Cooter says, epistemologically neo-positivist and therefore vulnerable to all sorts of theoretical critiques, still, both *Emperor* and *The Gene* deserve recognition for re-establishing the relevance and utility of the past to clinical medicine and scientific research today, the latter in ways that are formally innovative. Both books have their limitations, of course, but they also push limits. As history practiced from the inside of medical practice and research, Mukherjee's work—especially *Emperor*—does not cultivate extensively sociological, cultural, or political aspects of medical research favored in humanist and social science discourse. The focus on scientific developments in cancer or genetics research, entwined with biographical sketches of researchers and surgeons, admittedly resemble traditional doctor-driven histories. The inclusion (albeit limited) of patients' and doctors' experiences also gives Mukherjee's history a bit of the savor of an older medical humanities approach Cooter dismisses.

Still, *Emperor*'s historical retrospective of the conceptual and treatment history of cancer does productively estrange the book from the tired tropes and paradigms of first wave medical humanities. As for *The Gene*, family stories of illness cleverly interrupt and animate the review of developments in genetic science, creatively infusing fresh meanings and culturally thickening the "intimate history" of a radical idea. Far from flawless, these hybrid performances are available to historians, oncologists, geneticists, and everyone in between interested in the biological mechanisms that determine normalcy and its intimate other. Without overstating Mukherjee's "intention" to create a bridge between history of medicine and physicians-scientists in his writings in general, it is safe to say these longer books capture the spirit of French physician and historian Jacques Poirier's words: "If it concerns everyone, the history of medicine belongs to no one; doctors, philosophers … anthropologists … literary artists, historians (whether they are of science, technology, religion …culture) must consider themselves at home" in it.[66]

Literary science writing and the possibility of beauty

If Mukherjee's longer work raises questions about hybrid narrative form, academic disciplines, and the perils of reception for doctor-writers located in between the historical and the scientific, his literary science writing in short essay form outlines a slightly different problematic centered on science and literature as cognate modes of knowing and speaking. As indicated, *The Gene* is infused by a strong literary impulse to play with form, specifically to experiment with science writing rather than remain safely within its conventions. But it is in a tight, elegantly crafted essay like "Tenderness" that we get quite another view of the literary dimension of Mukherjee's science writing as he steers away from both patient stories and history of scientific concepts mode. In this final section, I consider two essays that attest to his attempts to forge through small-scale industry a rapprochement between literary-aesthetic and medical-scientific modalities of seeing and speaking.

"On Tenderness" recounts a visit to Gregor Mendel's monastery in Brno, "the birthplace of genetics."[67] In a garden in front of the abbey where he grew his pea-flowers, Mendel had stumbled on "the most seminal discovery of modern biology"—that "hereditary information is transmitted from one generation to the next in the form of discrete particles of information—genes."[68] Mukherjee begins with wry narration of his exchange with the custodian, a ghost from Mendel's "own stifling times" now still guarding as it were the abbey where Mendel spent 40 years as a "disciplined, deferential, and dull" monk: "How on earth did *this* man, in *this* place, unlock the mystery of genes?" Mukherjee asks.[69]

Buffeted by disappointment, like James Joyce's boy-narrator on a quest-pilgrimage to Araby-in-Dublin, Mukherjee returns empty-handed from his own quest for "something magical: an insight into the *soul* of the man who had revolutionized biology."[70] But, as it turns out, he does carry *something* back from dull Brno. A quick tour of the rooms at the Abbey reveal to him a vision: a "monk in wire-rimmed glasses tend[ing] plants—stooping, with paintbrush and forceps, to transfer the orange dust of pollen from the stamen of one flower to the pistil of the next."[71] The overgrown garden thus flowers into an epiphany and an essay on the essential nature of work in science (as in writing, I would add): slow, tactile labor. Building on an extended metaphor of the garden and gardening, "On Tenderness" implicitly develops into an *apologia pro vita suovo* of the scientist's life of careful/caring labor. Mendel became *Mendel* not because he exhibited courage or wit in extraordinary measure; rather, Mukherjee wants us to believe that it was "merely" a certain quality of tenderness that marked the monk and that marks countless other anonymous laborers in the vineyards of modern science, past and present.

Not exactly a word that leaps to mind as a descriptor for science or scientists, "tenderness," in Mukherjee lexicon, suggests a "certain intimacy between humans and nature—a nourishment that must happen before investigation can happen; the delicacy of labor that must be performed before the delicacy of its fruits can be harvested."[72] Science begins with tending. Meticulously caring for cell cultures, knowing when to coax, when to leave alone, when to add or subtract; in science as in gardening such fine calibrations constitute tending. In his own lab, Mukherjee writes that when he "witness[es] science in action, [he] see this tenderness in abundance"; the best researchers have "a gardener's instinct."[73] Spelling the opposite of indifference, of carelessness, and inattention, Mukherjee's choice certainly has the virtue of surprise. His modest rhetoric continues to push back more than two centuries' worth of critiques of modern science as dismal, impersonal, and destructive (epistemically and materially). The reference to the hand, an important motif carried over from the figure of the Mendelian gardener, and the emphasis on the tactile aspect of fingers and instincts working together, coaxing, pulling, letting be, turns scientific labor into a sort of guild-like craftsmanship.

This *apologia pro vita suova* for science is a strange (but lovely) late modern recuperation of late Victorian-era apprehensions of terrain lost to dehumanizing technology. In place of "science and technology"—that overfamiliar domineering couple humanists have come to fear—Mukherjee offers us "science and humanism," as he reinflects the practice of science as a "process by which scientists extract ... facts from the grim soil, roots and tendrils intact, to glean knowledge about the inner workings of nature."[74] This organic reframing of "real" science which delinks it from the forces of anonymization and dehumanization brings contemporary science down to earth, to the scale of a garden and of the human hand. What is refreshing about "Tenderness" is not just the essayist's eloquent advocacy of science, but the precise modes and manner of that advocacy.

"Love in the Time of Numbness; or, Doctor Chekhov, Writer" leads us down a different path, as Mukherjee turns to Anton Chekhov's time on Sakhalin Island, a Russian penal colony.[75] An oncologist's meditation on how literature might counter desensitization, the essay begins not in Russia but with the author's maternal grandmother whose neurological illness deprived her of her sense of taste. The consequences of that gradual numbing for her family's own taste buds are initially searing: "The lentils [she cooked] exfoliated the tongue."[76] With time, tongues became numbed. As he moves between varieties of numbness (those begotten at the table and those acquired in the cancer ward), Mukherjee launches his rumination on the function of writing in numbing times. Without specifying the contemporary sources of numbing world-sorrow, he asks how one might continue to write under such anesthesia or numbness of one's senses *and* one's sense of beauty. A moment in the life of Chekhov offers clues. Itself a deadening test of endurance, Chekhov's journey to Sakhalin Island, home to criminals of various stripes, took him across steppes, tundra, rivers, and seas. Infected with tuberculosis, Chekhov worried even more about "the stagnation in [his] soul"; Mukherjee's reading of the Russian physician-writer's motives for making what would seem a thoroughly ill-advised journey from Moscow to the Sea of Okhotsk is that he wished to get away from the "deadliness" of Tsarist Russia post-Emancipation and "un-numb the numbness," that is, avoid ennui through an encounter with life in extremis.[77] Mukherjee believes Chekhov teaches us not how to feel pity or to whip up outrage but to cultivate a wakeful form of seeing or a response we might characterize as *esthesia*, a term with medical and aesthetic significations.

Mukherjee charts Chekhov's internal journey as a passage from observation, description, diagnosis to empathy, and compassion that "moves us beyond numbness toward healing."[78] The word "tenderness" occurs twice although without the same kind of punch it carries in the Mendel essay. The term is differently nuanced here and gives way to the central concept of esthesia and, on the other modern end of the spectrum of its meanings, to beauty. Tenderness, esthesia, beauty: these words give Mukherjee as doctor/scientist/writer some leverage as he reaches for a way to define in a rawer, greener, less rehearsed way, what he calls, "clinical humanism."[79] Dried-out and brittle, the frozen terms "empathy" and "compassion" have been encountered so frequently in the medical and health humanities literature that we are numbed to whatever freshness and ethical energy they might once have possessed. It is against this context that Mukherjee's revisiting of a moment in the life of physician-writer Chekhov can be considered as in effect an exploration of possibilities that remain after the shift away from the numbing repetition of these clinical desiderata.

Warning emerging writers against making a parable out of Chekhov, Mukherjee himself does so. Similarly, I am tempted to make a parable out of his essay. I suggest his reading of Chekhov on Sakhalin Island in 1890 asks us to rethink the antidotal effectiveness of outrage, indignation, and piety, widely consumed in the academic humanities and in the world at large. So, what will move us to alertness beyond the state of anesthesia that this standard pharmacopoeia fails to dispel? What can make us perceive and feel again? The essay posits beauty as the antidote to anesthesia. At first blush, this call to return to the aesthetic—"beauty, in all its myriad forms"—sounds a bit vague, apolitical, and outdated, especially to literary critics and scholars who have put in time toppling aesthetics or beauty to insist that literature is more than a playground for the *homines ludentes* of humanist aesthetics. But what if we give the benefit of the doubt to this doctor-scientist-writer's call for "beauty," issued from terrain on which literature and medicine/science converge? Can his call for "beauty" from somewhere in this border country be construed as a call to renovate the tired and re-articulate the familiar in tough times when both the humanities and the sciences are losing their purchase on policy and the public? Perhaps, we could say about Mukherjee's "quiet manifesto for our times"—the creation of "beauty"—what the limited-omniscient narrator at the end of J.M. Coetzee's *Disgrace* intones about the notion of trying to be a good person after *apartheid*: "A good person. Not a bad resolution to make, in dark times."[80] "Beauty": not a bad thing to keep at recuperating in numbing times?

Beauty of course is neither a thing nor a nomination for an agreed-upon object, nor a cause—political, religious, or even intellectual. And it is certainly not offered here as a neat conclusion that gives us the long and the short of this essay or of Mukherjee's literary science writing. Following the philosopher, Agnes Callard, we might say rather that beauty or aesthesia (the opposite of anesthesia, numbness) is contemplation, contemplation that does not "squeeze its value into the language of justice or dignity or basic human rights ... for humanists, contemplation is not a cause. It is a calling."[81] Alternatively, we can, in the spirit of Coetzee, construe Mukherjee's invocation of beauty as a resolution of effort, or as the writer's necessary performance of a promise to herself rather than a reference to some distinct, already-known end or solution. Beauty, one infers from all that Mukherjee writes about Chekhov, his exemplary writer-physician, names whatever antidote bypasses numbness on one hand and anger or self-righteousness on the other. It is a restorative perhaps that allows one to write tenderly, tentatively; it is the answer to the question of how the writer, whether physician or not, administers the aesthetics of cure that can keep us living (on), awake and alert.

Notes

1 Siddhartha Mukherjee, *The Emperor of Maladies: A Biography of Cancer* (New York: Scribner, 2011).
2 Siddhartha Mukherjee, *The Gene: An Intimate History* (New York: Scribner, 2016).
3 Ibid., 757.
4 Ibid.

5   Alexander Linklater, "The *Emperor of All Maladies: A Biography of Cancer* by Siddhartha Mukherjee – review," *The Guardian*, January 2011, https://www.theguard ian.com/books/2011/jan/23/emperor-maladies-biography-cancer-siddhartha-mukh erjee-review.

6   Ibid.

7   Siddhartha Mukherjee, "Same and Different," *The New Yorker*, Annals of Science Issue, (2016), https://www.newyorker.com/magazine/2016/05/02/breakthroughs-in-ep igenetics.

8   Siddhartha Mukherjee, "The Letting Go," *New York Times Magazine*, August 2011, https://www.nytimes.com/2011/08/28/magazine/lives-the-letting-go.html.

9   "A Conversation with Siddhartha Mukherjee, MD, DPhil," interview by Tony Cosgrove, Cleveland Clinic, November 2017, video, 1:13:31, https://www.youtube. com/watch?v=Kc4-3E9g6ps.

10 Ibid.

11 Sathnam Sanghera, "My Family Secret," *The Times* (London, UK), May 2016, https:/ /www.thetimes.co.uk/article/siddhartha-mukherjee-my-family-secret-r09drnfv6.

12 Chadi Nabhan and Siddhartha Mukherjee, "Episode 14: Physician, Scientist, and Author Siddhartha Mukherjee," May 28, 2019, in *Outspoken Oncology Podcast*, *Journal of Clinical Pathways*, audio, 49:41, https://www.journalofclinicalpathways.com/mul timedia/episode-14-physician-scientist-and-author-siddhartha-mukherjee.

13 Corinne Doria, "The Right to Write the History: Disputes over the History of Medicine in France – 20th–21st Centuries," *Transversal: International Journal for the Historiography of Science* 27, no. 3 (2017): 26–36. doi: 10.24117/2526-2270. 2017. i3.03.

14 Mukherjee, *Emperor*, 337–338.

15 Listing *aesthesia* as a rare medical term, the *OED* defines it as "sensory capacity or ability of an organism, organ, etc.; an instance of this. Also: a physical sensation (nor-mal or abnormal)." Visit https://www-oed-com.unh.idm.oclc.org/view/Entry/3230. As we'll see, in Mukherjee's meditation on Chekhov, an opposition is set up between anesthesia and esthesia.

16 Mukherjee, *Emperor*, 3–5.

17 Mukherjee, *The Gene*, 30. In an interview prior to *The Gene*'s publication, Mukherjee expressed his interest in "more experimental forms of nonfiction … somewhere between memoir and fiction." See: https://www.nytimes.com/2016/05/22/books/revi ew/siddhartha-mukherjee-by-the-book.html.

18 Jerry Coyne, "*The New Yorker* screws up big time with science: researchers criticize the Mukherjee piece on epigenetics," *Why Evolution is True* (blog), May 5, 2016, https://whyevolutionistrue.com/2016/05/05/the-new-yorker-screws-up-big-time-with -science-researchers-criticize-the-mukherjee-piece-on-epigenetics/; Chris Woolston, "Researcher under Fire for *New Yorker* Epigenetics Article," *Nature* 533, no. 7603 (May 9, 2016): 295–295.

19 The echo of the plot of *Midnight's Children* in this detail of the twin birth is hard to miss.

20 Coyne followed up his initial blog entry with others: "Dreadful science journalism at *Vox*: all interpretations of science are equal, but some are cuter than others," May; "The End of the Mukherjee Affair: He "clarifies" in response to a critical letter," May 24, 2016; and "Mukherjee corrects his new book in light of epigenetics kerfuf-fle, still defends his mischaracterization of gene regulation," July 30, 2016. See, too, Michael Eisen's analysis of the controversy, "The Imprinter of All Maladies," *It Is Not Junk* (blog), May 10, 2016, http://www.michaeleisen.org/blog/?p=1894; Jennie Dusheck offers a different view of the case in "An Evolving View of Cancer: It May Not Always Start with a Mutation," *Stanford Medicine*, Winter 2017, https://stanmed .stanford.edu/2017winter/how-epigenetics-is-changing-our-understanding-of-cancer -biology.html.

21 Tabitha Powlege, "That Mukherjee Piece on Epigenetics in *The New Yorker* (blog), May 13, 2016, PLoS Blogs Network, https://blogs.plos.org/blog/2016/05/13/that-m ukherjee-piece-on-epigenetics-in-the-new-yorker/.

22 Mukherjee, *The Gene*, 543–544.

23 Ibid., 12.

24 Ibid., 13.

25 Ibid., 20–21.

26 Ibid., 30.

27 Ibid., 31.

28 Mukherjee, *Emperor*, 113.

29 Ibid., 1.

30 Ibid., 7.

31 D. Ross Camidge, "A Chronology of Cancer," *BMJ: British Medical Journal* 342, no. 7802 (2011): 878–878.

32 Mukherjee, *Emperor*, 307–308.

33 Mukherjee, *Emperor*, 5.

34 Ross, "A Chronology," 878.

35 Anne Whitehead, Angela Woods, Sarah Atkinson, Jane Macnaughton, and Jennifer Richards, eds., *The Edinburgh Companion to the Critical Medical Humanities* (Edinburgh: Edinburgh University Press, 2016), 1–5.

36 Mukherjee, *Emperor*, 337.

37 Ibid., 6.

38 Ibid., 7.

39 Ibid., 3.

40 Mukherjee, *The Gene*, 23.

41 Ibid., 28.

42 *Emperor*, 448–449.

43 Ibid., 459.

44 Ibid.

45 Ibid.

46 Ibid., 6.

47 Atul Gawande, *Being Mortal: Medicine and What Matters in the End* (New York: Henry Holt, 2014).

48 Roger Cooter, *Writing History in the Age of Biomedicine* (New Haven, CT: Yale University Press, 2013), 161, 271.

49 Janet Maslin, "Cancer as Old Foe and Goad to Science," *The New York Times*, November, 2010, https://www.nytimes.com/2010/11/11/books/11book.html.

50 Anna Wagstaff, "Siddhartha Mukherjee: Explaining Cancer," *Cancerworld*, September 1, 2012, https://cancerworld.net/cover-story/siddhartha-mukherjee-explaining-ca ncer/.

51 Mukherjee, *Emperor*, xvii.

52 "A Conversation," Cleveland Clinic, video.

53 Charles McGrath, "How Cancer Acquired Its Own Biographer," *The New York Times*, November 8, 2010.

54 Cooter, *Writing History*, 164–166.

55 Philip Teigen, "The Global History of Rabies and the Historian's Gaze: An Essay Review," *Journal of the History of Medicine and Allied Sciences* 67, no. 2 (2012): 320.

56 Ibid., 327.

57 Cooter, *Writing History*, 162.

58 Michael Stolberg, "Metaphors and Images of Cancer in Early Modern Europe," *Bulletin of the History of Medicine* 88, no. 1 (2014): 48–74.

59 James Wright, "The Radicalization of Breast Cancer Surgery: Joseph Colt Bloodgood's Role in William Stewart Halsted's Legacy," *Bulletin of the History of Medicine* 92, no. 1 (2018): 141–142.

60 Agnes Arnold-Forster, "A Pathology of Progress? Locating the Historiography of Cancer," *The British Journal of the History of Science* 49, no. 4 (Dec. 2016): 627.

61 Doria, "The Right to Write," 27.

62 P. Prioreschi, "Physicians, Historians, and the History of Medicine," *Medical Hypotheses* 38, no. 1 (June 1992): 97–101.

63 Ibid., 97.

64 Ibid.

65 Mukherjee, *Emperor*, 16, 343, 362; Sherwin Nuland, "Doctors and Historians," *Journal of the History of Medicine and Allied Sciences* 43, no. 2 (April 1988): 137–140.

66 Quoted in Doria, "The Right to Write History," 35.

67 Siddhartha Mukherjee, "Introduction: On Tenderness," in *The Best American Science and Nature Writing*, ed. Siddhartha Mukherjee and Tim Folger (Boston, MA: Houghton Mifflin Harcourt, 2013): xvii.

68 Ibid., xiv.

69 Ibid., xvii.

70 Ibid., xvi.

71 Ibid., xvii.

72 Ibid., xviii.

73 Ibid.

74 Ibid., xx.

75 Siddhartha Mukherjee, "Love in the Time of Numbness; or, Doctor Chekhov, Writer," *New Yorker*, April 11, 2017, https://www.newyorker.com/culture/cultural-comment/love-in-the-time-of-numbness-or-doctor-chekhov-writer.

76 Ibid.

77 Ibid.

78 Ibid.

79 Ibid.

80 J. M. Coetzee, *Disgrace* (Harmondsworth: Penguin, 1999), 216.

81 Agnes Callard, "What Do the Humanities Do in a Crisis?" *New Yorker*, April 11, 2020, https://www.newyorker.com/culture/annals-of-inquiry/what-do-the-humanities-do-in-a-crisis.

15 Arthur Kleinman

Professional caregiving narratives become personal

Carol Levine

Introduction

To have achieved so much in so many different areas, as a Harvard psychiatrist, researcher, writer, and educator, even with lots of help along the way, Arthur Kleinman seems to be a one-man multidisciplinary team. He has played a major role in creating not one but two subspecialties—medical anthropology and narrative medicine. He is a specialist in global health, Chinese and other cultural responses to illness and suffering, healthcare delivery, the moral basis of medicine, and more. In each of these areas, he has been a prolific, passionate, and elegant writer, producing monographs and edited books, research articles, and reflective essays. In many of these works, he writes about his own experiences as a professional caregiver. His most recent book, *The Soul of Care*,[1] describes, in often harrowing detail, his experience as a caregiver for his late wife and collaborator, Joan Kleinman. Building on all that went before, the memoir articulates his view that care is the critical, and often missing, element in healthcare today.

Before turning to that book, this chapter will summarize three prior books that covered some of the topics that bear on the memoir. As the caregiver for 17 years for my late husband, who was left quadriplegic and brain-damaged after an automobile accident, I have a personal interest in this area. I have also spent over 20 years researching and writing about family caregiving, particularly family relationships with healthcare professionals in the care of a person with a chronic illness or disability. From both perspectives, I find in Kleinman's writing many aspects to admire and support and a few others that raise questions.

The Illness Narratives: suffering, healing, and the human condition

The Illness Narratives[2] is probably the most well-known of Kleinman's books. It gave me a metaphor that helped me understand my life as a family caregiver. Published in 1988, the book did not come to my attention until the mid-1990s. By then I had been struggling for several years, not only with the demands of constant caregiving, but, even more challenging, also with the uncaring attitudes of doctors, nurses, and administrators who saw me only as the person who was

DOI: 10.4324/9781003079712-15

supposed to do everything but ask for nothing. I lost my identity as a writer, researcher, mother, grandmother, and daughter. Even my role as wife was transformed from loving partner to The Wife, as in "Tell The Wife to do it." One impatient hospital nurse told me, "Your life is over. Get used to it." Then I read *The Illness Narratives*, in which Kleinman wrote:

> The chronically ill are like those trapped at a frontier, wandering confused in a poorly known border area, waiting desperately to return to their native land. ... This image should also alert us to the social nature of chronicity: the entrance and exit formalities, the visas, the different language and etiquettes, the guards and functionaries and hucksters at the border crossing points, and especially the relatives and friends who press their faces against windows to wave a sad goodbye, who carry sometimes the heaviest baggage, who sit in the same waiting rooms, and who even travel through the same land of limbo, experiencing similar worry, hurt, uncertainty and loss.[3]

Nothing I read before or since captured my experience so accurately and poetically. I borrowed this image for the title of an anthology called *Living in the Land of Limbo: Fiction and Poetry about Family Caregiving*,[4] with credit to Kleinman's book.

The main themes of *The Illness Narratives* are now familiar: the importance of understanding illness from the patient's (Kleinman uses the term "sick person," more commonly today just "person") and family's perspective, and distinguishing it from the concept of disease, the biomedical explanation for symptoms and diagnosis. Symptoms and disabilities create illness problems in work, family life, social interactions, and other areas. It is the clinician's responsibility to explore and interpret the meanings of illness to the person and family and to collaborate with them on a treatment plan that addresses the disease but also the illness.

This is not a task that can easily be accomplished in a 15-minute office visit or hospital stroll-by conversation. It needs time and the right skills. Kleinman uses detailed case examples—the illness narratives—from his clinical practice. He is not only a master storyteller but also a master listener and observer of gestures, movements, and verbal responses. Eleven chapters of the 16-chapter book are case examples of extended interviews over time. If Kleinman is interested in yet another career, he might try fiction.

While all are gripping narratives of people in physical and emotional distress, three describe people with chronic pain, a particularly relevant subject in the current opioid epidemic in which poorly treated chronic pain has led to unprecedented increases in addiction, overdoses, and death. Kleinman noted that at the time he was writing the book, chronic pain was a major public health concern. Even without the indiscriminate marketing and prescribing of opiates that flourished with the introduction of OxyContin, he saw that

> Medical care fosters addiction to narcotic analgesic drugs, polypharmacy (the use of multiple drugs) with medications that exert serious side effects,

overuse of expensive and risky tests, unnecessary surgery that can produce serious damage, and obstacles to leaving the disabled role.[5]

Consider the case of Howard Harris (like all the people profiled in this book and others mentioned in case examples in this chapter, this is a pseudonym), which describes the difficult life of a small-town police lieutenant who has severe chronic pain that limits his work and family life. Kleinman observes the manifestations of pain.

> Howie sits bolt upright, both feet on the floor about one foot apart, his lower back and upper torso rigid. Every few minutes he grimaces, and every twenty to thirty minutes he stands up stiffly and gently moves his spine from side to side while firmly gripping the back of the chair he has previously judged to be the steadiest.[6]

Financial pressures prevent Howie from retiring on disability; and his fellow officers cover for him. Yet he knows his situation is only going to get worse.

His wife and sons feel left out of his life, which is controlled by pain and work. They wonder at times if the pain is real. His wife Ellen says: "I know he's in pain. But every day? Can it always be that bad?"[7] Howie had a troubled childhood with an absent alcoholic father and a mother who suffered from frequent backaches. Kleinman says that Howie Harris meets the official definition of major depressive disorder but his depressive mood "represents demoralization from the life of pain more than anything else," and Kleinman asserts that what is needed is "a kind of care that is radically different from that now routinely available."[8]

In interpreting Howie Harris's case, as he does with all case examples in the book, Kleinman recommends new approaches. For Harris this means

> treatment that would address simultaneously his behavior impairment, the distress in his social relationships, and his demoralization and self-defeating personality patterns. Treatment should begin with the systematic evaluation of the psychosocial crises in his experience. It should include therapeutic interventions directed at each of the major problems and integrated within a comprehensive clinical approach to pain. Such an approach would seek not merely to control the pain but particularly to prevent chronicity and disability.[9]

When Kleinman wrote *The Illness Narratives*, he said that this kind of approach was not routinely available. Nor does it seem to be routinely available today.[10]

Women are especially vulnerable to the effects of chronic pain, but treatment programs have largely been based on problems in men's lives. Carolyn Mazure, a physician-researcher on women's health, has argued that women need a treatment approach that recognizes their lower thresholds to pain and sensitivity to drugs, and particularly their social roles as mothers and nurturers. Treatment programs that address women's issues are rare, although increasing.[11] Kleinman does not address gender differences explicitly.

The final chapter of *The Illness Narratives* outlines a method—a mini-ethnography—for exploring problem areas in illness. With coauthor Peter Benson, Kleinman published in 2006 a list of seven questions for clinicians to use with their patients.[12] This explanatory model is an interviewing technique to open communication channels and elicit the patient's or family's understanding and explanation of the illness.

Asking the questions, of course, is only the first step. The clinician must then listen carefully and respectfully to the answers. The main thrust should be to

> focus on the patient as an individual, not a stereotype, as a human being facing danger and uncertainty. ... [I]t is an opportunity for the doctor to engage in an essential moral task, not an issue in cost-accounting.[13]

This method is not the same as cultural competency, which all too often assumes that all people with similar cultural or ethnic backgrounds have the same beliefs and practices.

Kleinman and Benson conclude that

> what clinicians want to understand through the mini-ethnography is what really matters—what is really at stake for patients, their families, and at times, their communities. ... Even the busiest clinician should be able to find time to routinely ask patients (and where appropriate, family members) what matters most to them in the experience of illness and treatment.[14]

What really matters

Kleinman's emphasis on finding what really matters to patients leads directly to a summary of his book *What Really Matters: Living a Moral Life Amidst Uncertainty and Danger*.[15] In this book, Kleinman takes the questions in the mini-ethnography to a level beyond the illness experience. Like the pain case histories, the issues it raises feel even more relevant in today's troubled world than when it was written. It chronicles, in Kleinman's words, "moral experience and how individuals and groups come to grips with dangers and uncertainty."[16]

The stories in *The Illness Narratives* are based on situations that are part of ordinary modern life. The stories in *What Really Matters* extend to situations created or exacerbated by political, economic, religious, and social trends. There are six stories in which names and details have been changed, and one story about a historical figure—W. H. R. Rivers, an anthropologist and psychiatrist who treated British Army officers traumatized by their experiences in World War I. Rivers is the central figure in Pat Barker's novel *Regeneration*.[17]

Some of the people in these stories are participants or former participants in major wars or humanitarian missions. Winthrop Cohen, for example, joined the US Marine Corps in 1942. He was shipped to the Pacific, where he was on active duty in the invasion of four islands and was twice decorated for bravery. After the war, he returned to New York, attended college on the GI Bill, and became a lawyer. He joined a large law firm on the West Coast and had a successful career. He married a woman from the wealthy Protestant business class. (In a footnote, Kleiman notes the distinction between Winthrop Cohen's anglophile first name and his Jewish surname and lower-class background and calls him by his full name throughout the book.)

Winthrop Cohen believes that the war made him a killer. He killed more than once, but the event that haunted him and that is at the core of his major depressions occurred when he encountered a Japanese medic at a small field hospital. The man did not offer any resistance and held up his hands in what Winthrop Cohen saw as a "Christlike" gesture. Nevertheless, Winthrop Cohen shot him. As he told Kleinman: "It was me, Winthrop Cohen, who killed him. In cold blood. Without any threat. There is no other word for it. I murdered him. I murdered a doctor while he tended to his wounded men. Pure and simple."[18]

Winthrop Cohen responded to a short course of depression therapy and returned to work. He was able to put away the horrifying memories but not the underlying realization that he had acted against his core beliefs—his soul. And Kleinman feels uneasy.

> He [Winthrop Cohen], a Jew on his way to success in the Christian world, had killed a "Christlike" figure. He said that. And my thoughts now completed the charge: he had thereby enacted a vicious myth that has been immensely destructive over so many generations.[19]

In recounting this chilling incident, Winthrop Cohen described the Japanese medic holding up his hands in surrender as a "Christlike gesture," although nothing about the common gesture of surrender is inherently "Christlike." Perhaps Winthrop Cohen saw it as a reminder of the Crucifixion. It is unlikely that the Japanese medic was a Christian; the most common religions in Japan are Shinto and Buddhism. Most depictions of Jesus with arms extended are blessings, not surrenders. Wilfred Cohen describes what he did as cold-blooded murder. In his even more devastating comment, Kleinman links the two elements by interpreting Winthrop Cohen's understanding of his wartime experience as a Jew who killed Christ, the myth that has been at the root of generations of anti-Semitism. Surely this says as much about Kleinman's own experiences as a Jew in a Christian world as it does about Winthrop Cohen's.

Winthrop Cohen faced real danger in war. Other stories in *What Really Matters* involved people in situations in which their core identities were challenged. Dr. Yan Zhongshu, for example, a Chinese physician who had lived through the political persecutions of the Cultural Revolution, was betrayed by a colleague to whom he had confided personal information. The colleague publicly called for his dismissal and attacked him physically. Yet when Dr. Yan later had the opportunity to exact revenge by recommending that this colleague be assigned to an outlying province where he would probably not survive, he chose instead to speak out against the policy rather than the person. Reflecting on the many choices that Dr. Yan had to make to survive and practice medicine, Kleinman says that "Rather than a stark story of good and evil, Dr. Yan's account speaks to the gray zone of survival, the banality of moral compromise leading to untoward outcomes, and the unmasterable features of moral life."[20]

The seventh chapter in the book is titled "Bill Burt/Simcha Adler"; these two people have no connection to each other, but they are linked by their association with the author. This chapter is about Kleinman's own background and moral experiences. In a compelling example, Kleinman did not act according to his moral beliefs. This occurred in 1967 when he was an intern at Yale-New Haven Hospital, overseeing the care of a teenager with a rare liver disease. When the boy died, Dr. A., a well-known senior professor, "bluntly orders me [Kleinman] to immediately ask the family for permission for an autopsy" so that the liver can be examined microscopically. Kleinman suggested giving the grieving family time to see the body and share their feelings. Instead, Dr. A. "brutally" informed the family that "for the sake of science there needs to be an autopsy performed immediately before their son's liver begins to rot."[21] This request produced anger and adamant refusals.

Dr. A. then rushed back to Kleinman, pushed him against the wall, and "in a commanding voice, his hands shaking with anger, orders me to take the three biopsy needles that nestle in his laboratory coat pocket." While he distracts the family, he says, Kleinman will run back into the hospital room, lock the door, and take multiple biopsies of the boy's liver.

Facing an angry superior, Kleinman acceded to the request, quickly jabbed the biopsy needles into the liver, and ran from the room. He rushed past the family, who were still complaining to Dr. A. Kleinman says, "I am too anguished to look or speak to them, even though I know them far better than he does."

This episode, Kleinman says, "occupied altogether less than an hour of my professional life … yet it moves inside me still, like a deep flow of hot lava." This episode bothers him

> most in that I did something that I knew at the time was unethical, that what I did was coerced out of me, in a cultural ethos where this was a normal experience, and that I was unable to express my revulsion or any criticism but had to "eat the bitterness," as Chinese people put it.[22]

This episode is not unique in medical training and other situations in which a powerful person demands something unethical or at least ambiguous. What is unusual is the deep and lasting impression it made on Kleinman, and his willingness to share his feelings of shame.

And what of Bill Burt and Simcha Adler, whose names are in the chapter title? They are both characters from Kleinman's adolescence. Before entering Stanford Medical School, he spent a summer as a manual laborer in the New York City sewer system. Bill Burt was his boss and protector from the supervisor who berated and humiliated all the workers. When Kleinman considered dropping out of medical school after one semester, he wrote to Bill Burt that he could find a good life without being a doctor. Bill Burt disagreed, and wrote a long, impassioned letter that ended: "You don't need to write back until you have an M.D. after your name."[23]

Simcha Adler was an Israeli Kleinman met on a summer trip to Europe after his first year of medical school. Kleinman had a stunning experience in France (described in *The Illness Narratives*), in which he asked a receptionist at an inn why all the tombstones in a small cemetery bore the same date of death. The receptionist, mistaking him for a German, told him angrily that they were all Jews killed by Nazis on the same day. Kleinman changed his plans, flew to Tel Aviv, and met Simcha Adler who was the leader of a new kibbutz (commune). Adler invited him to visit, with the goal of joining the kibbutz. Adler, a Holocaust survivor, appealed to Kleinman's Jewish heritage. But Kleinman realized his future lay in being an American Jew and a doctor. Throughout his writing, Kleinman refers to his Jewish background, suggesting that it is important to him but also a source of ambivalence.

Bill Burt and Simcha Adler had only brief times with Kleinman. Yet their influence was long-lasting. In them, as in later mentors, Kleinman says,

> I came to see the pressing need for father figures in my own self-building. And this led to a further recognition of why I so urgently needed to be a mentor and healer to others, and perhaps also to why I initially searched for moral heroes.[24]

Writing at the Margin: discourse between anthropology and medicine

Published in 1995, *Writing at the Margin*[25] is Kleinman's exploration of his own role in the two fields with which he is most strongly associated. The metaphor refers, he writes, "to the margin between anthropology and medicine as well as the boundary of Chinese and North American societies where, since 1968, I have lodged my intellectual project."[26] In a strict sense, he continues,

> the usage is accurate, even overcoded. Medical anthropology is at the margin of medicine; it is also at the margin of anthropology. A medical anthropologist in the field of China studies is also at the edge of the mainstream disciplines and professional interests, and in the 1990s, when health insurance reform was widely debated [as it is today], being a medical anthropologist puts one at the margin of medicine.[27]

As a Jew, Kleinman also feels a different kind of marginality, which he describes in *What Really Matters* and elsewhere.

Although Kleinman refers to his childhood in many of his writings, his statement in this book is perhaps the most candid connection between autobiography and scholarship. He writes:

My own fate was to possess what connects us yet is utterly separate—sealed as a son who never met his father, a grade school student who bore two utterly separate family names, from two opposed sub-ethnic factions, one in public school [Kleinman], the other in religious school [Spier]; a scion of a mysterious past about which his Victorian family was silent or whispered inarticulately, so that I had the extra developmental task of figuring out by myself, yet not announcing to others, lest they be hurt, what identified me, which therefore could not be authorized (or denied). ... Hence, the margins I seek are unfinished, even already overstepped, and become something altogether different out of interaction.[28]

Oddly, he does not comment on the irony that both surnames mean "small man" in German, an attribute that does not apply to him in any way.

The book is divided into three parts: the culture of biomedicine; suffering as social experience (also the title of another of Kleinman's books)[29]; and the state of medical anthropology. Some of the chapters are coauthored. For the purposes of this chapter, I will focus on Chapter 3, "Anthropology of Bioethics," a critique of mainstream bioethics and its role in the culture of biomedicine. This chapter is a version of Kleinman's entry in the 1995 *Encyclopedia of Bioethics*, called "Anthropology of Medicine."[30] (The article appears without changes in the 2004 edition as well.[31])

Kleinman makes a distinction that appears in several other works between what is "ethical" and what is "moral."

Whereas ethical discourse is a codified body of abstract knowledge held by experts about "the good" and ways to realize it, moral accounts are the commitments of social participants in a local world about what is at stake in everyday experience.[32]

In this view, the subordination of the self to social relationships is at the heart of morality. This is the Chinese view, he says, as well as that of other non-Western cultures.

In this calculus, mainstream bioethics does not emerge a winner. His list of criticisms of bioethics starts with its Western emphasis on the "individuated self," in which "the autonomy of the person is claimed to be a paramount value along with the idea of justice and benevolence."[33] For non-Western societies such as China, Japan, and India, "social obligation, family responsibility, and communal loyalty outweigh personal autonomy in the hierarchy of ethical principles."[34] Furthermore, bioethics discussions take place in hospitals, research institutes, philosophy departments, and other specialized locations, not in doctors' offices, clinics, homes, and communities.

He goes further: "The very idea of ethics privileges the Western view of the individual. ... Simply comparing individualism to sociocentrism can never be sufficient. It is essential to make the critique of individualism central to a cross-cultural approach to ethics."[35] If that were not enough, he adds that there is a deeply troubling question in the philosophical formulation of an ethical problem as rational choice among abstract principles, because the problem is always the burden of a man or woman's particular world of pain and possibility. ... The patient's experience is appropriated by the rational technical categories of professionals.[36]

There is more, but this is enough to convey Kleinman's position, stated in black and white, he says, to emphasize the importance of an anthropological view in understanding what really matters in decision-making.

My experience of the early and influential years of modern bioethics leads me to a somewhat different conclusion. During my years at the Hastings Center, as Managing Editor and then Editor of the *Hastings Center Report* and Managing Editor of *IRB: A Review of Human Subjects Research* (now called *Ethics and Human Research*), I spent many hours listening to the founders of modern bioethics debate serious issues. To me the main reasons bioethics focused on individual autonomy was that physicians, the center of medical power, made decisions without consulting their patients; or if they did, without giving them options. This occurred in medical practice, and especially in research. The infamous Tuskegee experiments of untreated syphilis among Black men followed for years, even when a reliable treatment was available, lives on in the collective memory of Black people today.

Kleinman does not subject the social-centric view to similar criticisms. Yet how do individuals fare in a world in which they are subject to family, religious, and community goals? Not very well, especially if they are female. Much of Kleinman's writing about social suffering describes clearly unethical and inhumane treatment of individuals by the ruling group (the Holocaust is just one example). If he were updating this work, he might look at the well-documented disparities in healthcare that exist for minorities and poor people and that have become a defining feature of the coronavirus pandemic. The social-centric view is often determined by power relationships, and those with less power predictably fare less well.

Perhaps Kleinman could be encouraged to re-examine bioethics today to assess whether forces that were only beginning when he wrote in 1995 are making a difference. One example is feminist ethics, in which care is a primary theme. Another is the growing number of international bioethics institutes, staffed by local experts familiar with cultural norms. He might also think about autonomy, not as an individual apart from family and society, but as a value that enhances both and protects the individual from being exploited by powerful forces or being the subject of unwanted interventions.

Another chapter in the book discusses "The Social Course of Epilepsy" in interior China.[37] In a research study, Kleinman and his coauthors interviewed epilepsy patients and their families to ascertain the impact of the disease. Individuals experienced stigma, isolation, and other losses, but what was more notable to the authors was the way the family suffered from the individual's disease, especially the challenges in finding a marriage partner. Concealing the disease was one tactic; even worse was not to marry, threatening the centrality of the family in Chinese society.

It is one thing to understand the way different societies address illness and suf-fering, and the importance of family and social structures in an individual's life, but quite another to see the ill person as shameful. Is Kleinman here suggesting that we in the West adopt Chinese practices and hand over all power to families, whatever their structure and history? Not likely to happen. Or is he just suggest-ing that bioethics in the West pay much more attention to social context and the ethnography of the situations? How do we reconcile this view with Kleinman's keen observation of families as living in the same land of limbo as patients?

The importance of filial piety in Chinese society may be waning today. As China becomes more industrialized and capitalism flourishes, adult children are moving away from their birthplaces to find a better life in cities. In 2013, the Chinese government went beyond encouraging filial piety and enacted a law requiring adult children to keep in touch with their aging parents. The law, called "Protection of the Rights and Interests of Elderly People," contains nine clauses outlining the duties of children and their obligations to tend to the financial and spiritual needs of the elderly.[38] The law had no specific penalties, but in 2016, the government issued a new set of regulations that could make it more difficult for children who fail to visit or phone their parents regularly to get a bank loan. They may even lose their library privileges. Parents can sue their children for failure to support them. A new version of the classic text that teaches the importance of respecting and pampering one's parents—"The 24 Paragons of Filial Piety"—includes advice to children to buy health insurance for their parents and teach them how to use the internet.[39] I have to wonder: what would Confucius say?

The Soul of Care: the moral education of a husband and a doctor

Kleinman's most recent book, *The Soul of Care*, is an illness narrative from the perspective of the person's caregiver and partner in work and life. It is also a memoir of the caregiver's childhood, medical career, and changing perspective on his life's work understanding illness and caregiving. The two parts do not exist seamlessly, although each is compelling in its own way.

The dramatic Prologue describes an incident in which Joan Kleinman screams at her husband, believing him to be an imposter invading her home. As a psy-chiatrist, Kleinman realizes that this is an episode of Capgras syndrome, a delu-sional state in which the person perceives everyone and everything around her as a sham. For a husband and caregiver, however, it is a devastating experience, even though the next day Joan denies that this even happened.

The Prologue presages the theme of the book:

> Caregiving is hard, sometimes tedious, unglamorous work, but it resonates with emotional, moral, and even religious significance. ... I believe we are living through a dangerous time when high-quality care is seriously threat-ened among families, in the health care professions, in our hospitals and

aged care homes, and in our society at large. Amid the hardness, hate, violence, and cynicism that fuel politics today, an anti-caring ethos prevails, and undermined by funding that scarcely touches the need, care can be wrongly portrayed as softness and sentimentality. It is neither. Care is the human glue that holds together families, communities, and societies. But it is being ... sacrificed on the altar of economy and efficiency, demanding more and more of families and health care professionals with fewer and fewer resources, and threatening to displace meaning in healthcare. The moral language of human experience, of people's suffering and healing—the bedrock of or common existence—is being stifled, and at worst will be lost.[40]

After this passionate plea, to which Kleinman returns at the book's end, he spends the next six chapters describing his unhappy childhood, troubled adolescence, university and medical school, and the experiences that led him to his ultimate specialties. Several of these themes have appeared before in previous books but are described in more detail.

Like many good writers, Kleinman was a good and voracious reader. He read groundbreaking scholars like Clifford Geertz, but also writers like Camus, Marx, Conrad, Shakespeare, and many others. In 1974, he published four articles that he says "defined the next forty-plus years of my work on caregiving."[41] To begin with, he writes:

> The practice of medicine was only one example of the far broader practice of care. Second, care itself was based on what truly mattered in the illness and treatment experience for patients and practitioners. And what mattered differed for professional, personal, and social reasons. And third, this more patient-oriented approach applied not just to healthcare in Boston and the rest of the United States, but to what I had observed and studied in Taipei and, later still, Chang-sha.

He found that it was "*experience* [italics in original] I wished to explore and shape—experiences of pain, injury, and suffering and their makeover in therapy and care—and how to approach these as a healer and writer."[42]

The second half of the book centers on his life with Joan. They met in Palo Alto at the movies, and married a year later. He notes that Joan was from a different world. Her California family was middle class and Protestant, while he had grown up in Brooklyn in a Jewish neighborhood. His family was well-to-do but fell into financial distress because of his grandfather's ill-chosen business choices. Joan had studied in Europe and spoke French fluently. He alludes to but does not write more about these differences except to say that they "overcame the resistance from both our families"[43] to marry. From that point on, Joan's family, whoever they were, do not appear in the book, even at her death.

Joan introduced him to the Chinese aesthetic and moral traditions that she studied and that formed the foundation of their family ethos. He explains:

The Chinese worldview centered on the here and now, on incorporating a moral and ethical responsibility into everyday life. To live a good life, you needed to cultivate the self and the relationships that made you and your world more human.[44]

Joan Kleinman emerges from these pages as a truly remarkable woman, mother, daughter-in-law, and collaborator. The story of her illness begins in Chapter 7, when, in her late 50s, she begins to have vision problems. Referred to an ophthalmologist, Kleinman says,

I have a vivid memory of him casually turning his back to us in the examination room as he filled in information on the computer screen. He didn't seem to see us as real people with real lives—an unsettling sensation we were to have often, in many doctors' offices, over the coming weeks and months.

A second ophthalmologist had no better idea of what was going on, and a neurologist "mumbled his way through a lengthy list of potential diagnoses, which he could neither confirm nor deny."[45]

Each new expert required their own test results, and then referred the Kleinmans to still other experts. Much of the time was spent waiting. Many readers will recognize this statement:

Patients and families wait endlessly in waiting rooms, which of course only ratchets up their anxiety and frustration. … Mostly they wait for answers. For people caught in the grip of this cruel cycle, waiting represents lost time, time needed for all the other things that enable us to cope, to carry on, and to prepare.[46]

Waiting is often more distressing than hearing bad news, which is at least news. Eventually they went to see a senior colleague at Harvard famous for his diagnostic skills. "We remained silent as my usually dry and witty colleague gravely marshaled the unmistakable evidence that Joan's troubling symptoms were caused by early-onset Alzheimer's disease."[47] Joan was in the 5% of people in whom Alzheimer's begins in the brain's occipital lobe. Having made the diagnosis, the colleague "could not be drawn out on the prognosis; what we could expect and in what kind of time frame. He had, in fact, no recommendations at all to make about how we should proceed."[48]

The details of her decline (with periods of relative calm) are at times shattering and at times inspiring. During the increasingly difficult times, Joan's rages and visual and difficulties navigating spaces at home took over. Kleinman, formerly dependent on her to take care of him and their two children and all the household management, was now her caregiver. He is frank about his prior lack of participation in ordinary chores.

I was not quite as spoiled as in my childhood—because I did wash dishes and set the table—but my privilege was still incredible, in hindsight. I never made the bed, paid a bill, or tended to the house. I knew where our washing machine was, but I certainly had no idea how to use it, or the dryer.[49]

Yet he approaches the changed situation confidently. And sometimes this works. How many people could manage to take a person with advanced dementia from Boston to China for a three-month research trip? But there were also excursions that didn't work, such as a trip to the opera in New York. Among the anecdotes are reflections that may spark recognition among caregivers of people with different chronic conditions. For example, in the early years, "Some friends dropped away. Others became closer to us ... long-trusted friends would disappear and disappoint, only to resurface during a later crisis."[50]

As long as it was possible (and Harvard provided aides to help), he took Joan to his office. Their two adult children helped, as did Marcia, Kleinman's mother, who was then in her 90s and whom Joan had encouraged to live near them, first in Seattle and then in Boston. In retrospect, Kleinman believes he waited too long to take necessary but unwelcome steps. The first was to hire a homecare aide named Sheilah (a pseudonym) to take care of Joan during the day. Joan initially refused to acknowledge Sheilah, but after a few months she accepted her help gratefully.

The final step came in the last period of Joan's life, which she spent first in an assisted living facility and then in a nursing home carefully chosen by Kleinman and their children. While there, Sheilah and another aide provided 24-hour care to supplement the nursing home staff's care. There she died quietly on March 6, 2011. From first signs to end of life took over ten years.

What was missing in the book for me was Joan's own illness narrative, or at least an approximation of it. Kleinman doesn't report any specific conversations with Joan about writing about her illness—what to include, what not to include. An elegant, fastidious person, perhaps she would have placed some restrictions on the personal details. Or as a long-time collaborator, she may have trusted her husband to tell this story as he had told so many others. I faced this dilemma when writing about my husband, especially the medical error that led to the amputation of his forearm. I read what I had written to him; he had not known (or didn't remember) the series of events. He was firm in his desire to see this essay published, and that made me feel more confident that it was right to ask him to relive a terrible event.[51]

The last section of the book is an argument that caring for each other is essential, not just for individuals and families, but for communities and society. A series of articles in *The Lancet* outline his views cogently. For example, he writes,

The great failure of contemporary medicine to promote caregiving as an existential practice and moral vision that resists reduction to the market model or the clarion call of efficiency has diminished professionals, patients, and family caregivers alike. ... If caregiving is absent from the political and economic discourse on health care, then nothing but institutional and monetary issues seem to matter.[52]

The main thrust of *The Sold of Care*, however, is personal, not political. "The soul is who we are in an existential sense of what we mean to ourselves and others, what we stand for, what we do." Kleinman concludes,

> I found my soul in that elevating and frustrating work. That the soul I discovered or remade—both seem true—is damaged and scarred seems to me evidence that caregiving is an imperfect project ... the multifaceted and unwieldy reality of living a human life.[53]

Accepting that ambiguity is a challenge for each of us as caregiver or care receiver.

Conclusion

Arthur Kleinman's life and work are explorations not just of medicine or anthropology but of humanity at its core. He brings the person and the family to their rightful place at the center of medical care. He sees both the specifics of a person's life and situation and the larger world in which they live. This emphasis is as essential for bioethics as it is for medical care.

Kleinman has challenged us to create a better world for caregivers, the people they care for, and the professionals who serve them. Are we ready for this challenge? Or are we trapped in the political land of limbo, where caregivers, like the people they care for, "travel through the same land of limbo, experiencing similar worry, hurt, uncertainty and loss?"

Notes

1 Arthur Kleinman, *The Soul of Care: The Moral Education of a Husband and a Doctor* (New York: Viking, 2019).
2 Arthur Kleinman, *The Illness Narratives: Suffering, Healing, and the Human Condition* (New York: Basic Books, 1988).
3 Ibid., 181.
4 Carol Levine, ed., *Living in the Land of Limbo: Fiction and Poetry about Family Caregiving* (Nashville, TN: Vanderbilt University Press, 2014).
5 Kleinman, *The Illness Narratives*, 57.
6 Ibid., 61.
7 Ibid., 67.
8 Ibid., 69.
9 Ibid., 73.
10 See, for example, Travis Reider, *In Pain: A Bioethicist's Personal Struggle with Opioids* (New York: HarperCollins Publishers, 2019).
11 C. M. Mazure and D. A. Fiellin, "Women and Opioids: Something Different Is Happening Here," *The Lancet* 392, no. 10141 (2018): 9–11.
12 Arthur Kleinman and Peter Benson, "Anthropology in the Clinic: The Problem of Cultural Competency and How to Fix It," *PLoS Medicine* 3, no. 10 (October 24, 2006): e294.

13 Ibid.

14 Ibid.

15 Arthur Kleinman, *What Really Matters: Living a Moral Life Amidst Uncertainty and Danger* (New York: Oxford University Press, 2006).

16 Ibid., 1.

17 Pat Barker, *Regeneration* (New York: Viking Press, 1991).

18 Kleinman, *What Really Matters*, 32.

19 Ibid., 38.

20 Ibid., 120.

21 Ibid., 168.

22 Ibid., 169.

23 Ibid., 186.

24 Ibid., 231.

25 Arthur Kleinman, *Writing at the Margin: Discourse between Anthropology and Medicine* (Berkeley, Los Angeles, CA, 1995).

26 Ibid., 1.

27 Ibid.

28 Ibid., 3–4.

29 Arthur Kleinman, Veena Das, and Margaret Lock, eds., *Social Suffering* (Berkeley, Los Angeles, CA: University of California Press, 1997).

30 Warren T. Reich, ed., *Encyclopedia of Bioethics*, revised edition (New York: Simon & Schuster Macmillan, 1995).

31 Bruce Jennings, ed., *Encyclopedia of Bioethics*, 4th edition (New York: Macmillan Reference, 2014), 1667–1674.

32 Kleinman, *Writing at the Margin*, 45.

33 Ibid., 46–47.

34 Ibid., 47.

35 Ibid., 48.

36 Ibid., 49.

37 Ibid., 147–172.

38 Edward Wong, "A Chinese Virtue Is Now the Law," *The New York Times*, July 2, 2013.

39 Andrew Jacobs and Adam Century, "As China Ages, Beijing Turns to Morality Tales to Spur Filial Devotion," *The New York Times*, September 5, 2012.

40 Kleinman, *The Soul of Care*, 4–5.

41 Ibid., 101.

42 Ibid., 59.

43 Ibid., 45.

44 Ibid., 46.

45 Ibid., 132–133.

46 Ibid., 133.

47 Ibid., 135.

48 Ibid., 135–136.

49 Ibid., 128.

50 Ibid., 140.

51 Carol Levine, "Life but No Limb," *Health Affairs* (July/August 2002): doi: 10.1377/hlthaff.21.4.237.

52 Arthur Kleinman, "Caregiving as Moral Experience," *The Lancet* 380 (November 3, 2012): 1551.

53 Kleinman, *The Soul of Care*, 244.

Index

Printed in the United States
by Baker & Taylor Publisher Services